Morphometrics is the statistical study of biological shape and shape change. Its richest data are landmarks, points such as "the bridge of the nose" that have biological names as well as geometric locations. This book is the first systematic survey of morphometric methods for landmark data. The methods presented here combine conventional multivariate statistical analysis with themes from plane and solid geometry and from biomathematics to support biological insights into the features of many different organs and organisms.

MORPHOMETRIC TOOLS FOR
LANDMARK DATA

Morphometric tools
for landmark data

Geometry and biology

FRED L. BOOKSTEIN

Center for Human Growth and Development
The University of Michigan

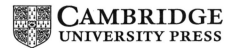
CAMBRIDGE
UNIVERSITY PRESS

PUBLISHED BY THE PRESS SYNDICATE OF THE UNIVERSITY OF CAMBRIDGE
The Pitt Building, Trumpington Street, Cambridge CB2 1RP

CAMBRIDGE UNIVERSITY PRESS
The Edinburgh Building, Cambridge CB2 2RU, United Kingdom
40 West 20th Street, New York, NY 10011-4211, USA
10 Stamford Road, Oakleigh, Melbourne 3166, Australia

First published 1991
Reprinted 1997
First paperback edition 1997

Library of Congress Cataloging-in-Publication Data is available.

A catalog record for this book is available from the British Library.

ISBN 0-521-38385-4 hardback
ISBN 0-521-58598-8 paperback

Transferred to digital printing 2003

Contents

isotropic in its coverage of directions within each of these subspaces. Such methods have been available for landmark data only since the middle 1980s.

Changes of landmark configuration may be imagined as deformations of the tissue in which the landmarks are embedded. The thin-plate spline, which represents the mapping as a pair of thin metal sheets relating the landmark sets, is a convenient tool for that visualization. The algebra and graphics of this visualization are explored.

A discussion of Sewall Wright's path-analytic approach to factors, joint causes of whole collections of observed variables, and a generalization, Partial Least Squares, for analysis of multiple blocks of variables.

Two other types of biological shape data are briefly reviewed, curving outlines and histological textures, and connections or conflicts with the landmark-based style of analysis are noted.

Three reading lists are set out: earlier overviews of morphometrics, introductions to the statistical analysis of multiple measurements in the natural sciences, and the classic literature of nineteenth-century analytic geometry.

This chapter explains the usefulness of landmark data for the analysis of biological shape change and introduces the specific data sets that will be the objects of exemplary analyses in subsequent chapters.

In landmark-based morphometrics, the analogy between "distance" among cases and Euclidean distance in a vector space of arbitrarily high dimension is replaced by a much more careful treatment of ordinary distance as measured between landmarks by ruler.

A variety of characterizations of the notion of "landmarks." They link three separate scientific thrusts: the geometry of data, the mathematics of deformation, and the explanations of developmental or evolutionary biology.

There are three principal types of landmarks, corresponding to three basic ways of grounding the explanations they entail: discrete juxtapositions of

tissues, maxima of curvature or other local
morphogenetic processes, and extremes of algebraic
functions of other data at some distance.

landmarks when the other two are each fixed in position. In the vicinity of a mean triangular form, any shape measure of a triangle of landmarks can be identified with a direction in the plane of the shape coordinates.

Preface

No book about methodology is ever finished, really. But after 10 years of major developments in morphometrics, each published (or unpublished) as a separate article, it was time for a coherent overview. My "introductory lecture," for which there was no text available, would take four hours at the podium. Students complained that my lecture notes, even when not handwritten, were unreadable. I was beginning to mislay some of the explanations of lovely patterns from the earliest examples, while other early work needed triage: Certain changes of position were so blatant as to be embarrassing. And I had grown weary of the endless cross-referencing between papers: Bookstein (1989*q*) citing (1986*x*), (1987*w, y, z*), and (1990*v, k*, and forthcoming) – many of which cited each other incestuously as well.

Yes, it was time for a 10-year retrospective, if only to simplify the indexing. Yet the principal stimulus for the writing of this book was none of these general intellectual aches and urges, but instead a specific crisis. In 1987 the National Science Foundation instituted a series of workshops on morphometrics for systematic and evolutionary biology. The first took place in Ann Arbor, Michigan, in May 1988. Each instructor was to distribute a text in advance of his lecture. (Most of these are collected in Rohlf and Bookstein, eds., 19C).) As they arrived at Michigan through the spring of 1988, these notes ranged from 15 to 40 pages in length; but mine ran to 224. It was thus relabeled the "zeroth edition" of the manuscript for this book. Only a partial draft, it covered Chapters 4 through 7 of this text, without *any* of the introductory material – without even a bibliography. "That's all right," I quipped, "most of tł e references are to my own work anyway."

In other words, by 1988 there existed a synthesis of the landmark-based morphometric methods, but no associated pedagogy. For this teaching task there is simply no substitute for a bound volume. I have endlessly shuffled too many slides into the 20- to 40-minute versions of the obviously necessary "four-hour introduction" without ever quite managing to set these techniques in an accessible context. My apologies to any of my listeners who were baffled by my experimental lectures at AAAS, AAPA, AIBS, ASA, ENAR, ICSEB, IMS, IPMI, or ISM meetings; apparently the expositions were uniformly more obscure than these initials. This experimentation might have continued indefinitely except that (1) another NSF workshop was approaching (Stony Brook, New York, June 1990), for which I needed another text to distribute, this time one that would be self-contained, and (2) Cambridge University Press had accepted this volume for publication, "pending satisfactory completion."

Hence the edition you hold in your hand. The newest material is found in the simpler Chapters 1 through 3, while the more technical expositions in Chapters 4 through 7 date from up to eight years ago. Historically, the statistics of simple tensors were developed first, in 1982; then the shape coordinates that linearize them (1983); then the critique of distance-based analyses (1984); then the serious pursuit of feature spaces, both the uniform and the nonuniform (1985); then underlayment of the statistical and geometrical points of view by the spectrum of bending energy of the thin-plate spline model (1987); finally, only yesterday, the language of Chapters 1 through 3 and 8, which speak directly to this unification.

The publication of this book is intended to declare the existence of a new specialty: *morphometrics*, the biometry of shape (for a more focused definition, see the beginning of Chapter 1). Morphometrics as a discipline should be of interest to anyone in statistics, image analysis, or quantitative biology whose work involves the contemplation of living or fossil form, its causes or its effects. Those are also the fields from which I expect readers to come: professionals and preprofessionals in any of these areas whose problems bear them broadly across the boundary of their own discipline toward one of the other two. Biologists interested in the processes regulating shape over ontogeny or phylogeny need tools for coherent quantitative reports that do not waste data. Computer scientists pursuing features of solid medical images ought to use quantitative form comparisons to guide their parameterizations. Statisticians who have always suspected there might be more structure to some sets of variables than their names and covariances will be challenged by a style of data for which that suspicion is justified. Surgeons, cardiologists, and neurologists need to test and understand covariates of the disproportions they see or correct. All these research purposes, and many, many others, can benefit from the tools taught here.

The new discipline thus deserves a place in several graduate curricula. In biology, it should be required of the student proposing a dissertation in any aspect of morphology. In statistics, it should be offered, like psychometrics, econometrics, or log-linear modeling of tables, as an elective in applied multivariate analysis. In image processing, it should be strongly urged upon anyone proposing to specialize in medical imaging. In paleobiology, it should be required, period. This book is intended as a main text and reference for such courses in morphometrics and as a supplemental text for lower-level surveys of biomathematics, biometric statistics, quantitative paleobiology, and the like. The examples are not restricted to any single field, but draw widely from medical studies of normal growth and of congenital syndromes and from comparative and evolutionary studies.

To the breadth of coverage intrinsic to the morphometric theme corresponds a commensurate breadth of background. Mastering the material in this book requires that the reader have at least moderate expertise in three different subject areas – geometry, statistics, and mathematical biology. A short course in morphometrics, for which some of this background might be waived, would include Chapters 1 through 3 (except for Section 1.3) and about half the rest of the book: Sections 4.1–4.3 5.1, 5.3–5.5, 6.1–6.5, 7.2–7.3, 7.5.1, and 7.6. For the remainder of the text, the background needed is perhaps the equivalent of a two-semester upper-level undergraduate sequence in multivariate statistics or biomathematics, or the equivalent of a one-semester course in advanced analytic geometry. Of these, only the first, the statistics sequence, is at all common in the American college curriculum. Selections from the reading lists in Section 2.5 can substitute for the syllabus of any of these prerequisites that the aspiring morphometrician has unaccountably missed, but in that case two or three of the books must be *read*, not browsed, not skimmed.

Beyond this background, the way to learn morphometrics is to think closely and skeptically through dozens of applications, as varied as one can find. Whether beginner or advanced, the student of morphometrics should be careful never to specialize in a particular organism or human organ or particular form of question, but should instead master a large number of specific techniques, such as those emphasized in this book. New morphometric methods introduced for particular applications, like the landmark methods that arose in roentgenographic cephalometrics, usually apply broadly to make sense of data in a variety of biological contexts. It is a good tactic to tailor a method for a particular problem, then see how far afield it can be pushed. In the effort to understand which attempts at generalization succeed and which fail, one may arrive at a clear statement of the tacit assumptions that actually bore responsibility for success in the original context. Exceptions to this metastatic pattern – D'Arcy Thompson's notion of transformation grids, or Blum's invention of the medial axis, each proposed as a general method right from the start – have hitherto not found many specific applications to problems of measurement. Rather, methods carefully developed for particular contexts (growth gradients, for example, or the rubber-sheet techniques for recognizing chromosomes) have proved quite protean. Any model that leads to verifiably meaningful biological explanations in any morphometric application should be tentatively considered for every morphometric application, no matter what the literature of the subject finds respectable; but a model must work first in *some* application, must improve on the routine use of the methods currently "standard" there, before it is worth considering anywhere else.

Many colleagues inadvertently helped me write this book. Those who collaborated on the projects or expositions here include Bernard Crespi, Court Cutting, Barry Grayson, Lewis Holmes, Robert Moyers, Richard Reyment, F. James Rohlf, Paul Sampson, and Elena Tabachnick. Among the many others who asked good questions or supplied good answers are Miriam Zelditch, Richard Skalak, David Ragozin, Stephen Pizer, James Mosimann, Kanti Mardia, Pat Lohmann, William D. K. Green, Colin Goodall, and the late Harry Blum. It is time for me to thank Stephen Jay Gould and Joel Cohen for suggesting, way back in 1973, that it might be possible to be an academic morphometrician. (That phrasing is anachronistic, of course – the vocation of "morphometrician" had not yet been invented.) Two editors – James Tanner of *Annals of Human Biology* and the late Morris deGroot of *Statistical Science* – invited me to publish large chunks of not terribly well digested morphometrics when it was still quite unprecedented to do so. Elena Tabachnick made hundreds of suggestions to improve the comprehensibility of the manuscript. When figures show evidence of balance, the hand is usually Teryl Lynn's, my illustrator since my dissertation days.

Besides the NSF workshops, two other small groups have borne the brunt of my early attempts at explaining the more technical parts of this material: the Ninth, Tenth, and Eleventh International Conferences on Information Processing in Medical Imaging (Bethesda, Maryland, 1985; Zeist, The Netherlands, 1987; Berkeley, California, 1989), and the two Wilks Workshops on Shape Theory organized by Colin Goodall at Princeton University in 1987 and again in 1990. Thanks to all of you for your patience during the question periods dealing with the thin-plate splines, and special thanks to Goodall and to Kanti Mardia for answering some of the questions, especially those dealing with the ties to Kendall's shape space, more adeptly than I could. I am grateful to Mardia, also, for so elegantly and expeditiously working out the exact distribution of the complex normal model, Section 5.6, in collaboration with his student Ian Dryden, and yet graciously naming the coordinates after me anyway.

Principal support for the development of the methods reported here has come from NIH grants DE-05410 and GM-37251 to the University of Michigan, each for the explicit purpose of such development. Other support has derived from NIH grants DE-03610 and NS-26529 to the University of Michigan and DE-03568 to New York University and from NIAAA grant AA-01455 to the University of Washington. The two morphometric workshops at which earlier "editions" of this text were first distributed were due *Preface* entirely to the enthusiasm of David Schindel of the Systematic Biology Program at the National Science Foundation. Jennifer Kitchell and Bill Fink urged me to prepare that monstrous hand-out for the 1988 meeting, and F. James Rohlf was similarly tolerant of an inordinate Xeroxing bill in 1990. My own computer programs run mainly on MTS, the Michigan mainframe. Rohlf has devoted too much time to packaging the spline routines for easy access by the ordinarily perseverant quantitative biologist (see the program TPSPLINE in the disk pack of Rohlf and Bookstein, 1990, and also Rohlf's 1991 program TPSRW); Paul Sampson, the same for the statistician; and Leslie Marcus and Richard Reyment have been spreading the word that there is something in land-mark-based morphometrics worth the frustrations of learning it early in its evolution. I thank all of you for your trust that someday these ideas would be not only demonstrated but also explained.

Ann Arbor, Michigan
June 10, 1991

1
Introduction

Morphometrics is the study of covariances of biological form.

The objects of morphometric study are not the forms themselves, but rather their associations, causes, and effects. This book treats the theory and practice of such studies in their most important special case, the application to **landmark data**. Most of the text introduces and exemplifies a diversity of modern geometric tools that increase the sensitivity and specificity of biological explanations of form. In this introductory chapter I tersely present the four main design principles of these tools and lead the reader through a typical example to demonstrate their interplay. The example is followed immediately by a second introduction aimed at the reader more conversant with statistics than with biology. The chapter closes with a brief sketch of the organization of the rest of the book.

1.1. FOUR PRINCIPLES

Many logical and methodological themes recur throughout this book. I have collected them here in the guise of "principles," tenets the meanings and implications of which will echo again and again in the theorems, constructions, and examples to follow. The principles appear together in this section and the next and then go their separate ways throughout the next six chapters. Chapter 8 draws them together again to serve as a framework for the summary of the techniques recommended here as "routine." Their limits, also mentioned many times in Chapters 2 through 7, will suggest the closing speculations of Chapter 8 on new tools for the next edition of this tool kit.

1.1.1. First Principle: landmark locations

In many biological and biomedical investigations, the most effective way to analyze the forms of whole biological organs or organisms is by recording geometric locations of **landmark points**. These are loci that have names ("bridge of the nose," "tip of the chin") as well as Cartesian coordinates. The names are intended to imply true homology (biological correspondence) from form to form. That is, landmark points not only have their own locations but also have the "same" locations in every other form of the study and in the average of all the forms of a data set (see Section 5.4).[1] An explanation of findings based on covariances of landmark locations usually will be phrased as an argument either that particular processes "push landmarks around," "push them apart," "deform substructures," and so forth, during part or all of ontogeny, or else that evolution has been induced to arrange similar changes over phylogeny.

Chapter 3 is devoted to the lore of landmarks: theory, practical hints, and introduction of the five extended examples that underlie most of the worked analyses later in this book. Section 2.4 will briefly touch on other styles of data concerning biological form, such as textures or outlines. In general, these other styles sustain explanations not in terms of relative displacements (often there is nothing to point to as undergoing "displacement") but only using different semantics of much weaker force: bulges form or do not (but how does one know the locations are comparable?); cells cluster linearly or circularly (but how can we describe the locations, orientations, or directions of the clusters?). An example later in the book will indicate how information from curving outlines can be analyzed effectively once the landmarks are dealt with.

1.1.2. Second Principle: shape coordinates

Measurement of the shapes of configurations of landmark locations reduces to multiple vectors of **shape coordinates**. These come in pairs that represent the shape of one triangle of landmarks in a manner completely independent of size. That is, the study of covariances of landmark configurations *begins* when the configurations are represented by multiple triangles. This is equally true in two dimensions or in three. For two-dimensional data the triangulation can be managed by locating all other landmarks with respect to two in particular that are held fixed at points with coordinates $(0,0)$ and $(1,0)$ of an abstract "common digitizing plane."

---

[1] The organization of this book is lexicographic by chapters, sections, subsections, and sub-subsections. Thus Section 5.4 is the fourth section of Chapter 5. Figures, tables, and equations are numbered serially within each *section*. Thus Table 3.4.2 is the second table in Section 3.4, and Figure 7.3.5*a* is panel *a* of the fifth figure in Section 7.3.

That triangles are sufficient to represent landmark data for the purpose of studying their associations of shape is the subject of Chapter 5. I am not claiming that the shape coordinates are likewise sufficient for *reporting* the findings they generate; the form of these reports is the subject of the Fourth Principle. The reduction of landmark configurations to sets of shape coordinates is the most pictorial of a few statistically equivalent ways (see Section 5.6) to circumvent all further arbitrary choices of coordinate systems or of "variables" once a selection (itself unavoidably arbitrary) of landmarks has been made.

1.1.3. Third Principle: the form of questions

All the main styles of biometric investigation can be realized upon landmark data by submitting the shape coordinates to multivariate statistical analyses. Although the analyses may be nearly standard in form, the questions to be asked need not be standard at all. They may refer to individual diagnoses, individual forecasts of future form, planning of individual treatment, detection or description of group differences, effects of growth or age or size difference upon form, covariances of outside factors with form, ecophenotypy, covariances of form with its nonmorphometric consequences (such as function or survival), treatment or selection effects upon growth or form, detections of patterns of systematic variability of form at diverse geometric scales, or any of a number of other possibilities.

Most of these questions can be posed in two semantically distinct variants: not only "*Is* there (statistical evidence for) a covariance between the landmark data and (the putative factor or covariate)?" but also "*What is* the nature of the covariance between the landmark data and (the putative factor or covariate)?" These interrogative forms exclude the questions typical of earlier applications of morphometrics in numerical taxonomy. Questions about "similarity" or "common ancestry" are not easily phrased in terms of covariances and have no particular meaning in the context of landmark data.

1.1.4. Fourth Principle: the form of answers

The most unusual of this book's themes is the form I recommend and exemplify for reporting answers to these morphometric questions. Findings usually are best represented not in conventional statistical tabulations but instead via geometric diagrams superimposed over a picture or drawing of a typical form. Ordinarily, a single data analysis will exploit several different diagrams *each of which corresponds to one part of the covariance signaled by a single statistical analysis*. The "parts" are size change and shape change, or size variation and shape variation; the shape part is further subdivided at a diversity of geometric scales. The diagrams graphically express formulas for particular "variables" – distances and ratios – aligned with the pattern of covariances or effects uncovered by one of these parts of the analysis.

For instance, an effect on the shape of a single triangle of landmarks may be drawn as a vector attached to any one of its vertices; the same effect usually can be drawn as an ellipse – a tensor – the axes of which refer to ordinary distance measures. The two reports have identical multivariate statistics but correspond to rather different sorts of biological explanations or metaphors. A size effect can be incorporated in the picture of the ellipse, but that is graphically separate from the depiction of the same shape change as displacement; which will be the more suggestive of biological insight will depend on the phenomenon under study. The application of either of these diagrams may be to any single triangle or instead to an "average triangle" – the *uniform component* of shape difference or shape variation, to be introduced in the next section. Likewise, effects on configurations of more than three landmarks might be reported as "displacements," "growth gradients," or "deformations" that are, in turn, either "global" or "local," and in which size change is variously a parameter or a covariate. In fact, in landmark-based morphometrics, the exploration of multiple interpretations of overlapping findings is the model for good reporting.

1.2. A TYPICAL EXAMPLE: THE "PHENYTOIN FACE"

1.2.1. A study of prenatal exposure to phenytoin

Dr. Lewis B. Holmes, M.D., director of the Embryology–Teratology Unit at Massachusetts General Hospital, has kindly permitted me to reproduce an example drawn from his long-term study of phenytoin effects. Phenytoin is an anticonvulsant (specifically, antiepileptic) agent often prescribed for adults in the form of a maintenance dosage. Recently it has been suspected of being teratogenic to fetuses when administered through the mother. In a manner typical of explorations in teratology, this suspicion was founded on a psychological, not a biological, finding: A trained dysmorphologist often can classify children as "exposed" or not – that is, can characterize certain children as having "the face" (of phenytoin) – without being able to report in words or diagrams exactly what it is that generates that recognition. (A similar "feeling" led to the discovery of Fetal Alcohol Syndrome, the most prevalent avoidable birth defect.)

Once a dysmorphologist spots a reliable similarity among faces in association with a common insult, it becomes possible to mount a sustained investigation of dose–response relationships, covariances between morphological and functional aspects of teratogenesis, and the like. Holmes's project, of which this example is a small part, is designed in this spirit: The facies corresponding to prenatal damage will be used as proxy for effective dose in studies of neurologic sequelae. One of the principal running examples of this book, treated recurrently in Chapters 5 through 7, is the report of a prospective study involving the morphological consequences of prenatal exposure to moderate levels of alcohol. Here, too, the larger intention is to use the face as proxy for measures of specific brain damage.

1.2.2. The data: sample, photographs, landmarks

For preliminary analysis, Holmes selected a sample of 45 older children, all of whom appeared to have "the face" of phenytoin. Of these, 31 had been exposed to phenytoin *in utero* in typical dosages. (Thirteen of these children had also been exposed to phenobarbital, but there appear to have been no additional effects of that exposure upon the data we explored.) Each of the 45 was photographed from the front in a manner that, because ours was a no-budget pilot study, was uncontrolled. Not much attention was paid to issues of head position, and no information about absolute scale is available (camera-to-subject distance was not monitored, nor is there a ruler visible in the photographs). Thus we can study only shape, not size, for these faces. The landmarks selected for this project numbered 16 on each frontal photograph. Although they were digitized directly from the photographs, it is simplest to display them schematically in outline drawings of "typical" forms from the two groups (Figure 1.2.1).

For the analysis here, four landmarks from the midline and six pairs of lateral landmarks were located by pinholes through actual prints and digitized at a conventional digitizing tablet to the nearest 0.1 millimeter. This is in accordance with the First Principle, which suggests the thoughtful reduction of pictorial data to named landmark locations as the first step in any analysis of organic form above the tissue level. These landmarks are discussed further, along with other facial landmarks, in Section 3.4.4;

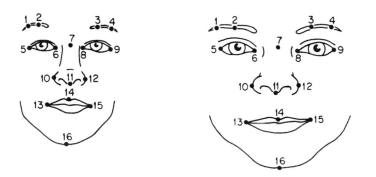

Figure 1.2.1. Typical frontal forms from the phenytoin face study. Tracings of typical unexposed (left) and exposed (right) subjects have been altered between landmarks to conceal subjects' identities. The 16 landmarks of the morphometric analysis are indicated by serial numbers (see Table 1.2.1).

Table 1.2.1. *Landmarks for the phenytoin study*

Landmark name	Number(s)	Description
Midline landmarks		
Nasal bridge	7	Bridge of the nose
Columella	11	Bottom of the columella where it springs from the upper lip
Upper vermilion	14	Midpoint of Cupid's bow, upper vermilion border
Chin	16	Lowest midline point of symphysis
Bilateral landmarks		
Eyebrow central	2, 3	Intersection of the eyebrow curve with a vertical line through the midpoint of the pupil
Eyebrow lateral	1, 4	Intersection of the eyebrow curve with a vertical line through exocanthion
Exocanthion	5, 9	Lateral intersection of upper and lower eyelids
Endocanthion	6, 8	Medial intersection of upper and lower eyelids
Nasal ala	10, 12	Most lateral points on alar curvature
Lip commissure	13, 15	Lateral intersection of upper and lower vermilion borders; also known as Cheilon

see also Farkas (1981). Holmes adapted this particular set of landmarks from Clarren et al. (1987).

Following the Second Principle, the archiving of these landmark locations is quickly followed by a reduction to the descriptor space of shapes: their expression as shape coordinates to some convenient baseline. The appropriate formulas, such as equations (5.1.1), will be explained *in situ*. In this approach, two relatively reliable landmarks are fixed in position on the page (by a combination of scaling, translating, and rotating); the resulting locations of all the other landmarks express their positions "with respect to" that fixed pair. (However, the "size variable" that would have been associated with any of these shapes had the photographs preserved scale information is *not* the scale factor divided out in the course of this construction; see Section 5.5.) For nearly symmetric forms, it is better to choose a baseline along the axis of putative symmetry. Of the four landmarks along the midline (Table 1.2.1), the most reliable are the first and third, Nasal bridge (#7) and Upper vermilion (#14), and so that segment serves as our baseline for this first exemplary analysis (Figure 1.2.2*a*).

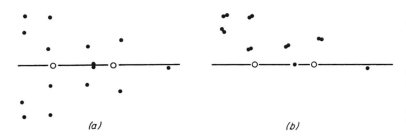

(a)   (b)

1.2.3. Questions

Figure 1.2.2. Construction of the
hemiface (symmetrized frontal
view). (*a*) Fourteen shape coordinates to a baseline from #7 to
#14. (*b*) Reflection across a con-
venient midline, to be followed
by averaging (not shown).

Each shape coordinate that results from this construction may
be interpreted as a legitimate, though often rather odd-sounding,
ratio of distances, that is, a conventional shape variable. The
vertical shape coordinate (horizontal in Figure 1.2.3) is the more
familiar; doubled, it represents the distance between the inner
corners of the eyes in this coordinate system normalized to the
"upper facial height" from Nasal bridge to Upper vermilion, and
so it is actually the ratio of intercanthal distance to that version of
upper facial height. The other coordinate in the same plot is the
proportional height of the inner canthi upon that same upper
facial baseline. Whereas these may seem to provide an odd and
arbitrary foundation for any study of the corner of the eye, the
theorems in Chapter 5 ought to convince you that they are
sufficient. No set of shape measures of a landmark configuration
can be more powerful than the corresponding set of shape coordinates for detecting or diagramming group differences or other
covariates pertaining to "aspects of shape" not specified or restricted in advance of the analysis. That is, there is nothing to lose
by proceeding via these coordinates, but a great deal to gain in
terms of multiplicity of feature spaces, availability of alternate
interpretations, and the like.

Although the data were digitized on both sides of the face, it is
more efficient to analyze the landmarks in a symmetric form.
Geometrically, one might imagine picking up the left side of the
face, reflecting it over a "midline" to superimpose on the right,
then averaging the sides. The effect of this operation is not much
changed by small deviations in the actual midline locus chosen for
this exercise. Following the Second Principle, we carry out the
symmetrization using the shape coordinates just created. We
"reflect" the left side over the midline that is used as the baseline
(Figure 1.2.2*b*), then average the shape coordinates of left and
reflected right landmarks. Algebraically, this is the same as averaging the coordinates after the second (anatomically horizontal)
coordinate of one side has had its sign reversed.

1.2.3. Questions

The question asked of this sample of 45 symmetrized forms is
exactly in accordance with the Third Principle. It deals with the
covariance between form (landmark configuration) and an exoge-

7

nous variable (exposure to phenytoin or not). Specifically, we inquire whether or not there are statistically significant differences between the group mean forms and, if so, which biological process(es) might account for these differences. Underlying this mode of explanation is the epidemiological/teratological supposition that those truly exposed were systematically affected by the prenatal insult, whereas those not truly exposed have come to resemble "the face" in unpatterned, haphazard ways.

1.2.4. Findings

1.2.4.1. A shift "at" Endocanthion. —

It is customary to submit a set of shape coordinates to one single multivariate test for some large general hypothesis (group difference, size or age effect, etc.) at issue. This proved unnecessary for these data, as the difference between the group means proved adequately significant for one of the shape-coordinate pairs by itself: Endocanthion (inner corner of the eye), as shown in the scatter in Figure 1.2.3. In the lateral coordinate of this plot, which is the ratio of endocanthal width to an "upper facial height," the 16 highest values [relatively most hyperteloric (widely set) eyes] pertain without exception to children who were, in fact, exposed. The difference in mean ratio is about 12%: 0.549 for the 14 unexposed children, 0.613 for the 31 exposed children. The appropriate T^2-test (not a t-test, in light of the full plane of directions of shape change from which we were free to choose; see Section

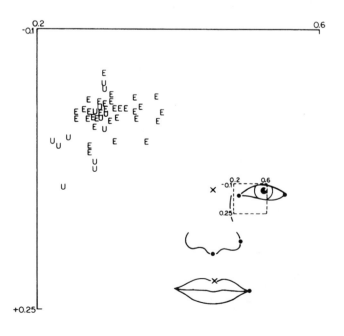

Figure 1.2.3. First finding of the phenytoin-face study. Scatter of shape coordinates for Endocanthion. Shape space has been rotated back to anatomical vertical. U, unexposed; E, exposed. (Recall that all cases appeared subjectively to have "the face" of phenytoin.)

6.5.1.3) is conventionally "significant" at about $p \sim .007$. These shape coordinates seem quite well behaved, without obvious sub-clusters or outliers.

From this single figure, one cannot yet tell how to interpret the finding. Although extracted by manipulation of one set of shape coordinates, it actually expresses the change of shape of one entire triangle (Nasal bridge–Upper vermilion–Endocanthion). Furthermore, we cannot yet say whether the "effect" (the recon-figuration of landmarks within the criterion of having "the face") is specific to this triangle or is instead distributed somehow over the whole photograph in a less focused fashion. That is, in accordance with the Fourth Principle, its "effect" must be construed wholly independently of arbitrary choices in the course of carrying out the statistical analysis. Reporting the difference, then, must wait until we have thoroughly explored all the other feature spaces that are relevant to a biological interpretation under the Fourth Principle.

1.2.4.2. A uniform shear. —

The diagram in Figure 1.2.4, explained further in Section 7.2, is a serviceable exploratory display style for the pursuit of certain large-scale explanations. I have enlarged the relative displace-ments of all the intergroup mean shape coordinates 10-fold so as to highlight the deviations of these mean differences from a particularly simple geometry, the "linear" or "uniform" model. In the model, all shape change is by the same ratio of increase in length as a function of direction, regardless of location. In this application, as applied to symmetrized data, it represents a trans-formation of the two sides of the face outward and upward from

1.2.4. Findings

Figure 1.2.4. Second finding of the phenytoin-face study: the in-tergroup displacements, enlarged 10-fold, between mean landmark locations to the upper facial base-line. (The origins of the vectors are not altered; they spring from the mean landmark locations for the unexposed group.) Solid lines: Observed mean landmark shifts. Dashed lines: Best-fitting uni-form (linear) transformation be-tween these means, under the "null" probability model ex-plained in Section 7.2. Note the discrepancy between dashed and solid lines at Endocanthion: The intergroup divergence there is double what would be predicted from the others. Inset right: Sketch of the uniform transfor-mation fitted by the dashed dis-placements, no longer multiplied 10-fold.

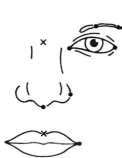
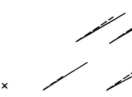
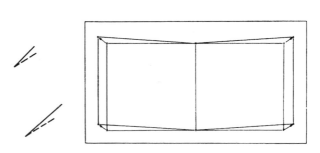

9

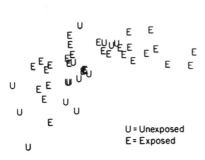

U = Unexposed
E = Exposed

Figure 1.2.5. Third finding of the phenytoin-face study. The uniform component of shape variation, case by case, resembles that for Endocanthion alone (finding 1), but with greater group overlap.

the midline by parallel vectors all proportional to the original bilateral width landmark by landmark.

We can report the fit of this model by a quantity analogous to the "fraction of variance explained" in ordinary regression: 72% of the observed mean shift of shapes between the landmark configurations is summarized in one single global pattern, the change in width ratio by about 6% together with an upward cant of about half that extent. Most of the remaining 28% of this generalized sum of squares is the additional upward-outward expansion (amounting to 12%, not 6%) at Endocanthion.

1.2.4.3. Scatter of a uniform component. —

Using equation (7.2.2) we can express this linear component of the group difference in a scatter having one point for every child, an "estimated linear component." Information from Endocanthion has been *omitted* from this estimate. That scatter (Figure 1.2.5) resembles what we have already seen for the most sensitive landmark, Endocanthion, separately. The difference between the exposed group and the unexposed is aligned with the displacement from the vaguely elliptical scatter of U's to the somewhat differently shaped ellipse of E's. The separation is not perfect: some of the exposed children were not characterized by this upward-outward shear of the lateral landmarks. A similar observation applies to the scatter of the shape coordinates for Endocanthion alone (Figure 1.2.3). Apparently the dysmorphologist misidentified some nonhyperteloric subjects as having having "the face" on the basis of a different feature or combination, but he was right in all sufficiently hyperteloric cases. There is variability of expression of the effect within the "exposed" ellipse, but its coefficient of variation, in comparison with the mean difference from the "unexposed" group, seems under adequate control.

1.2.4.4. Summary. —

There is a better way to explain this combination of features than "a linear term plus hypertelorism." Looking again at Figure 1.2.4, we see that the four points of the orbital region are not changed much in shape. What we see might better be described as changes in the *positions* of those landmarks with respect to a baseline that is also changing its own relative scale. Visualizing this interpretation is much clearer with reference to a baseline on one of the rigid components of the rearrangement (see Section 7.4.4.1). At the left in Figure 1.2.6 is a display of the same group comparison (this time the changes multiplied by a factor of 5) to a baseline across the eye from inner to outer corner. The small changes in the positions of the eyebrow points can be ignored. Notice that Nasion appears to move relatively *downward*, the entire lip area

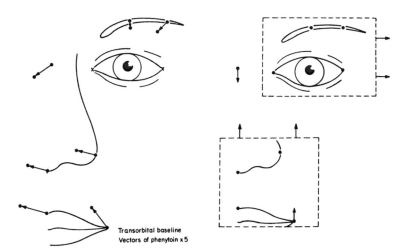

Transorbital baseline
Vectors of phenytoin x 5

Figure 1.2.6. Findings of the phenytoin-face study. Tentative summary explanation (all vectors of comparison × 5). Left: Group difference to a transorbital baseline. Right: Summary in terms of rigid motions suggesting a deformation above Nasion.

upward – this massive shortening of what we had used before as the baseline accounts for the complexity of Figure 1.2.4.

By assigning points with similar displacements to "compartments," still following the Fourth Principle, we summarize this set of three interrelated findings by the schema of Figure 1.2.6 (right). The upward cant of the upper bilateral landmarks is consistent with displacement of the nasal bridge slightly downward with respect to lateral structures and displacement of the upper vermilion point slightly upward. A net reduction in upper facial height would have the effect, in the shape-coordinate formalism, of driving all landmarks away from the midline (the lateral components of the dashed lines in Figure 1.2.4). The additional disproportion specific to the segment between the inner canthi is best interpreted, in our view (Holmes and myself), not as the change of a ratio but as an actual hypertelorism: displacement by some millimeters of additional interorbital bone. It is very tempting to combine the findings "at Nasal bridge" – the hypertelorism and the downward displacement both – in a hypothesis of additional neural mass above and inside the nasal bridge, that is, interior to the lower middle forehead. From these landmarks we cannot check this hypothesis directly, but it corresponds to the effects of other known neuroteratogens upon central structures in the frontal lobe.

This explanation must not be thought of as having been statistically tested. It is a selection from a great variety of alternate biological processes consistent with the observed group differences. Only to those differences, not to the explanations, does there correspond a multivariate statistic.

1.2.5. Generality of the example

The rhythm by which Principles 1–4 interact with each other, with the data, and with the biologist's wisdom is typified quite well in this little example. The reduction of data to those 16 landmark points, in accord with the First Principle, is done once and for all; and yet at the end of the analysis our findings suggest that interesting things appear to be happening behind the nasal bridge, where one might mine more assiduously (as from a side view) for additional anatomical information – if not in the present study, then in the next. The Second Principle, too, requires attention only once in most studies. In the phenytoin study it suggested a simple symmetrization, reducing the effective number of landmarks from 16 to 10. Otherwise it was present mostly behind the scenes, guaranteeing that the features we reported at the end of the statistical exploration would characterize the landmark configurations per se, not merely the accidental coordinate system(s) in which we chose to report them. The shape coordinates are not unique in freeing the morphometrician from this risk of relativism, but they are unique in supporting the full range of reportable features within a single formal notation.

By comparison, the Third and Fourth Principles are most commonly part of a cycle of interaction between computation and contemplation: Compute a diagram (i.e., difference of mean forms, Figure 1.2.4), and notice a biologically suggestive feature (the linear term); compute another diagram (answer another question – now, the scatter of individual "linear components," Figure 1.2.5), and notice another biologically suggestive feature (the combination of separation and overlap); recall the local intensification of Figure 1.2.5 seen earlier in Figure 1.2.3, and combine these multiple findings in a single composite hypothesis (Figure 1.2.6); find a way of testing *that* using the machinery of shape coordinates (not shown – I must reserve some methods for current grant proposals, after all!); and so on. Although the immediacy of recourse to the shape coordinates may at first seem arbitrary and artificial, they actually serve to conceal statistical machinery quite effectively from the biologist's view. Under the Second Principle, interaction with one's data becomes primarily a synthesis of the geometric and the biological, with hardly any explicitly numerical quantities intervening.

1.3. SHAPE FEATURES AND MULTIVARIATE ANALYSIS

Not every reader will come to this text in search of tools to solve already-nagging biometric problems or as intellectual prophylaxis prior to beginning a well-formed investigation. Some will instead be encountering these ideas in advance of applications, as part of a professional education in statistical or biometric method. Indeed, morphometrics is not only a discipline for explanation in quantitative biology but also an interestingly specialized application of multivariate statistics, analogous to variants for other fields wherein data are highly structured, such as computer vision or weather prediction. The reader having more training in multivariate statistics than in quantitative biology may find useful a second overview that emphasizes the statistical strategies involved, rather than, as before, the connections between geometric patterns and biological factors or processes. For this reader, the First Principle becomes the assertion that landmark data support a joint language for talking about geometry, homology, and multivariate statistics all at once. (The word "homology" here refers to the primitive notion of biological correspondence between two biological forms; it will be analyzed in Chapter 3.) The common object of all this language for K landmarks is a shape space of $2K - 4$ dimensions (for planar data; for spatial data, $3K - 7$ dimensions) ordered both statistically and geometrically and so supporting a great diversity of interesting subspaces. The elements of each subspace may be thought of as parameterized families of "maps" moving landmarks about in accordance with control mechanisms that we cannot observe but that probably would make biological sense if we observed their consequences as regular features covarying with explanatory factors.

That said, it surely does not follow that multivariate morphometrics is the application of textbook multivariate methods to a geometrically disorganized data base of sizes or ratios. Especially in light of the Second and Fourth Principles, "multivariate morphometrics" should comprise not the syllabus of books currently referred to by that phrase (see Section 2.5) but instead the following few themes (Bookstein, 1990*e*).

(1) Size is a central factor in most morphometric explanations. (The word "factor" here is used in a somewhat technical sense; see Section 2.3.) Whereas "size-and-shape space" and "shape space" differ by only one degree of freedom (compare the spaces of size variables and size ratios to be constructed in Chapters 4 and 5), this discrepancy should not be thought of as the result of "partialing out" or "dividing out" any one single measurement (Mosimann, 1970; Bookstein, 1989*c*). Rather, any representation of the single "missing" dimension correlates, in general, with all aspects of shape and must be maintained as a separate explicit factor in all analyses. Should a single size variable be required, it is often usefully taken as the net second moment of the landmark configuration about its own centroid (the "Centroid Size" score, Chapter 4).

In practice one often encounters shape changes or covariances that can be described with only a very few parameters applying to the form or to large regions of it. Among these most-global transformations is **(2)** the **uniform component of shape change** introduced in connection with Figure 1.2.4. A geometrically appropriate "distance" for forms compared or scattered via this model is often the log ratio of diameters of the ellipse into which a circle is taken by the transformation (log anisotropy, Section 6.2.4). Another global transform is **(3)** the **rigid motion** of one subset of landmarks with respect to another (translation and rotation without change of shape of either separately). The best description of rigid motion is by the parameters of kinematics, but we shall not go into that here (Karger and Novák, 1985).

A special case of rigid motion is the displacement of a single landmark point over a background of a configuration of many others not changing their shape. Many different approaches to the morphometrics of landmarks are capable of handling this special case, but most do not generalize to the other equally important feature spaces. Among these inferior approaches are Procrustes superposition (Section 7.1) and analysis of extreme ratios of interlandmark distances (Section 6.4.3). Still other approaches, such as finite-element analysis, do not handle single landmark displacements well (Section 7.3.3.2). The only formalism known to me that handles all the special cases, along with the general case of correlated differences in size and arbitrary aspects of shape, is the method of shape coordinates emphasized in this book.

In the general shape change, one that is not the same over the whole form or the identity over most of it, the correspondence between homologous landmarks usually can be imagined as having arisen by discrete sampling from a **homology map**, a smooth transformation, which is then expanded in an orthonormal series of functions defined over the form.

(4) *Some functions underlying a decomposition of homology maps incorporate no information either from the actual form under study or from its observed variation.* These include, for outline data, Fourier expansions (in three dimensions, spherical harmonics); for landmark data, these are the *growth-gradient models* fitted by projection methods, as in Section 7.4. The uniform maps (category **2**) may be thought of as a special case of growth gradients, having gradient zero.

Each of the methods **1–4** mentioned thus far is a projection into a feature space defined a priori, before the onset of computation. All these should be computed as statistical fits (by least squares, robust least squares, or, if one is extremely optimistic about the "truth" of one's models, maximum likelihood) in a manner conscientiously independent of all arbitrary assumptions beyond the list of landmarks involved. The spaces involved in these features often correspond to "nested" hypotheses in the usual statistical sense. For instance, the "feature space" of no shape change, the arena of analysis by the Procrustes methods, is the one-dimensional space of size changes; features **5** and **6** live in a space complementary to that of the uniform component (**2**) and so may be considered to seek features among the latter's "residuals"; and so forth.

(5) *Other functions into which homology maps may be decomposed incorporate information about the "typical" form under study, but not about its variability.* Although this seems a useful sort of feature in principle, the only example known to me is my technique of principal warps (eigenfunctions of the bending-

14

energy matrix), to be introduced in Section 7.5. The partial warps, products of principal warps by a single 2-vector representing a magnitude and a direction in the picture plane, are geometrically orthogonal dimensions of displacement of many landmarks at the same time. These features underlie the "nonlinear" or "regional-izable" part of a landmark rearrangement (the null space of the uniform changes); their orthogonality is with respect to summed-squared landmark displacement at optimal superposition (the so-called *Procrustes distance*). **Bending energy** is a quadratic form for one metaphorically reasonable notion of "distance" specific to this subspace. The central presence of this mean-dependent quadratic form is one way in which the geometry of landmark data makes itself felt in modifications of textbook multivariate algebra: In conventional multivariate statistical theory there is no obvious analogue to any quadratic form other than the covariance matrix itself. This second quadratic form, which is not of full rank, is introduced in Section 2.2 and explored late in Chapter 7 as the feature spaces it grounds are explained.

(**6**) *A third useful class of functions, presenting a different anal-ogy to ordinary principal components, are orthogonal statistically as well as energetically*, and so depend upon the covariance matrix of shape differences under study as well as upon the mean landmark configuration. This class of decompositions includes eigenshapes for outlines (see Section 2.4.1), the (computationally trivial) factor analysis of a scatter of shape coordinates for triangles (Figure 1.2.3; see also Section 5.3.3) or of the uniform component derived from more numerous configurations (Figure 1.2.5; see also Section 7.2), and the *relative warps* introduced in Section 7.6 for the variation remaining in the space complementary to the linear (uniform) changes. Just as different principal components are both uncorrelated and orthogonal in the quadratic form that is the identity matrix, so the relative warps are both uncorrelated and orthogonal in the quadratic form that is bending energy. Whereas the principal warps (feature style **5**, no reference to variances) are obtained from a joint diagonalization of the bending-energy ma-trix and the identity (Procrustes) matrix, these nonlinear compo-nents are extracted via simultaneous diagonalization of bending energy and the observed covariances of the landmark locations. Each relative warp expresses the summation of correlated dis-tributed effects of larger or smaller geometrical scope. The rela-tive warp of largest scale for a set of landmarks typically has the appearance of a growth gradient or other systematic disproportion graded one-dimensionally across some transect of the form; the last few are highly local. For an example, see Section 7.6.4.

A "zeroth" pair of these relative warps, having *no* bending energy, will be the ordinary principal components of a sample scatter of uniform components, as we noted them informally in Figure 1.2.5. The combination of these components with the first few relative warps and with size, all by correlational methods (see

15

Section 2.3.1), is intended wholly to supplant principal-component analysis of arbitrary variables of extent as applied to landmark data.

When all these features have been computed and inspected, they empower the usual two grand multivariate strategies, the study of patterns of covariation *within* and *between* domains of measurement.

(7) *Analysis of the covariances among the separate morphometric feature spaces.* There is no single distance measure for morphometric analysis, and there is no single feature analysis of any landmark data set. After a set of landmarks is analyzed or ordinated according to the methods **1–6** separately, one combines the analyses as one would any other collection of incommensurable information: by the study of two-dimensional and higher-dimensional scatter plots of the features with respect to each other and in the light of known biological regulatory possibilities. For instance, allometry is the examination of correlations of size change with components of uniform and nonuniform shape change.

(8) *Analysis of the structure of covariation of all of these morphometric descriptors with other measurement schemes exogenous to morphometrics,* including descriptions of group differences, ecophenotypy, changes over evolutionary time, changes over ontogenetic time, apparent selective value, known biomechanical constraints, properties of cell division, and so on. The covariances among multiple "blocks" of variables, morphometric or otherwise, should be pursued via the method of Partial Least Squares, reviewed in Section 2.3.2. These analyses include the relation of different sets of landmarks in multiple views (see Tabachnick and Bookstein, 1990*a*) and the relation of sets of shape coordinates to lists of ecological or functional covariates. The principal import of morphometric analyses in the larger context of quantitative biological science is borne by the covariances of morphometric descriptors with measurements outside the domain of morphometrics.

1.4. PROSPECTUS

After this Introduction, the main text of this book is divided into six chapters. Chapter 2, "Preliminaries," briefly surveys the history of the developments to be reported, then introduces two important borrowed technologies that will underlie most of the logical strategies for ties between data and explanation: interpolation of scattered data via thin-plate splines, and simplification of blocks of covariances via least-squares factor models. These technologies seem ideally suited to the applications to which I have assigned them here, and so they deserve an introduction more extended than that for other techniques I have borrowed, techniques more algebraic than conceptual. The chapter ends with two auxiliary reading lists: the main themes of morphometrics for data other than landmark locations, topics omitted from this book, and other resources for morphometrics and related statistical methods that might profitably be consulted by the reader seeking additional enlightenment (but that must not be expected to have anticipated the point of view put forward here).

Chapter 3 is about landmarks. I begin by reviewing their role in linking morphometrics to other forms of biometrics. In assigning coordinates to one form based on locations upon another, they serve also as instructions for where one should put down one's ruler. Landmarks are better used, however, if they are treated as discrete samples of a continuous underlying process the biological terminology for which refers to "homology," the geometric to "deformation" or "transformation." Neither language directly refers to "variables" or other statistical machinery. That is, landmarks are quite a bit more than instructions for measurement; they are the places at which one's explanations of biological processes ought to be grounded. At the same time, they are "less than" measurements, in that the transition from their locations to proper statistical variables must be made with great care. The chapter goes on to review the three main categories of landmarks commonly encountered in practice: anatomical points (discrete juxtapositions of distinct tissues), maxima of curvature or other relicts of local morphogenetic processes, and more ambiguous records of processes at a distance – extremal diameters, centers of circles that are tangent to the outline at more than one point, and the like. The principal data sets underlying most of the examples of the later chapters are then introduced: provenance of the samples and operational definitions and meanings of the landmarks involved. (Most of these landmark data sets are explicitly tabulated in Appendix A.4.) The chapter concludes with a discussion showing how Blum's technique of *medial-axis analysis*, expressing a geometry wholly different from the deformation model, can supply information when curvatures are smooth and landmarks consequently lacking.

Chapter 4 is a brief, backward-looking consideration of the analysis of distance data, hitherto the main stuff of morphometric statistical analysis, but now, in my view, obsolete. I construct the statistical space in which the distances reside and demonstrate some appropriate applications to distance data of conventional multivariate techniques – true factor analysis, analysis of covariance – but argue that one cannot really expect to understand biological shape by statistical manipulations of size measures. Chapter 5 turns to a better basis for landmark-based shape analysis, the technique already introduced here: the *shape coordinates* to any baseline. These may be thought of as having "already transformed" the space of interlandmark distances into an algebraic form suited to the great variety of biological explanations typically sought in shape studies. The chapter introduces the fundamental algebraic and geometric properties of the shape coordinates and the purposes to which they may be applied without any reference to subspaces: computation and comparison of averages, size allometry, and other simple phenomena. Chapter 6 introduces the interpretation of effects upon the shape coordinates in the simplest case, the triangle of landmarks. I explain the geometric core of this interpretation, the shape-change *tensor*, both algebraically and geometrically, and exemplify all conventional multivariate biometric strategies in this special case. In particular, shape distances between triangles, like uniform distances among the general landmark configuration, often are best measured by the log anisotropy of this tensor; the chapter explains the nature of this approximation and the reasons it is so compelling.

Most morphometric questions beyond the existential ("*Is* there an effect?") will be found to have multiple answers, one for each style of "explanation" to which these geometric features can be put. The latter part of Chapter 6 and all of Chapter 7 review the geometric algebra of these descriptions one by one and explain their relationships to the shape coordinates that encapsulate the data. The sorts of interpretations that can coexist, that *simultaneously* apply to the same observed covariances, include size differences and size allometry, uniform changes of shape, gradients across whole diameters of the organism, regional rearrangements at a scale distinctly smaller than that of the whole organism, and displacements of single landmarks. The multiplicity of these findings is enriched, in turn, by a covariance structure of their own, among themselves or with exogenous factors or consequences of form.

Chapter 7 is thus different from those preceding. It consists of material mostly unpublished and untaught prior to the 1988 draft of this volume. (I fondly consider my difficulty in publishing it piecemeal to testify to its seamless intellectual coherence.) If morphometrics is the empirical fusion of geometry with biology, then this chapter is my most explicit attempt to supply a common language. Though it is the last substantive chapter, it really lies at the core of the tool kit, the locus (to change metaphors) at which real biometric leverage (in the form of wisdom about promising feature spaces) is applied to geometric data in order to further biological understanding. All these techniques strenuously take advantage of the geometric ordering of the data as well as the statistical. I begin with the "zeroth-order" shape feature (the Procrustes fit) in the application to asymmetry, the only context I know where the associated distance measure makes sense. The chapter then turns to the simplest subspace of shape space per se, the linear (uniform) component already exemplified in the phenytoin study. This ramifies into two series of spatially ordered extensions: one based in polynomial functions of the Cartesian coordinates, the other in expressions of the spacing of the landmarks among themselves. Both lead to hierarchies of descriptions of a steadily increasing complexity; the scientist may pursue these as far as they prove fruitful. As the shape coordinates supersede analysis by size and shape variables, so these features, beginning with the simple single shape-change tensor of the preceding chapter, are intended permanently to supersede the representation of form change by lists of "coefficients."

The concluding Chapter 8 returns to the concerns of this Introduction, reviewing all the intervening material in the light of Principles 1–4 underlying the phenytoin face study. I summarize the routine steps for their realization that will have been illustrated repeatedly in the course of the exemplary data analyses, and then expand on issues that I hope will enspirit an efflorescence of dissertations or research aims in this new morphometrics. My experience to date with Principle 1, the primacy of landmarks, leaves open many issues in the generalization of this notion to more subtle forms of data. Principle 2, on shape coordinates, leaves open the visualization and modeling of their probability distributions, especially in three dimensions. Principle 3, "the form of questions," deserves extension in several directions: alternatives to the particular interpolation mapping function relied on here, new kinds of optimal biometric descriptions, and the relation of geometrical-statistical orderings of form to other reasonable orderings, such as the developmental or the geographical. Finally, to the extent that the 200-odd figures in this book attest to Principle 4, variety in "the form of answers," these pages themselves are certain to be superseded and made obsolete by the new technologies of high-speed computer workstations. All books like these will be supplemented and then supplanted by videotapes and, ultimately, by interactive animated imagery of creatures growing, adapting, or evolving.

Reverting to Gutenberg's medium, the mathematically beautiful topics that do not result in "features" – the pessimism of the random-walk model, the non-Euclidean geometry of simple (uniform) tensors, applications of bending-energy minimization to image analysis – have been placed in Appendices, along with listings of data and a useful fragment of the spline programs.

2
Preliminaries

This chapter assembles miscellaneous topics that underlie the statistical, geometrical, and biological reasoning about morphometric data and morphometric explanations put forward in this volume. Section 2.1 deals with the progression of insights by which the synthesis reported here emerged in the 1980s out of a creative but disorganized earlier literature spanning most of the century. Two dogmas – that one should analyze landmark coordinates without specifying particular size or shape measures in advance, and that such analyses should be no less symmetric than the Euclidean plane or space of the data – underlie the development and dissemination of Principles 1–4 of Chapter 1. The core of this chapter, Sections 2.2 and 2.3, is a review of two very useful techniques I have borrowed from other disciplines for applications in morphometrics. The **thin-plate spline** is an interpolation function originally developed for computational surface theory and computer graphics; here I am suggesting it as the most appropriate formalism currently available for D'Arcy Thompson's old theme of biological homology as a geometric mapping. By the end of Chapter 7 the reader may be convinced that in its algebra and its geometry these interpolants have exactly the right flexibility for the interplay with biological explanations at many different physical scales. In particular, the nonnegative-definite quadratic form of deficient rank that was referred to in the preceding chapter as "bending energy," which drives the regional analysis of shape change, is copied verbatim from the spline literature. The second major borrowing is from Sewall Wright's model for biometrical explanation as **path analysis**. In morphometrics, most models that in other fields would be computed by ordinary regressions will refer instead to dependence of suites of observed variables, such as shape coordinates, upon explanatory factors, I shall review the manner in which path models "decompose" observed covariances and explanatory schemes.

Following these explanations is a review of some traditional types of morphometric data not conformal with the landmark-bound methods – outlines and textures. It is no criticism of these other techniques to point out that the tactics so useful for landmarks, such as homology maps or bending energy, do not work so far afield; other methodologies have been, and continue to be, developed where landmarks cannot tread. The chapter closes with auxiliary reading lists covering a bit of statistics, other approaches to morphometrics, and, most important, the classic analytic geometry of real planes and real space, which underlies all the accommodations of ordinary multivariate algebra to the rich geometric ordering of morphometric data.

2.1. A BRIEF MODERN HISTORY

It is only recently that morphometrics has been considered its own branch of statistics. Up through the mid-1970s it was viewed instead as a standard application of multivariate analysis (Blackith and Reyment, 1971; a comparison of that volume with its own second edition, Reyment, Blackith, and Campbell, 1984, is itself interesting). Back then, the multivariate analyses of morphometrics dealt with "size measures" and "shape measures," often distances and angles, presumed to have derived from biological forms in some unsupervised way. Their principal thrust, now almost abandoned, was the conversion of their multivariate patterns into "distances" of another sort, analogues to Mahalanobis distance between specimens or groups, on which the newly emerging methods of numerical taxonomy could operate. (The first use of the word "morphometrics" that I have been able to find is in this sense: Blackith, 1965.) Those approaches, now termed "traditional morphometrics" (cf. Marcus, 1990), tended to ignore the origins of data in the geometry of biological specimens or their images. Other approaches to morphometrics of that time selected other tools of measurement than applied multivariate analysis, but combined them with biological data in a similar spirit, for instance, the clever borrowings from image analysis reviewed, again as "morphometrics," by Oxnard (1978).

So insouciant a dilettantism is no longer possible. Today, in all the areas of morphometrics, automatic borrowing of techniques from other metrologies has been replaced by careful scrutiny of foundations. This is true equally of methods for outlines and methods for landmarks, the two great classes of organismic data to which morphometric methods are applied. This book is concerned primarily with data of the latter class. For a review of the outline methods in a similar spirit beyond the brief discussion in Section 2.4.1, see Rohlf (1990a) and Straney (1990).

The transition of morphometrics into a discipline in its own right, the synthesis of geometry, statistics, and biology, can be traced back as far as D'Arcy Thompson's *On Growth and Form* of 1917. Thompson suggested there that changes of biological form be both modeled and described as mathematical diffeomorphisms (deformations that are smooth and that have smooth inverses). He called these "Cartesian transformations." I have reviewed the vicissitudes of Thompson's suggestion elsewhere (Bookstein, 1978). Beginning in the 1930s there appeared a long series of attempts to pursue the implications of his suggestion for biometrics – that statistical analysis of form should likewise be carried out upon these descriptions of "Cartesian transformation" – but the efforts were fragmentary and did not often benefit from the advice of statisticians. Huxley (1932) noted the relevance of polynomial and axial models of growth rate; Richards and Kavanagh (1943) were the first to display these transformations as tensor fields; Sneath (1967) fitted them as bivariate polynomials, but only in order to reduce them to a net "distance" for application in numerical taxonomy.

Suddenly, without any premonitory ferment, this particular biometric barrier was surpassed in the late 1970s and early 1980s in several centers at once. Bookstein (1978) provided difficult algorithms for crossed systems of principal strain trajectories, or "biorthogonal grids," representing transformations between single forms, and went on to suggest that an appropriate morphometric statistical method would be based on the same algebraic features represented somehow as vectors rather than curves. By 1982 (Bookstein, 1982 a,b) there existed a method for the informal testing of some simple hypotheses about these derivatives in samples of forms or growth series. The computations were based on means and variances of selected strains in triangles of landmarks. It was not yet known how the analyses of separate triangles might be combined, but several of us suspected that a better multivariate statistical analysis would wrestle with the landmark locations directly, rather than in the form of the nonlinearly derived lengths, length ratios, principal strains, and so forth. This better synthesis emerged between 1983 and 1986 as an essentially complete framework for the analysis of landmark locations as raw data.

The important contributions during that brief period when the discipline was synthesized included a paper of mine (Bookstein, 1984a) reducing the difference of a pair of pooled principal strains to a modified t-ratio (rather than the correct T^2) and permitting the first general test of differences in growth changes; another paper of mine (Bookstein, 1984b) introducing the "shape coordinates" for triangles and showing how shape differences can be weighed by a formal T^2-test; Goodall's 1983 dissertation, deriving the equivalent F-ratio while avoiding any size standardization; and Kendall's announcement (1984) of the global shape spaces to which Goodall's and my methods inadvertently applied as statistical metrics in tangent spaces (linearized feature spaces). Our joint publication in the first volume of *Statistical Science* (Bookstein, 1986a, with commentary) proudly announced the convergence of all three of these approaches on one single foundation for the morphometrics of landmarks. This core of material has since been formalized further, in a different notation, in Goodall (1991). I am not aware of any serious problems with this synthesis or of any informed attacks upon it.

Beyond the biological theory of landmark points supplying our data, this disciplinary core can be reduced to two basic statistical dogmas whose realization results in Principles 1–4 of the preceding chapter. First, a fully efficient approach to the joint distribution of any number of labeled point locations in two dimensions or three can be constructed in terms of a feature space referring only to those point locations themselves, without the necessary intervention of any particular distances, angles, or other prior size or shape variables. Second, whenever the hypothesis of "isometry" (no effects on shape) is rejected by the appropriate significance test, one should proceed to detect and describe specific features of effects upon shape in a manner likewise invariant against choices of "variables" or "directions" a priori. Mardia and Dryden (1989a) have shown that the particular normal approximation underlying these linearized feature spaces is asymptotically maximum-likelihood, and hence asymptotically fully efficient in spite of the linearization. Their demonstration is based on a presumption of i.i.d. (independent, identically distributed; see Chapter 5) circular noise at the landmarks, but the extension to the general case (cf. Goodall, 1991) is immediate. The principal work guaranteeing the extension to three dimensions is Kendall's (1984); such analyses are exemplified in Grayson et al. (1988) and later in this volume. The explicit comparison of the new methods with the "traditional" is treated here and in Bookstein and Reyment (1989) and Rohlf and Bookstein (1990).

The consensus involving these new methods is important to note because of three shared formal properties that, collectively, obviate most of the arbitrariness that had bedeviled earlier approaches to the same data. The crucial features of the morphometric core are *efficiency*, *complete coverage of feature subspaces*, and *directional symmetry of embedded distributions*.

2.1.1. Efficiency of coverage of shape space

One corner of this common foundation is the demonstration by elementary theorem (Bookstein, 1986a) that the "shape space" common to these schools incorporates the linearized multivariate statistics of all possible "traditional" shape measurements of the same landmark locations. This theorem, for instance, leads to the demonstration (Bookstein, 1987a) that the so-called finite-element methods, which display particular nonlinear transformations of biologically somewhat arbitrary linear manipulations of the landmark coordinates, must lose statistical power against any general alternative hypothesis, so that the diagrams by which their findings are reported are seriously misleading in most applications (see

Section 6.6). That critique applies to my own early work with grids as well as to later efforts by Cheverud and Richtsmeier (1986), Richtsmeier (1988), and others. Other applications of the same fundamental theorems have been to the extraction of shape features most indicative of specific anomalies (Grayson et al., 1985, 1987; Clarren et al., 1987), to the description of large-scale effects upon shape (Bookstein, 1987a; Bookstein and Sampson, 1987, 1990), and to the devising of a principal-component-like decomposition of within-sample shape variability in an invariant fashion (Bookstein, 1989b; see also Section 7.6), as well as many other threads.

This guarantee of efficiency "in all directions," "in all linearizable features" is perhaps the most important practical consequence of the methodological consensus. Methods have been created for translating these equivalent techniques from one notation to another and for detecting the ways, often subtle, in which other sets of variables *lose* information or efficiency with respect to these optima. (Section 6.4.3 provides a "worked example" of that sort of critique.) For instance, Sections 4.1 and 7.6 compare analyses of the same data set, eight calvarial landmarks for 21 growing rats, first using only size variables (landmark distances) and then shape coordinates together with a single size factor. The information content of the data sets is shown to be the same, but the shape coordinates support diagrams that are far clearer; an analysis using ratios of conventional distance is worse than either. The inequivalence obtains mostly because of the strong geometric ordering of the space of alternate distance measures, an ordering inaccessible to studies of ratios one at a time. The theorem in Section 6.4, originally published in 1986, notes that the extremes of strain ratio (ratio of corresponding distances between weighted averages of landmarks) from one mean landmark configuration to another may always be expressed along *transects of triangles*, distances measured from single landmarks to the weighted average locations of two others. The net T^2-statistic for a test of group mean shape difference, however (see Section 5.4), does not reduce to the comparison of two suitably selected exemplars of these transects, one of largest ratio, one of smallest. That net T^2 instead pertains to an appropriately rank-reduced multivariate test for a vector of ratios among themselves of *all* edge lengths within the configuration. Note, too, that the extreme ratios are typically omitted from the basis for the vector space supporting the T^2. It is the joint distribution of the edge ratios that supports the correct statistical interpretation, not their comparisons separately.

2.1.2. Coverage of feature subspaces

When a shape change is detected by this single T^2-statistic, or the equivalent F-ratio (Goodall) or likelihood (Mardia and Dryden), the morphometrician's task becomes the specification of features by which this change may be tied to biological explanation. As effects upon shape are of indefinitely wide variety, so, too, are the types of features to be inspected should the hypothesis of isometry (no shape difference) be rejected. Many of these emerged years or decades ago as isolated methods all their own; the advantage of the synthesis is their joint expression as multiple estimations, often statistically nested, in a common format. For configurations of K landmarks, the variants of current interest include the rigid motion of certain subsets of the landmarks with respect to the remainder (each such possibility is associated with a descriptor lying in a subspace having dimension 3 for planar data, and there are $2^{K-1} - K - 1$ such subspaces), the individual displacements of similar lists of landmarks (having the same number of subspaces, each now of dimension twice the count of "moving" points), the two-dimensional subspace of uniform shears (Section 7.2), the eight-dimensional subspace of quadratic growth gradients (Section 7.4), and the scale-specific features of nonlinearity themselves linearized in the principal warps (a mean-dependent rotation of the single subspace of features complementary to the uniform transformations). These are all phrased as group comparisons or exogenous covariances. There are also methods available for studying intragroup morphometric covariances, including the single-triangle or uniform factor models of Section 7.2 and the relative warps of Section 7.6 (a different, covariance-dependent rotation of the complement of the linear feature subspace). A particularly interesting factor, either exogenous or endogenous, depending on the space in which the analyst is working, is size. As there is often *allometry* (effects of size upon shape), whenever groups differ or vary in size it is helpful to test for that possibility (Bookstein, 1986a) before attempting to invoke further explanatory factors exogenous to morphometrics. Whenever allometry is present, the detection of other effects on shape proceeds with greater power if applied to residuals from the allometric model. Examples may be found in Section 4.3 (for distance data) and Sections 6.5.1 and 6.5.2.

2.1.3. "Circularity" of shape with respect to individual landmark shifts

In all these applications there is a geometry of features inherited from the geometry of landmarks. In developing the methods in this book, great care was taken at all times that they be circularly symmetric in their weighing of directions in shape space and in all the natural subspaces. By this I do not mean that the data must be modeled as somehow circularly *distributed* – though such models are available to be tested or rejected (see Section 5.3) – but that since the publication of the synthesis in Bookstein (1986a), a sound method must explore all directions of variation in shape space using the same metric that applies to the construction of shape space per se, prior to consideration of any covariances. Kendall (1984) shows how this metric is an embedding of the natural Euclidean metric that would be applied to the landmark locations prior to their reduction to equivalence classes of shapes. (Small, 1988, explains the far-reaching implications of this geometry for interpretations of uniform shape changes.) On a background of $n - 1$ landmarks unchanging in position, the variation of "shape" in the standard construction of shape space is circular (isometric with Kendall's metric) whenever the variation of the real location of that nth landmark is circular in its own picture plane. In other words, in the standard construction the geometry of shape space does not distort displacements of single landmarks as a function of direction.

Beyond this geometry of single point displacements there are many other subordinate geometries that may be nested as hypotheses under the standard shape-space construction; methods for these more specialized applications must be circularly symmetric as well. *Uniform shears* of equal extent, for example, result in displacements to an equivalent distance in the appropriate invariant subspace of shape space, regardless of the principal directions of the shear. (Here, "extent" is measured by log anisotropy, log ratio of the diameters of the ellipse into which a circle is taken by the transformation; see Section 6.2.4 or Appendix A.2.) In the limit of small changes, these are exact Euclidean circles about the identity transformation in that subspace. Thus, all such changes are detected by the common T^2 or F with the same full efficiency, regardless of direction.

The shape coordinates, and the feature space of the uniform transformations, are now nearly a decade old, having been introduced in manuscripts written in the early 1980s. Their extension to the more complex subspaces has occupied me considerably since then. This book is the first presentation of all this material in coherent survey form.

2.2. THE THIN-PLATE SPLINE

Although the biologist is comfortable referring to landmarks as "homologous" (see the next chapter), no such construct as "the" homology mapping can be observed from finite data. It would, nevertheless, supply a useful language for the description and presentation of changes of landmark locations, the actual data under consideration, if we could draw these maps rather flexibly and suggestively, however tentatively, as visible, legible deformations. Thus, from time to time in the methods and presentations that follow we shall have need of a general-purpose **interpolation function** expressing by explicit formula *one* of the mappings that might model a particular biological homology sampled by pairs of points. The technique of thin-plate splines is adequate for the

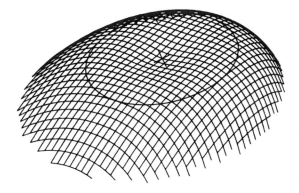

Figure 2.2.1. Fundamental solution of the biharmonic equation: a circular fragment of the surface $z(x, y) = -r^2 \log r^2$ viewed from above. The X is at $(0, 0, 0)$; the remaining zeros of the function are on the circle of radius 1 drawn.

purpose of visualizing statistical analyses, and it suggests many biometrically productive insights (see Sections 7.5 and 7.6). A Fortran subroutine carrying out the interpolation may be found in Appendix A.1. A lengthier, more technical discussion of all these matters is given in Bookstein (1989a). Generalizations to include other types of information, such as blurring of landmark locations, can be found in Bookstein (1990a,g), and a three-dimensional version of the algorithm shown here two-dimensionally is the subject of active investigation at this time.

2.2.1. The function $U(r)$

At the root of the spline analysis is the special function sketched in Figure 2.2.1. This is the surface

$$z(x, y) = -U(r) = -r^2 \log r^2,$$

where r is the distance $(x^2 + y^2)^{1/2}$ from the Cartesian origin. The minus sign is for ease of reading the form of this surface: In this pose, it appears to be a slightly dented but otherwise convex surface viewed from above. The surface incorporates the point $(0, 0, 0)$, as marked by the X in the figure. Also, the function is zero along the indicated circle, where $r = 1$. The surface in Figure 2.2.1 has contact with a horizontal tangent plane all along a circle of radius $1/\sqrt{e} \sim 0.607$ concentric with the circle of radius 1 that is drawn.

The function $U(r)$ satisfies the equation

$$\Delta^2 U = \left(\frac{\partial^2}{\partial x^2} + \frac{\partial^2}{\partial y^2} \right)^2 U \propto \delta_{(0,0)}.$$

The right-hand side of this expression is proportional to the "generalized function" $\delta_{(0,0)}$ that is zero everywhere except at the origin but has an integral equal to 1. That is, U is a so-called *fundamental solution* of the *biharmonic equation* $\Delta^2 U = 0$, the

27

equation for the shape of a thin steel plate lofted as a function $z(x, y)$ above the (x, y)-plane.

The reader may be wondering just how arbitrarily this particular function $U(r)$ was chosen. In fact, its identity will be determined virtually completely – up to the exponent of r – by the requirements that we shall eventually place upon the maps to be built up with its aid in Section 2.2.4. Up to this exponent, $U(r)$ is the only possibility known to me that will support the analysis of localizable features – principal, partial, relative warps – by reference to quadratic forms operating on coordinate data, as introduced in Chapter 7. That exponent, the single remaining arbitrariness, is discussed in Section 8.3.2.2.

2.2.2. Bounded linear combinations of terms $U(r)$

Figure 2.2.2 is a mathematical model of a thin plate of steel or other stiff metal that should be imagined as extending to infinity in all directions. Underlying the plate (actually, passing through it) is a rigid armature in the form of a square of side $\sqrt{2}$, drawn in perspective view as the rhombus at the center of the figure. The steel plate is tacked (fixed in position) some distance above two diagonally opposite corners of the square, and the same distance below the other two corners of the square. In the figure, this

Figure 2.2.2. Part of an infinite thin metal plate constrained to lie at some distance above a ground plane at points $(0, \pm 1)$ and the same distance below it at points $(\pm 1, 0)$. The rhombus at the center represents the rigid square armature enforcing these constraints by fixing the positions of the X's, which all lie on the surface above the corners of the square. Far from the armature, the height of the plate approaches a multiple of the cosine of the double central angle.

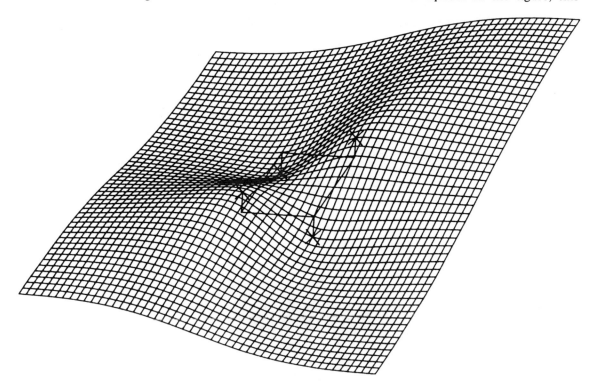

tacking is indicated by the X's, which are to be taken as lying exactly upon the steel sheet but also as rigidly welded, via their "stalks," to the corresponding corners of the underlying square.

The surface in Figure 2.2.2 corresponds to a visually satisfactory multiple of the function

$$z(x, y) = U\left(\left[x^2 + (y - 1)^2\right]^{1/2}\right) - U\left(\left[(x + 1)^2 + y^2\right]^{1/2}\right)$$
$$+ U\left(\left[x^2 + (y + 1)^2\right]^{1/2}\right) - U\left(\left[(x - 1)^2 + y^2\right]^{1/2}\right)$$
$$= \Sigma(-)^{k+1} U(|(x, y) - i^k|) \quad (i = \sqrt{-1}),$$

a straightforward linear combination of the functions $U(r)$ based at each of the four corners of the square. The functions $U(r)$ are taken with coefficients $+1$ for the ends of one diagonal, -1 for the ends of the other.

It can be shown that this function $z(x, y)$ is, indeed, the solution of the biharmonic equation $\Delta^2 z = 0$ consistent with the tacking of a previously flat infinite plate to points alternately above and below the corners of the square as shown. Physical steel takes this form, as long as the displacements are small, because the function $z(x, y)$ is the configuration of lowest physical bending energy consistent with the given constraints. For a thin plate subjected to only slight bending, the bending energy at a point is proportional to the quantity

$$\left(\frac{\partial^2 z}{\partial x^2}\right)^2 + 2\left(\frac{\partial^2 z}{\partial x\, \partial y}\right)^2 + \left(\frac{\partial^2 z}{\partial y^2}\right)^2,$$

and the net energy is proportional to the integral of this quantity – the **quadratic variation** – over the whole plate. That is to say, $z(x, y) = \Sigma(-)^{k+1} U(|(x, y) - i^k|)$ minimizes

$$\iint_{\mathbf{R}^2} \left[\left(\frac{\partial^2 z}{\partial x^2}\right)^2 + 2\left(\frac{\partial^2 z}{\partial x\, \partial y}\right)^2 + \left(\frac{\partial^2 z}{\partial y^2}\right)^2\right]$$

over the class of all functions z taking the values $(-1)^{k+1}$ at i^k, as drawn.

As one travels far away from the origin, this plate takes on a most interesting configuration. In all directions it is asymptotically flat and level (though not coplanar, for the levels are different at infinity in different directions). In Figure 2.2.2 this is particularly visible outboard of the splined corners themselves. For instance, the corner of the plate facing the viewer in the diagram apparently has become nearly level somewhat underneath the level of the constraint at the nearest corner of the armature, and likewise the other three corners. For large $r^2 = x^2 + y^2$, $z(x, y)$ reduces to

$$z(x, y) \sim \frac{4(y^2 - x^2)}{x^2 + y^2 + 1},$$

together with terms that drop to zero as $1/r$ or faster. Except for the term $+1$ in the denominator, this value is just -4 times the cosine of the double angle $2 \tan^{-1}(y/x)$. Thus, a long way from $(0, 0)$ our metal sheet takes the form of a very slowly rising and falling circuit of the armature, *of bounded variation*: 4 units above the armature at points far out along one diagonal, 4 units below the armature at points far out along the other.

At the points of the armature itself, this particular plate is at heights

$$\pm z(1, 0) = \pm \left[-2U(\sqrt{2}) + U(2) \right]$$
$$= \pm \left[-2(\sqrt{2})^2 \log 2 + 2^2 \log 4 \right] = \pm 2.77.$$

The variation in the height of the plate at infinity is larger than that of the armature – larger than the constraints upon the plate.

The thin-plate spline and the energy that it minimizes have been wonderfully generalized to other kinds of data than points for application to problems in computer vision and animation. This development began with Terzopoulos (1983, 1986) and has continued in collaborations with Witkin and Kass (Witkin, Terzopoulos, and Kass, 1987; Kass, Witkin, and Terzopoulos, 1987). Bookstein (1989a) explains the differences in the implementations consequent upon this divergence of application areas. For other applications of spline methods in statistics, see Wahba (1990).

2.2.3. Displacements in the coordinate plane

In Figure 2.2.2 the displacement of the thin plate lies in a direction orthogonal to the lie of the plate itself. This orthogonality is not necessary (of course, we are no longer modeling a physical plate; that applied only for bending of small extent normal to the coordinate plane of x and y). We may imagine the displacements $z(x, y)$ to be applied directly to one of the coordinates x or y of the plate with which we started. Thus, we may interpret the scheme of Figure 2.2.2 as the **interpolation function** shown in Figure 2.2.3. The four points begin in the form of a square; then one diagonal is displaced with respect to the other diagonal until there results the form of a kite. Over the square on the left there is superimposed a grid of points so that we can visualize the effect of this transformation on the elements of area

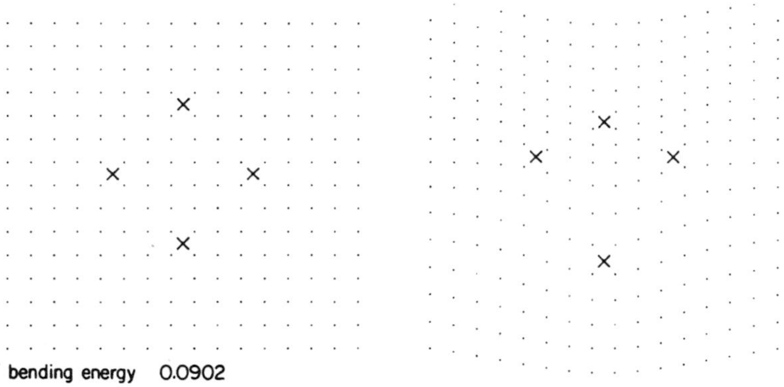

bending energy   0.0902

Figure 2.2.3. A multiple of the same function added to the *y*-coordinate of points of a square grid rather than lofted as a *z*-coordinate. There results an interpolation function between a square and a kite.

surrounding the X's. The *x*-coordinate is transferred from left to right without change, while the *y*-coordinate is altered by the value $z(x, y)$ that was the *z*-coordinate of the metal sheet in Figure 2.2.2. We thus arrive at the mapping function

$$(x, y) \rightarrow (x', y') = (x, y + z(x, y))$$

where $z(x, y)$ is the same function $\Sigma(-)^{k+1}U(|(x, y) - i^k|)$ we have been viewing in three dimensions.

In this manner the thin-plate spline we have been examining can be used to solve a two-dimensional interpolation problem, the computation of a map $\mathbf{R}^2 \rightarrow \mathbf{R}^2$ from data in the form of a square. In this special case, it represents the mapping consistent with the assigned correspondence of X's and adapted to their reconfiguration in the manner that *uniquely* minimizes a certain sort of "bending energy," namely, the (linearized) energy that would have been required had the landmark displacements in question been normal to the plane of the figure rather than within that plane. Compare the alternate interpolations of this same landmark set depicted in Section 7.3.

If physical steel sheets are merely *tilted*, changed from level to oblique, they need not bend: In tilting, energy does work against gravity, not against elasticity. To maintain the analogy between displacements of the plate normal to its plane and displacements of points in their plane, transformations of the landmarks that can be assigned the same effect as "tilting" should have no "bending energy." If we also allow the general increase or decrease of geometric scale (as by rerolling the physical plate), the class of these transformations is coextensive with the **affine transformations** or homogeneous shears, those that leave parallel lines parallel. We shall dwell at length upon such transformations in Section 7.2. Otherwise, to bend the plate requires energy; and the sharper the bending, the greater the second derivatives of the surface $z(x,y)$ and the greater the energy required. A pattern of "tacks" differing by a given height requires much less energy to install

31

when the points at which they constrain a metal plate are far apart than when they are close together.

2.2.4. Applications to arbitrary sets of landmarks

One can imagine the steel plate of Figure 2.2.2 to be fixed in position arbitrarily high or low above the base plane at any combination of points, not just the corners of a square as shown. Subject to whatever constraints are posed, the plate will still adopt the position of least net bending energy, and the description of its form will still be a linear combination of terms $r^2 \log r^2$ (Figure 2.2.1), fundamental solutions of the biharmonic equation, centered at each point where information (here, height) is specified.

The exploitation of the thin-plate equation to provide interpolatory splines in this way was originated by Duchon – *le principe des plaques minces* – in a series of reports in the middle 1970s (cf. Duchon, 1976) and was later formalized by Jean Meinguet (1979*a,b*, 1984) in a very general mathematical setting. To my knowledge these splines had not been considered for use in the analysis of plane mappings prior to my earlier papers (Bookstein, 1987*b*, 1988*a*, 1989*a*). The remainder of this section comprises a terse overview of the algebraic crux of the thin-plate method. For details, see the sources cited earlier.

Let $Z_1 = (x_1, y_1)$, $Z_2 = (x_2, y_2), \ldots, Z_K = (x_K, y_K)$ be K points in the ordinary Euclidean plane according to any convenient Cartesian coordinate system. We are concerned with functions f taking specified values at the points Z_i; should certain pairs or triples of Z's be closely adjacent, the effect is that of specifying derivatives of f as well as values. Write $r_{ij} = |Z_i - Z_j|$ for the distance between points i and j.

Define matrices

$$
P_K = \begin{bmatrix} 0 & U(r_{12}) & \cdots & U(r_{1K}) \\ U(r_{21}) & 0 & \cdots & U(r_{2K}) \\ \cdots & \cdots & \cdots & \cdots \\ U(r_{K1}) & U(r_{K2}) & \cdots & 0 \end{bmatrix}, \quad K \times K,
$$

$$
Q = \begin{bmatrix} 1 & x_1 & y_1 \\ 1 & x_2 & y_2 \\ \cdots & \cdots & \cdots \\ 1 & x_K & y_K \end{bmatrix}, \quad K \times 3,
$$

and

$$
L = \left[\begin{array}{c|c} P_K & Q \\ \hline Q^T & 0 \end{array} \right], \quad (K + 3) \times (K + 3),
$$

where ^{T} is the matrix transpose operator and 0 is a 3×3 matrix of zeros.

Let $V = (v_1, \ldots, v_K)$ be any K-vector, and write $Y = (V|0\,0\,0)^T$, a column vector of length $K + 3$. Define the vector $W = (w_1, \ldots, w_K)$ and the coefficients a_1, a_x, a_y by the equation

$$L^{-1}Y = \left(W|a_1\,a_x\,a_y\right)^T.$$

Use the elements of $L^{-1}Y$ to define a function $f(x, y)$ everywhere in the plane:

$$f(x, y) = a_1 + a_x x + a_y y + \sum_{i=1}^{K} w_i U(|Z_i - (x, y)|).$$

The role of the last three rows of L is to guarantee that the coefficients w_i sum to zero and that their cross-products with the x- and y-coordinates of the points Z_i are likewise zero. The function f is divided into two parts: a sum of functions $U(r)$ that can be shown to be asymptotically of derivative zero, like the example in Figure 2.2.2, and an affine part representing the behavior of f at infinity.

Then the following three propositions hold:

1. $f(x_i, y_i) = v_i$, all i. (This is just a restatement of the equations represented by the first K rows of L, those not involved in regularizing the function at infinity.) That is, the function f interpolates the correspondence $(x_i, y_i) \rightarrow v_i$; if we imagine the (x_i, y_i, v_i) as points in three dimensions, the surface $(x, y, f(x, y))$ is called the **thin-plate spline** on the *nodes* or *knots* (x_i, y_i, v_i).

2. The function f minimizes the nonnegative quantity

$$I_f = \iint_{\mathbf{R}^2} \left[\left(\frac{\partial^2 f}{\partial x^2} \right)^2 + 2 \left(\frac{\partial^2 f}{\partial x\,\partial y} \right)^2 + \left(\frac{\partial^2 f}{\partial y^2} \right)^2 \right]$$

over the class of such interpolants. Call this the **bending energy**. (This property derives from the interpretation of L as a projection operator; see the papers by Meinguet already cited.) This integral is zero only when all the components of W are zero; in this case, the computed spline is $f(x, y) = a_1 + a_x x + a_y y$, a flat surface.

3. The value of I_f is proportional to

$$WP_K W^T = V\left(L_K^{-1} P_K L_K^{-1}\right) V^T = V L_K^{-1} V^T,$$

where L_K^{-1} is the upper left $K \times K$ subblock of L^{-1}. This is the formula alluded to in Chapter 1; it will be explored thoroughly in Chapter 7. As a matrix, it is a function of the points (x_i, y_i) driving it via the kernel function U; applied to a vector $V = (v_i)$ of

33

displacements, it yields a scalar, the bending energy of an idealized metal sheet.

In the present application we take V to be the $K \times 2$ matrix

$$V = \begin{bmatrix} x_1' & x_2' & \cdots & x_K' \\ y_1' & y_2' & \cdots & y_K' \end{bmatrix},$$

where each (x_i', y_i') is a point homologous to (x_i, y_i) in another copy of $\mathbf{R}^2$. The application of L^{-1} to the first row of V specifies the coefficients of 1, x, y, and the U's for $f_x(x, y)$, the x-coordinate of the image of (x, y); the application of L^{-1} to the second row of V does the same for the y-coordinate $f_y(x, y)$.

The resulting function $f(x, y) = (f_x(x, y), f_y(x, y))$ is now vector-valued: it maps each point (x_i, y_i) to its homologue (x_i', y_i') and is the least bent (according to the measure I_f, integral quadratic variation over all $\mathbf{R}^2$, computed separately for real and imaginary parts of f and summed) of all such functions. These vector-valued functions $f(x, y)$ are the **thin-plate spline mappings** of this book. The whole procedure is invariant under translations or rotations of either set of landmarks, the (x, y) or (x', y'). If the pairing of points between the sets is in accordance with biological homology, the function f models the comparison of biological forms as a *deformation* and produces pleasant illustrations of the same. The statistical properties of f are, of course, precisely the statistics of the data matrices V and Q that drive its computation; those properties are the subject matter of Chapters 5 through 7, comprising two-thirds of this book. The net bending energy of a two-dimensional landmark reconfiguration is the sum of the bending energies of the x- and the y-parts separately; in this form, the quantity is independent of rotations of the coordinate system for either form.

The reader interested in working through the detailed computation of the example in Figure 2.2.3 is referred to Section 7.3.2, where this deformation is discussed in its biometric context. The disks associated with Rohlf and Bookstein (1990) include code for applying the thin-plate spline to arbitrary pairs of landmark configurations, suited for immediate execution on IBM PC's or their clones. Sections 7.5 and 7.6 rework this metaphor of bending energy, quite independent of the idea of deformation, into a reasonable analogue of principal-components analysis for landmark data.

2.3. THE STATISTICS OF "EXPLANATION"

Morphometrics is different from other biometrical methods. Its distinctiveness owes to the triple role played by landmarks. Their geometry supplies a language for describing individual forms, pairs of forms, and effects upon entire samples of forms. Morphometrics begins by exploiting landmarks under the first heading in gathering data, proceeds directly to the third heading to compute versions of all the classic path models, then reverts to the second as it interprets findings, wherever possible, as if they specified processes accounting for transformations of one "typical" form, perhaps a mean, into another.

It is useful to begin a discussion of the relations among morphometric statistics and morphometric explanations by examining one classic sort of statistical analysis that morphometrics does *not* resemble: It is not in any way a style of indirect measurement of "true parameters," whether morphological "distance" or anything else. The metaphor of estimating true values arises in the classic method of least squares, which already existed in recognizable form by 1810 (cf. Stigler, 1986). The method is designed for data in the form of "observations," such as the position of a planet at a particular time in the eyepiece of a telescope at a particular spot on the earth. Such observations are of no particular scientific meaning one by one. But in sufficient quantity, they may be combined in an "estimate" of the true orbital parameters of the celestial object(s) involved. First, the true Newtonian equations of motion of the planet are linearized in the vicinity of the true parameters, and the errors in all observed measurements are combined into one single error for each equation. Second, these equations are repeatedly summed after multiplication by the (known) coefficient of each (unknown) parameter in turn, yielding as many "normal equations" as there are unknowns. Third, the normal equations are solved to supply estimates of the true orbital parameters that have, under certain probability models for measurement errors, their own desirable properties. In summary, observations (positions in a telescope) are combined into parameters (invariants of motion – potentials, momenta, etc.) that are conceptually different and physically constant.

In the modification of this model for biometric use, at the hands of Francis Galton, Karl Pearson, and Sewall Wright, the conceptual separation of data (measures of organisms) from parameters (path coefficients) was maintained. But the tie between "parameters" and exact laws was replaced by a vague notion of causality. Recall that in the classic contexts for which least-squares methods were developed – principally celestial mechanics and geodesy – there was no mention of causality. Newton's laws do not "cause" the planets to take the orbits they take, but instead describe those orbits for all time, once "initial conditions" are set. By comparison, in Galton's equally classic analysis of the inheritance of height, there is no law regulating the height of offspring under any circumstances. Instead, we may believe that offspring height is "determined" by a collection of numerous "causes," of which parental height is one. The purpose of the biometric regression is to compute not a physical constant, like the orbital energy of Jupiter, but instead a path coefficient the value of which is subject to further explanations, such as by evolutionary argument or by an auxiliary computation based in gene frequencies. The regressions are based on a presumption of causality, but end up interpreted functionally instead, in terms of mechanisms (originally, to Wright, constant probabilities) rather than coefficients.

As applied to morphometrics, the incompatibility between these two invocations of least-squares methods went unnoted until Huxley's seminal work of 1932. At the crux of the problem is the manner in which explanations of these coefficients are eventually to refer back to the data they supposedly account for. Astronomers, after all, know exactly what object they mean by "Jupiter." They agree regarding the precise manner in which observations are to be compared from night to night, telescope to telescope, and regarding the roster of parameters relevant to celestial mechanics. Biologists must substitute contingencies for both of those intellectual luxuries; and while regression substitutes coefficients for constants, it is not at all obvious what substitutes for "pointing the telescope." Yet if we cannot say where we are pointing our measuring instrument, we cannot relate regression coefficients to meaningful explanations.

In Galton's analysis of height, for instance, by what principle can we assume that net height, from the floor to the crown, is the subject of regulation by any explicable biological process? Huxley reminds us that net height is actually the integral of all its *differentials*, its little elements, along the diversity of organs that make up the path taken by the yardstick. In principle, a different "parameter," a different covariance, should be computed for each infinitesimal segment of that path. To assert that we understand how a covariate of an epigenetic process affects "height" we must inspect the way in which it affects all the components of height; otherwise the explanation is wrong even when all regressions are computed correctly.

We need a language, then, whereby morphometric quantities are incorporated only as *lists* or *vectors of variables*, of arbitrary, preferably great, length. In principle, no factor can coherently account for changes in one variable of these lists – one distance of a network, or one shape coordinate for a configuration – without causing changes in them all. The nature of the "explanation" supplied by a factor for such a list is operationally construed as the picture corresponding to *all* the effects of the factor upon the variables of the list, each effect taken according to its own regression coefficient. Correlations among the separate regression "errors" are evidence for other explanatory factors, which are not relevant to the description of the effects of this one. The word "factor" here bears a rigorous technical sense: A **factor** is a joint cause of a collection of observed variables, a value such that when it changes, all the joint "effects" are affected (i.e., they change). We shall restrict our discussion, for the most part, to factors the effects of which are *linear*. Establishing the truth of factor models is not, at root, a specifically statistical task, but requires the observation of actual consequences of changes in factor scores in an experimental or quasi-experimental way. For instance, "size change" is a factor for shape, inasmuch as we notice that animals fed more chow and hence waxing larger change their shapes. Evolutionary time is not a factor in this sense, as regression coefficients upon time hardly ever make sense (see Appendix A.3). "Taxon" is a special case. We take the "effect" of a group name in an acausal sense: It is the mean difference of that group from the mean of a higher taxon.

In the applications of this book, the vectors of variables ordinarily will be lists of shape coordinates to a single baseline; in a few instances, they will be lists of interlandmark distances instead. These lists will not be mixed; in particular, all the variables of a list will be commensurate, in the same unit. The explanations of these lists in terms of factors will take two forms, as the factors do or do not have known values ("scores") prior to the statistical analysis. All models will involve *simple regressions only*. In my experience, contrary to the nearly universal recommendation of the textbooks (cf. Sokal and Rohlf, 1981), there are no sound applications of multiple regression in the biological sciences. Models that claim to be teasing out the "independent" effects of correlated predictors are simply ill-posed; such predictors presumably are themselves the consequences of independent higher-order factors that one has failed to measure. In the analysis of size-adjusted shape differences, Section 4.3, for example, a problem that appears at first to require a multiple regression of size variables upon Group and General Size is shown to supply meaningful coefficients only when the regression is recast to result first in coefficients for the regression coefficients of the Size measure upon Group (i.e., a single mean difference) and thereafter to supply another set of simple regression coefficients for the dependence of Size-adjusted length measures upon Group. See also Crespi and Bookstein (1989).

2.3.1. Explicitly measured factors

The simplest case of "factor analysis" arises when the variables of a morphometric measurement vector are to be explained by, or are to explain, a factor measured prior to the statistical analysis – even if the factor is temporally posterior to the form, as for "survival" in a selection study (Crespi and Bookstein, 1989). This is always the case for "exogenous" variables – taxon, environment, survival status. The relevant path diagram is that of Figure 2.3.1: *The correlations among the morphometric variables are irrelevant to the regressions.* The same path model applies to covariances with a size factor that has been measured in a space separate from the shape variables. Such a measure is Centroid Size (Section 5.5), but not General Size (Bookstein et al., 1985),

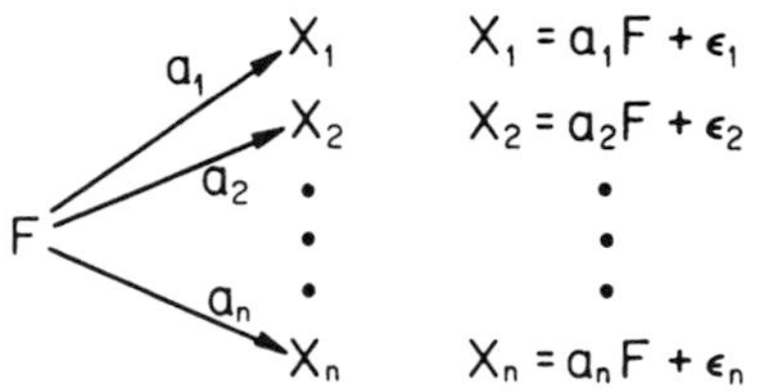

2.3.1. Exogenous factors

$$X_1 = a_1 F + \epsilon_1$$
$$X_2 = a_2 F + \epsilon_2$$
$$\vdots$$
$$X_n = a_n F + \epsilon_n$$

Figure 2.3.1. General scheme for explanations of morphometric data: F, an explanatory factor; $X_1, \ldots, X_n$, morphometric variables (interlandmark distances or shape coordinates); $a_1, \ldots, a_n$, regression coefficients of the X_i on F; $\epsilon_1, \ldots, \epsilon_n$, regression errors, uncorrelated with F and perhaps with one another as well.

which is the first principal component of a series of length measures that it predicts in a different way (Section 4.2).

The variables X_i of the morphometric vector may be any list of components computed in advance of the multivariate analysis: distances, shape coordinates, or their linear combinations into scores on the uniform components and the principal warps. For all these, the "effect" of the factor upon form is the transformation that alters each element of the morphometric vector according to its regression coefficient upon the factor. The pattern of these path coefficients on all the variables of the morphometric vector is ordinarily drawn as a diagram or projected into various relevant feature subspaces, as explained in Chapter 7. That is, the effect of any factor on shape is *computed* first, once and for all, and then *described* over and over by its projections into various subspaces. Again, the covariances of these subspaces – for example, of the "uniform part" of the change with the "nonuniform part" – are irrelevant to the description of the effect, except insofar as a separately computed size effect (regression) might be used to modify scale-sensitive shape diagrams appropriately.

2.3.2. Latent variables as factors

The logic of measurement becomes more intricate and interesting when the factors doing the predicting are endogenous to the space(s) of morphometric descriptors being "explained." This will be the case when the morphometric vector is a list of multiple interlandmark distances and the factor is General Size, which, by definition, "explains" all the distances (Bookstein et al., 1985: sect. 4.2), or when the factor is the Uniform Factor and the morphometric vector is a set of shape coordinates (Section 7.2 of this volume), or in the case of relations between shape feature spaces and multiple covariates (Section 6.5.2). In all these cases, factors are characterized by their property of providing best least-squares fits to the covariances that cannot initially be observed. That is, we estimate the factor *so that* the same quantities a_i serve at once as coefficients in the formula for the factor and as the path coefficients for the morphometric variables upon the factor so estimated. Earlier (Bookstein et al., 1985) we referred to this property as a *consistency criterion* by contrast with the *optimizing criterion* that normally drove expositions of factor analysis in the earlier biometric literature. The difference is crucial. "Optimizing" explanations presume the factor model to be true; the models I propose here make no such presumption, but only extract from the observed covariance structure the part that is consistent with the "explanation" proposed. **The morphometric methods proposed here provide no statistical test of "explanations."** They test only whether or not a vector of covariances with shape space is distinguishable from a list of zeros. To such a finding may correspond many different explanations. The important distinction here is actively obscured by Fisher's unfortunate choice of terminology in disseminating his methods for partitioning sums of squares. Either in analysis of variance or in regression, a linear model "explains" nothing whatever, neither variance nor anything else. Explanation is a scientific, not a statistical, activity, requiring strong foreknowledge of causation.

2.3.2.1. Least squares and latent variables. —

The approach to factor analysis presented here is derived from an original source, one of its earliest independent inventors: the great biometrician Sewall Wright (1889–1988). It is regrettable that Wright's crucial 1932 paper on the difference between component analysis and factor analysis, like the later exegeses (Wright, 1954, 1968), has gone uncited in most of the modern psychometric and biometric literature. His approach would have circumvented several confusions endemic to this area. Didactic expositions of this point of view are scarce; the following is a combination of ideas from Bookstein et al. (1985) and Bookstein (1990b).

Consider, first, the ordinary first principal component $A = (a_1, \ldots, a_n)$ of the covariance matrix $S = (\sigma_{ij})$ for a set of n variables $X_1, \ldots, X_n$. We are accustomed to characterizing A as the linear combination of the X's having greatest variance for coefficients whose squares sum to 1 – this criterion leads directly to the usual eigenanalysis, for example. It happens that A can be characterized as well by a least-squares property (Rao, 1973:63). It is the vector for which $A^T A = (a_i a_j)$, a matrix of rank 1, comes closest, as measured by the summed-squared differences $(\sigma_{ij} - a_i a_j)^2$, to the observed covariance matrix S. (The sum of squares of the a's now is not unity, but the eigenvalue of A.)

The least-squares fit to the covariance matrix S is at the same time a least-squares fit to each of its columns $(\sigma_{ik})|_{k=1}^n$. For the fit to these covariances to be itself optimal, $a_i a_k$ must be a least-squares fit to σ_{ik} as k varies. When we consider the problem for the ith row and the ith column together, this is equivalent to an ordinary simple regression problem with a_i for coefficient. The least-squares optimum is for $a_i = \sum_{k=1}^n \sigma_{ik} a_k / \sum_{k=1}^n a_k^2$. The numerator of this expression is the ordinary cross-product of the dependent variable in the regression (the column σ_{ik}) by the independent (the column A of coefficients). But in this instance it has an additional meaning: the ordinary covariance of the ith original variable with the abstract linear combination $\sum_{k=1}^n a_k X_k$ of the original variables. Because this combination can be thought of as a "score" case by case, we arrive at an interpretation of the elements a_i of these eigenvectors as proportional to covariances

39

between the original indicators and the so-called component "scores." Yet the generation of such scores was clearly superfluous. The formula for the component scores merely expresses the normal equations of the matrix optimization. The passage from the language of matrices to the language of factor "scores" and case values is a mathematical pun having no necessary empirical content.

One arrives at the simplest version of common-factor analysis by deleting the diagonal entries σ_{ii} from the domain of covariances to be fitted by this least-squares computation. *Factor analysis begins with least-squares fitting to the off-diagonal cells of S.* This is a good idea, as we could not fit the diagonals properly anyway: The products $a_i^2 a_j^2$ of the terms a_i^2 that approximate these diagonals must in reality be greater than the squares of the corresponding covariances modeled as $a_i a_j$. Wright's 1932 paper incorporates an elegant algorithm for the iterative solution of this slightly unbalanced least-squares computation, together with a normalization guaranteeing that the resulting elements of A still satisfy $a_i = \Sigma \sigma_{ik} a_k / \Sigma a_k^2$, if σ_{ii} is taken as a_i^2, and so still serve as path coefficients for regression of the observed variables upon an abstract "factor score." It is helpful to express the relation between the techniques in a diagram (Figure 2.3.2) showing their application to a covariance matrix for 10 variables. Whereas component analysis, panel *a*, fits products $a_i a_j$ to every element

Figure 2.3.2. Component analysis, common-factor analysis, and other techniques can all be implemented as least-squares low-rank fits to a covariance matrix or its parts. The square represents a covariance matrix for 10 observed variables. Wright's same iterative algorithm applies to all these cases; only the formulas for normalization change. (*a*) Least-squares fit to the entire matrix, including diagonals: case of principal-component analysis. (*b*) Fit omitting diagonals: case of common-factor analysis. (*c*) Fit omitting certain diagonal submatrices: Wright's method of general and group factors. The two group factors indicated here correspond to variables (1, 3) and (2, 4, 5, 8). (*d*) Fit to a wholly off-diagonal submatrix: the simplest case of Partial Least Squares. The least-squares analysis is again a component analysis.

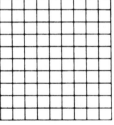
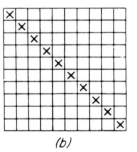

(a) *(b)*

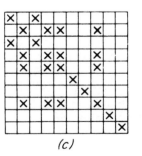
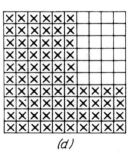

(c) *(d)*

of this matrix, common-factor analysis fits only to the off-diagonal elements, omitting the cells "crossed out" in panel b.

It should now be apparent why there is no systematic difference in usefulness between the findings of a component analysis and a factor analysis applied to the same data, a long-standing but rather fruitless controversy in psychometrics (cf. Velicer and Jackson, 1990). Hardly any information has been changed in the substitution of one technique for the other. The least-squares problems they attack differ only by n diagonal "cases" that, for highly correlated data, are very nearly functions of the off-diagonal elements.

A problem common to both component analysis and common-factor analysis is the typical emergence of bipolar components or factors after the first. In most fields that have theories strong enough to support quantitative expectations at all, path coefficients are expected to be positive; the scientist is forced to interpret these bipolar terms as "contrasts" or else to settle for some inscrutable rotation. Wright recommends suppressing these meaningless bipolarities by an iterative procedure that ultimately amounts to interactively specified, content-directed rotation. In terms of the least-squares fits of σ_{ij} to products $a_i a_j$, his suggestion is that not only the diagonals of the covariance matrix be omitted from the fitting procedure, but also the off-diagonal cells that belong to lists of variables sharing a priori or even a posteriori "group factors." (Scientific judgment is required at this step, which is why the technique is interactive.) Panel c of the figure shows a typical invocation of this fit. As the X's indicate, not only the diagonal cells are now ignored, but also the off-diagonal cells for submatrices on variables (1, 3) and (2, 4, 5, 8). The fit to these sequestered cells is not optimized in the primary computation; rather, the residuals $\sigma_{ij} - a_i a_j$ are to be analyzed subsequently by separate least-squares computations of their own, block by block. This 1932 algorithm has been programmed (Bookstein et al., 1985) and demonstrated upon some biological growth data.

But we are not yet done – the subsets of correlations that Wright fit by least squares still straddle the diagonal of the original matrix. *Even this constraint may be removed.* For instance, panel d of the figure shows a valid least-squares design ignoring all covariances except those relating variables 1 through 6 to variables 7 through 10. Subject to an additional normalization, even this hugely stripped-down least-squares problem has a well-defined solution: It is, in fact, one of the standard modes of Wold's (1975) Partial Least Squares (PLS: *L*east-*S*quares analysis of *P*art of a covariance matrix) in its simplest version. We are dealing in effect with two *blocks* of variables, some X's (old variables 1 through 6) and some Y's (old variables 7 through 10), to be represented by coefficients $a_1, \ldots, a_6$ and $b_1, \ldots, b_4$, and *two* latent variables, one for each block.

2.3.2. Latent variables

In the least-squares fit to the cross-covariance matrix of the X's against the Y's, suppose we already know one set of coefficients, let us say the a's. There would remain the least-squares computation of suitable b's. The coefficient b_1, for instance, would be derived via minimization of $\Sigma_1^6(\sigma_{i1} - a_i b_1)^2$. But this is an ordinary regression without constant term. From the usual formula, then, the value of b_1 minimizing the indicated sum of squares is $\Sigma\sigma_{i1}a_i/\Sigma a_i^2$. The numerator of this expression is exactly the covariance of the variable Y_1 with a **latent variable** $\Sigma a_i X_i$ combining the elements of the X-block with the a's for coefficients. At the actual least-squares optimum, then, each coefficient b_j will be proportional to the covariance of its Y_j with a single score $\Sigma a_i X_i$. Likewise, each a_i will be proportional to the covariance of its X_i with a fixed score $\Sigma b_j Y_j$. In this way, the least-squares fit to this part of a covariance matrix S can be interpreted, via this familiar mathematical pun on the normal equations, as the computation of **saliences** $a_1, \ldots, a_6$ each proportional to the covariance of its X with the latent variable $\Sigma b_k Y_k$ of the "opposing" block, and likewise the b's for the latent variable $\Sigma a_i X_i$. In this sense, each coefficient, a or b, is still derivable from simple (not multiple) regressions by a limiting operation. PLS is, at root, the extension of this least-squares logic to arbitrary superpositions of off-diagonal submatrices. Bookstein (1986*b*), Sampson et al. (1989), and Ketterlinus et al. (1989) argue the superiority of this least-squares technique over all other versions of structural-equations modeling, both LISREL and Wold's own implementations of PLS, in the context of examples from real behavioral data. That debate, though interesting, is beyond the scope of this book.

In any of these contexts, estimates of factor scores by weighted products of covariances by the constituent morphometric variables are invariant against the most common transformation of these spaces, *rotation of the coordinate system*. The rotation referred to here is not the rotation of a specimen on a digitizing tablet (that is long since corrected in the representation of data by invariants like size and shape) but the rotation of the shape coordinates induced by a change of baseline (see Chapter 5). When a pair of shape coordinates is rotated by an ordinary Euclidean turn, the factor loadings corresponding to any of these least-squares approaches rotate by exactly the same extent, so that the factor score $\Sigma a_i X_i$ is invariant under the transformation. (This is true only if analyses are carried out on covariance matrices, not correlation matrices; that will be the case for all the methods recommended here.)

In PLS, a block of centered variables $\{X_i\}$ accounts for another centered variable Y (observed or latent) not by the multiple-regression optimizing correlation but by the **net partial predictor** (Bookstein, 1986*b*) proportional to $\Sigma_i(\Sigma_{\text{cases}} X_i Y)X_i$ optimizing covariance for fixed sum of squares of the coefficients. This "prediction," too, is invariant under rotation of the X-block. If Y

is a latent variable for a block of variables $\{Y_j\}$, the relation between the two latent variables is invariant under rotation of either block, the X's or the Y's.

2.3.2.2. *Further notes on PLS.*—

The idea that one can analyze relations of two blocks of variables by the same principles that one uses to analyze single blocks is perhaps unfamiliar to the reader of this volume. You may perhaps have encountered the notion of *canonical correlation analysis*, the extraction of a "most-correlated" pair of variables from a pair of subspaces of measurements. Each score of a canonical pair is the predictor of the other by multiple regression upon the indicators of its block. To explain via PLS is to replace the word "correlation" in the preceding assignment by the word "covariance." *PLS begins with the extraction of a pair of linear combinations of two blocks of variables that have the greatest **covariance** under the constraint that both sets of coefficients sum in square to 1.* That is, the paired "factors" of a PLS analysis each optimally explain the cross-covariances with the other block. (In the general technique – see Sampson et al., 1989 – there is more than one "other block.") The tremendous advantage of this change is that the coefficients of the linear combinations are now meaningful; when the criterion was the correlation between scores, the coefficients had literally no meaning at all.

There are three other fundamentally different ways to understand what PLS is doing; perhaps one of these alternative explanations will make you more comfortable. Besides the optimization of covariance, there is the intuition via the "normal equations" of the previous exposition – each coefficient of a latent variable (each "salience") is proportional to the regression of that variable upon the score represented by the formula for the *other* block. In a third characterization, the paired latent variables of a PLS analysis are the loadings and scores of an ordinary principal-components analysis of the cross-block covariance matrix itself (not the data underlying!). This must be an analysis without centering – if that option is not available in the computer package with which you are familiar, duplicate every line of the matrix with all signs reversed, then compute principal components in the ordinary way with the "covariance, not correlation matrix" option specified. Yet a fourth characterization is the one with which this section began: the least-squares rank-1 approximation to the original covariance matrix. This one leads directly to the quickest algorithm (the singular-value decomposition) and the best informal figure of merit, namely, R^2 for the least-squares fit – the "fraction of summed-squared covariances explained" – rather than the correlation between the latent-variable scores, as mistakenly put forward by Wold and others. Informally, this R^2 is the extent to which the off-diagonal cross-covariance matrix is rank-1. There is no equivalent for analysis of a single block of variables. These last two interpretations are most congenial to the extension of PLS to "higher-dimensional latent variables" (higher-rank least-squares fits to the cross-correlation matrix); for an example, see Bookstein et al. (1990).

All PLS computations, like the simpler factor analyses preceding, are nearly invariant against changes of baseline in the shape-coordinate formalism as long as analyses are carried out using covariances rather than correlations.

In all these least-squares approaches, the latent variables, whether components or factors, have *no necessary reality whatsoever*; they are artifacts of the normal equations that specify successful convergence of the least-squares iterations. Component analysis and factor analysis are indistinguishable in their import because the maneuver by which they differ is nearly information-free, the suppression of the diagonal of the matrix before the least-squares step. Other techniques vary more crucial aspects of the least-squares setting. Treating entire diagonal submatrices of correlations as sequestered from the fit leads to a version of rotation to simple structure that should prove very useful in diverse areas of biometrics. Deleting the entire matrix, except for certain off-diagonal submatrices, is at the root of the PLS technique, which considerably clarifies the polluted waters of structural-equations modeling. This single family of procedures is sufficient for all the explanations essayed in this book.

2.4. OTHER KINDS OF MORPHOMETRIC DATA

This book is about what to do with landmark data. The many other invocations of geometry in biological measurement come into contact or conflict with the landmark-oriented praxes at several junctures. This section surveys two such areas: the study of curving outlines, and the study of replicated geometric objects without homology, such as textures, that can nevertheless hint at aspects of the regulation of biological form.

2.4.1. Outlines

At present, most studies of curving outlines of forms in two or three dimensions use landmark data relatively weakly: Only a point or two will be involved in specifying an interpolation rule extended to whole curves otherwise arbitrarily. Unlike the case in the study of landmarks, the statistics of most of these rules reduce to standard analyses of "distances" in a unitary and legible fashion. The distance between forms is usually an integral of a squared measure of Euclidean distance, Euclidean angle, or Euclidean curvature. One can thereby extract means or dimensions of a morphological space directly, by analysis of the full "interobject-distance" matrix. The mean, for instance, is that

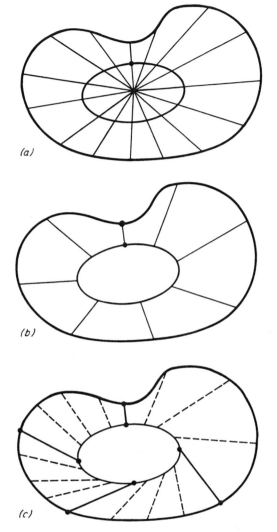

(a)

(b)

(c)

Figure 2.4.1. Variants of distance measures for curving forms: distances between "homologous" points. Once a computed homology is assigned relating a pair of outlines, their morphometric distance may be taken as the integral of the squared physical (geometrical) distance between homologous points around the outline. (*a*) Homology radial out of some center, ordinarily leading to radial Fourier analysis. (*b*) Homology linear in arc length from some starting point, ordinarily leading to elliptic Fourier analysis. (*c*) Hybrid algorithm (Bookstein, 1978): boundary homology linear in arc length between landmarks. (The correspondence is used to interpolate the homology map across the interiors, not to compute a "distance.")

pattern the distances to which are proportional to the first principal component of the matrix of all the interobject distances actually observed (Sampson, 1981). For the relation of these methods to the algebra of features, see Rohlf (1986, 1990*a*).

2.4.1.1. Distances between "homologous" points. —

The simplest versions of distance measures between curves rely on ordinary in-plane Euclidean distance between "corresponding" points on the forms. Figure 2.4.1 shows the two principal possibilities, as homology is computed out of a center or instead around the arc. The former possibility, but not the latter, can be directly generalized to three-dimensional surface data. The arbitrariness of these analyses is embedded in the unreality of the correspondence as it is actually presumed of the observed data. Whenever information is available, real organisms do *not* show correspondences that are uniform either in arc length around an outline or in angle out of a center. These interpolations are defensible only in the absence of all other information about homology: in particular, only in the absence of all additional landmark information. It is no accident that they work wonderfully for sand grains, which do not evolve by descent with modification, or grow.

There is a further problem with taking these distances to express specifically biological information. In most approaches the "homology" as executed is a function of the distance measure chosen, rather than vice versa. Forms are rotated and translated (the radius method), or relabeled (the arc-length method), to minimize the integral of squared distance computed between "homologues" over the family of all possible such maneuvers. Such a computation makes no sense when the purpose of morphometric analysis is to measure a *biological* homology that existed prior to the evolution of morphometricians. There exists no theorem that the evolutionarily correct homology is that which minimizes apparent morphological distance.

The legend for Figure 2.4.1 refers to "Fourier analysis." But, strictly speaking, the analysis of forms according to these distance measures is not any version of "Fourier analysis." Multivariate analysis of the integral squared distances between corresponding points of outline forms leads to ordinations that make no direct reference to Fourier coefficients or any other features of form. The Fourier analyses are, rather, devices for extracting features of a space of "variables" that may serve to describe the space(s) in which the forms described by these homology-free distances are ordinated. Then the Fourier coefficients have no particular claim upon our attention: The "features" they supply have no direct translation into the language of biological form correspondence. At best (Bookstein et al., 1982). Fourier coefficients may aid an ordination or numerical discrimination; they are no reliable guide to understanding homology or the biological processes that have modified form.

2.4.1.2. Derivatives. —

Two other variants of this general procedure are encountered in the literature of outline processing. Both involve taking *derivatives* of the outline curves and measuring dissimilarity between forms in terms of squared differences of those derivatives rather than distances between the original paired point loci. In one of these methods, Lohmann's *eigenshape analysis* (Lohmann, 1983; Lohmann and Schweitzer, 1990), it is the first derivative of the outline the squared differences of which at "corresponding" points are integrated to form a net distance. (The distances are then normalized by a correction for "shape amplitude" that does not

46

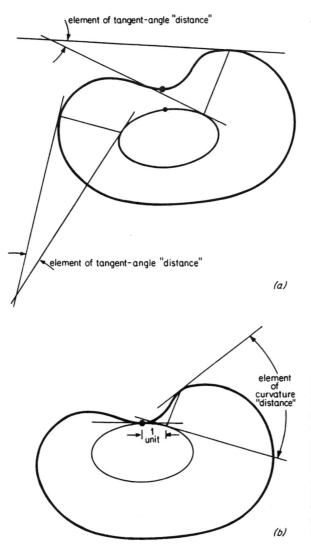

element of tangent-angle "distance"

element of tangent-angle "distance"

(a)

element
of
curvature
"distance"

1
unit

(b)

Figure 2.4.2. Variants of distance measures for curving forms: differentials. Each distance element has been visualized by a distance in the original physical space of the outline data, using a superposition upon one pair of "homologues" at a time. (*a*) Distances based on a function of first derivatives (the tangent angle): Lohmann's eigenshape analysis. (*b*) Distances based on a function of second derivatives (the curvature).

concern us here.) This method could be generalized to three-dimensional data, as the integral of squared angle between "corresponding" normals over a pair of surfaces. In another method, having historical priority by virtue of its usefulness in the early literature of computer vision, it is the curvature (essentially, the second derivative) of the outline whose differences are squared and integrated to generate a net distance between forms. In three dimensions, curvature is no longer a scalar, and this approach generalizes only with difficulty. Figure 2.4.2 illustrates these two possibilities by reexpressing each functional, the tangent angle or the curvature, as a geometric distance all its own.

It continues to be the case that these methods rely on an arbitrary assignment of "homology" underlying the subtraction. In

Lohmann's method, homology is taken linear in arc length; in the curvature method, it may usefully be taken, depending on the application (handwriting analysis, recognition of enemy aircraft), either as uniform in angle along radii out of a center or as linear in arc length.

In general, the distance that is based on curvature weights smaller-scale irregularities of perimeter much more heavily than large-scale features. The mismatching of these features is given a great deal of credence in the computation of distance, but the possibility that the small-scale features are merely misaligned under the arbitrary homology function cannot be dismissed (Bookstein et al., 1985: sect. 2.3). Distances based on simple positional separation of homologous points, measured either radially or by arc length, weight the largest-scale features most heavily, and so are less sensitive (though not wholly insensitive) to confounding by incorrect homology. Distances based on the tangent angle, such as underlie the method of eigenshapes, are intermediate in their sensitivity.

I am aware of no justification of either of these choices – the nature of the computed homology, the order of the derivation before subtracting and squaring – in any biological terms. Rather, all methods of this class seem badly in need of a device for taking homology into account in setting the correspondence of curves prior to computation of squared distances (compare panel *c* of Figure 2.4.1). In practice, such an accounting consists in the explicit *observation* of homology at a selection of discrete mathematical points. Then any computation of distances between curves ought to *begin* with the computation of relationships between landmark configurations, the principal theme of this book. (For another approach, which implicitly discards one coordinate as "missing," see the *Brizalina* example in the next chapter.) A tentative step in the computing of a curve-to-curve homology based on energy considerations is described in Appendix A.1.

2.4.2. Ordination

The usual applications of analysis of curving form (cf. Ferson, Rohlf, and Koehn, 1985; Rohlf and Bookstein, 1990) are limited to pattern recognition or clustering and "ordination," that is, the spreading-out of a sample of forms as points on a Euclidean plane or in a Euclidean space. Such procedures do not generally require the interpretation of the "dimensions" uncovered. This is just as well, inasmuch as the methods described earlier are not capable of supplying feature spaces in homologous form: We could not reliably use these features for biological explanations. Furthermore, ordination requires that we agree on "by how much" shapes differ; it will be argued throughout this book that that question is simply ill-posed. *In most investigations of landmark locations, no single distance measure is adequate*; then most ordination techniques applied to landmark data must destroy information (i.e., waste data). In particular, the method of "shearing," originally introduced as an ordination tool (Humphries et al., 1981; Bookstein et al., 1985), is better understood as a form of path analysis (Rohlf and Bookstein, 1987; Crespi and Bookstein, 1989; see also Section 4.4 of this volume). For a review of several older methods of ordination, see Sneath and Sokal (1973). Reyment, in earlier work (1990) and in his primer on quantitative paleontology (1991), presents advice useful to anyone who insists on pursuing landmark data to an ordination in spite of all the theoretical difficulties.

2.4.3. Data at or below the tissue level

The aspects of biological form that covary with explanatory factors are not restricted to the shapes of organs or organisms, the subject matter to which the landmark formalism seems best suited. Many measurements take place at levels of organization – tissues, cells, ultrastructure – to which the notion of deformation as biological homology clearly fails to apply. Historically, the first attempt at the quantification of a biological deformation was of this form; see the review in Bookstein (1978). Avery (1933) inked a square grid of dots on a tobacco leaf and photographed it thereafter at intervals. He measured areas of the resulting little quadrilaterals and displayed the pattern as a scalar field of growth rates. Richards and Kavanagh (1943, 1945) computed the principal axes of these deformations, by a rather ad hoc approximation, and proposed tying this description to other aspects of the anatomy, specifically, the directions of the vascular bundles. In other growing systems, the image stays constant even as marked points flow; mathematical treatments of these fields include that of Green and others reviewed in Bookstein (1978), especially the beautiful coordinate work of Schüepp (1966). Data in the form of traceable but unlabelable discrete points arise outside biology as well, in the calibration of imaging systems, as for remote sensing. Bookstein (1990*g*) points the reader to that context, and Wolberg (1990) reviews the applications from a computer-graphic point of view. Readers might also probe the literature of computer vision under the heading of "optical flow."

Beyond these models, there is the classic probability-based field called *stereology* or, especially outside the United States, *morphometry*. The field grew out of earlier work under the rubric of "geometric probability" or "integral geometry," comprising methods for the description of geometric patterns in images by numbers and functions. For a good review of this larger context, including a superb bibliography, see Stoyan, Kendall, and Mecke (1987); the digital mathematical treatments culminated in the work of Serra (1982). Stereology, as it arose from this general context, is the meaningful description of three-dimensional structures from

49

the properties of sectioned images. The main review in this area is by Weibel (1979–80). The specific praxis of three-dimensional measurement is apparently most advanced in neuroanatomy; the interested reader is referred to Capowski (1989) or Toga (1990).

Classic stereological methods suffered under a major limitation: One could not make inferences about true size distributions or counts of three-dimensional "inclusions," like cells, without the sheer tedium of reconstructing solid forms from serial sections. The situation has changed drastically with the advent of the confocal microscope, which permits direct observation of a (relatively) thick structure in a sampling volume between parallel planes. Two new developments, the "disector [*sic*]" and the "nucleator," have recently arisen to provide estimates of the mean and variance of particle size and particle surface area, estimates not previously available by image-processing methods. See Gunderson (1988) or Gunderson et al. (1988*a,b*) for enthusiastic explanations.

In the future, the methods of stereology may well merge with the techniques put forward in Section 6.2.6 for observation of deformation by direct statistical analysis of elliptical shapes. When true three-dimensional textures can be observed without sectioning, the techniques for truly homologous observations of scalar and tensor fields will become yet more powerful. For one experiment in this style, texture analysis of trabeculated bone, see Feldkamp et al. (1989) or Kuhn et al. (1990).

2.5. OTHER LITERATURE

The following paragraphs provide a terse bibliography of readings that might profitably be consulted by the student wishing to probe deeper into problems of geometry in biology. Items that are cited only in this section have not been incorporated into the main Bibliography at the end of the book.

2.5.1. Morphometrics

Many of the historically important articles have already been reviewed in Section 2.1. A good collection of approaches from the first half of the century, some of which proved fruitful and some not, is W. E. Le Gros Clark and P. Medawar, eds., *Essays on Growth and Form Presented to D'Arcy Wentworth Thompson* (Oxford, 1945). The earliest attempt to explain at length just what multivariate analysis might have to do with biological explanations was R. E. Blackith and R. Reyment, *Multivariate Morphometrics* (Academic, 1971); by 1984, the second edition (by Reyment, Blackith, and N. Campbell) was already a great deal less sanguine about the extent to which the standard methods could be applied in a routine manner. Neither edition takes the provenance of morphometric data at all seriously; in the first edition, there is only one "diagram," and that is a stick figure of an ant, with big black X's where the ruler supposedly was laid down. Another school of "borrowing" treats morphometric data as a special case of pictures – preserving the geometry but not the homology. Charles Oxnard's books, such as *The Order of Man* (Yale, 1983), are eclectic assemblages of examples of this style, often quite interesting. On allometry, the earliest modern exposition is the long article by S. J. Gould, "Allometry and Size in Ontogeny and Phylogeny" (*Biological Reviews*, 1966), followed by his more historical *Ontogeny and Phylogeny* (Harvard, 1977). The proceedings volume edited by Rohlf and Bookstein (1990), which overlaps somewhat in its text with this book, presents most of the elementary material in a form readily digested by postdoctoral students of evolutionary biology. It includes extensive discussions, absent from this volume, of image capture, imaging processing, and digitizing of both landmarks and outlines. Reyment's *Multidimensional Palaeobiology* (Pergamon, 1991) touches on many of the same introductory materials as does this book, though the emphases are just different enough to be interesting; it should prove useful for supplementary reading.

Bookstein et al., *Morphometrics in Evolutionary Biology* (Academy of Natural Sciences of Philadelphia, 1985), is a peculiar item, of rather more than historical interest. I am letting it go out of print because so much of it is obsolete: the sections on biorthogonal grids, on the truss method, and on "complexity." Other parts, such as the discussions of homology, of the medial axis, and of factor analysis after the fashion of Wright, remain quite up-to-date. Still, there have been too many changes at the foundation of morphometrics since 1983, when that book was drafted, to construe this volume as its "sequel," as was promised in 1985 and as was rashly claimed in the 1988 preprint of this text. Many earlier articles about specific multivariate tactics – by Jolicoeur, Hopkins, Burnaby – are reviewed in that earlier volume. Some of these were collected in a pair of readers: W. Atchley and E. Bryant, eds., *Multivariate Statistical Methods – Among-Groups Covariation*, and E. Bryant and W. Atchley, eds., *Multivariate Statistical Methods – Within-Groups Covariation* (both Dowden, Hutchinson & Ross, 1975).

2.5.2. Statistics

The *Encyclopaedia Britannica*, to which one should automatically turn for an overview of technologies, is oddly constrained in this area. Its main article on Statistics is much shorter than the article on Measurement, whereas they should properly be commensurate. The serious student should rather begin with the more approachable specialized encyclopedia, *The International Encyclopedia of Statistics*, ed. W. Kruskal and J. Tanur (Free Press, 1978). A newer encyclopedia, longer and more technical, is S. Kotz and N.

Johnson, eds.-in-chief, *Encyclopedia of Statistical Sciences* (Wiley, 1982–8).

Most existing textbooks of statistics are inappropriate for the student of quantitative biology, as they systematically pay no attention to issues of measurement or to the provenance of variables. A good, sophisticated introduction that does not fall into this trap is H. Jeffreys, *Theory of Probability* (Oxford, 1939). For the foundations of statistics in problems of measurement, see S. Stigler, *The History of Statistics* (Harvard, 1986), G. Gigerenzer et al., *The Empire of Chance* (Cambridge, 1989), or the classic by E. B. Wilson, *An Introduction to Scientific Research* (McGraw-Hill, 1952). D. Morrison, *Multivariate Statistical Methods*, third edition (McGraw-Hill, 1990), is a fine shorter survey of traditional multivariate techniques. More sophisticated overviews include C. R. Rao, *Linear Statistical Inference and Its Applications*, second edition (Wiley, 1973), A. P. Dempster, *Elements of Continuous Multivariate Analysis* (Addison-Wesley, 1969), and K. V. Mardia et al., *Multivariate Analysis* (Academic, 1979). A good guide to applications in a field not too distant from those at which this book takes aim is J. C. Davis, *Statistics and Data Analysis in Geology*, second edition (Wiley, 1986). An introduction to matrix notation simpler than any of these may be found in K. Jöreskog et al., *Geological Factor Analysis* (Elsevier, 1976; watch for a second edition with Reyment as first author). You should avoid books drawing their applications from the social sciences, as nothing there corresponds to the strong geometric ordering of variables that underlies all the efficient methods proposed here.

2.5.3. Geometry

The statistical reader will have come to this book deficient in a background of morphometrics; the biological reader, in statistics. Readers of either class are likely to be deficient in **geometry**. Since the time of Felix Klein (cited later), this has been considered to encompass not the "theorems" of your high-school class nor the pictorialization of vectors that is "linear algebra," but instead the *properties of figures under transformation*. It is difficult to find these items in the modern college curriculum, but anyone who intends to spend time doing morphometrics ought to assemble a small bookshelf of references never to be loaned out. (Accumulating the library will require years of browsing in used bookstores; most of these items are out of print most of the time.) Beyond the necessary introductions, this minimal library includes books on at least two great themes: the structure of space and the analytic geometry of the classic transformation groups. The intellectual beauty of all these leaves me breathless, but I must resist the temptation to divert the reader's attention to topics beyond those needed to explain some of the tactics used for morphometrics. Nevertheless, I cannot help recommending to all my readers – statisticians, biologists, or just interested bystanders – that before proceeding any further with this volume you obtain and peruse the best geometry book of all time, D. Hilbert and S. Cohn-Vossen's *Geometry and the Imagination*, which is still in print (original edition, 1932; Chelsea, 1952). Other good overviews of "modern geometry" include H. S. M. Coxeter, *Introduction to Geometry*, second edition (Wiley, 1969), M. Berger, *Geometry* (Springer, 1987), H. Behnke et al., eds., *Fundamentals of Mathematics*, *Volume 2*, *Geometry* (MIT, 1974), and D. Pedoe's *Course of Geometry for Colleges and Universities* (Cambridge, 1970; Dover, 1988).

2.5.3.1. The structure of space. —

C. Lanczos, *Space through the Ages* (Academic, 1970), is a splendid starting point. A grand old book still in print is W. K. Clifford, *The Common Sense of the Exact Sciences* (original edition, 1879). Before beginning any work with data from surfaces in three dimensions, you should study one of the older textbooks of differential geometry, such as J. Stoker, *Differential Geometry* (Wiley, 1969), or H. Guggenheimer, *Differential Geometry* (McGraw-Hill, 1963; Dover, 1977). A marvelous collection of historical aperçus on *visual* space, with a fine annotated reading list, is J. Koenderink, *Solid Shape* (MIT, 1990). (What you see is not what you get!) If you intend ever to teach this material, you will want to have the historical background presented in J. Coolidge, *A History of Geometrical Methods* (Oxford, 1940; Dover, 1963).

2.5.3.2. The classical transformations. —

The morphometrician should know about the simplest nonlinear transformations of the plane: projectivities, inversions, and quadratic transformations. The idea of concentrating on transformations was first put forward by Klein in 1872 and is best defended in F. Klein, *Elementary Mathematics from an Advanced Standpoint*, *Volume 2*, *Geometry* (Dover, 1939). Volume 3 of this same work, never translated, might be classified as an introduction to "practical geometry": Klein, *Elementarmathematik vom höheren Standpunkte aus*: *Präzisions- und Approximationsmathematik* (Springer, 1928). Some of the most useful basic formulas are surveyed in D. Struik, *Analytic and Projective Geometry* (Addison-Wesley, 1953). To understand the historical priority of log anisotropy as a distance measure for shapes of triangles, see H. S. M. Coxeter, *Non-Euclidean Geometry* (Toronto, 1965), or, better (at least, if you read German), F. Klein, *Nicht-euklidische Geometrie* (1928; Chelsea, 1959). Other books describe the parameterization of particularly interesting maps in the plane. Examine, for instance, the unexpected role of complex numbers and the square root of -1 in making sense of things in I. M. Yaglom's

2.5. Literature

Complex Numbers in Geometry (Academic, 1968) or his *A Simple Non-Euclidean Geometry and Its Physical Basis* (Springer, 1979). More advanced sources are G. Darboux, *Principes de Géométrie Analytique* (Gauthier-Villars, 1917), and H. Schwerdtfeger, *The Geometry of Complex Numbers* (Toronto, 1962; Dover, 1979). For the geometry of things that are not points – circles, lines – see E. Study, *Geometrie der Dynamen* (Teubner, 1903), F. Klein, *Vorlesungen über höhere Geometrie* (Springer, 1926; Chelsea, 1949), or F. Woods, *Higher Geometry* (Ginn, 1922; Dover, 1961). The classic literature of rigid motion in three dimensions is exposited in A. Karger and J. Novák, *Space Kinematics and Lie Groups* (Gordon & Breach, 1985). After you have examined all these, then go browse the appropriate shelves of your university's mathematics library. Books of analytic geometry are not much in demand; if your library owns these or any others, you will likely find them in place.

3
Landmarks

3.1. "DISTANCE" AND DISTANCE

The common thread of the morphometric tactics in this book owes to their common rejection of the metaphor, otherwise universal in multivariate analysis, wherein dissimilarities between objects are called "distances" and are drawn as such on the page or the computer display. Underlying all linear multivariate techniques is one single geometric device, the modeling of summed-squared differences down the arbitrary list of "variables" of a study as ordinary (physical) distances in simulated physical space. Indeed, the findings of most linear multivariate strategies can be restated without error in the purely geometric language of vectors and angles. Variances are squared lengths, correlations are cosines, and so forth. In this root metaphor, measured variables are considered to specify perpendicular axes of a Euclidean space of however many dimensions. "Distance" is computed by the ordinary extension of the Pythagorean theorem: The squared distance between cases having measured values $X_1, X_2, \ldots, X_k$ and $Y_1, Y_2, \ldots, Y_k$ is $(X_1 - Y_1)^2 + \cdots + (X_k - Y_k)^2$, just as for real points on real paper ($k = 2$) or in real space ($k = 3$). In this circumstance, both variables and cases are described by orthonormal sets of vectors of "loadings" linked by one diagonal matrix of *singular values*. Distances between cases derive from the cross-products of their loadings with respect to this diagonal matrix, and the covariances of the variables are the cross-products of *their* loadings with respect to the same matrix.

In most applications of multivariate analysis there is no other definition of "distance" at hand *except* this metaphorical one. In psychological research, for instance, one cannot observe the "distance" between two subjects' attitude profiles directly (not even in slices of brain tissue); the notion of the multivariate "distances" $\Sigma_i(X_i - Y_i)^2$ between profiles (along with the statistical machinery of whatever component analyses, cluster analyses, and the like are consequent upon them) is hence unambiguous. In nearly all applications of multivariate analysis outside morphometrics there is no possibility of confusion between the statistical notion of "distance" and any physical distance in the real world.

The situation is different for the morphometric data that are the subject of the analyses in this book. Because the objects of our analysis coexist with us in physical space, there is a prior notion of distance available that supersedes that embedded in the fundamental multivariate metaphor. The physical distances involved in morphometrics are not those between pairs of whole organisms (although distances of that sort sometimes enter into other forms of analysis, such as the ecological, by way of map coordinates). Morphometric distances instead express the patterns of relative location among the parts of one organism in comparison with those of another.

In this chapter I describe the fundamental role of landmarks in bringing real physical distances to bear upon multivariate analyses of biological form that are otherwise conventional in their algebra and execution. Indeed, the survey of these implementations for the fundamental metaphor of physical distance is *equivalent* to a complete survey of morphometric analysis as it applies to whole organisms: morphometrics above the tissue level. To know what quantity a morphometric analysis considers to be "the distance between two forms" is to know everything about the algebra and geometry of the ensuing computations. The analyses in this book, for instance, could be reconstructed in full simply from the fact that two incommensurate "shape distances" are involved, one "anisotropy" and the other "bending energy," as long as each name is accompanied by the formula by which it is derived from the sets of interlandmark distances as measured by ruler.

3.1.1. Homology biological and geometrical

All morphometric implementations of real physical distance within a multivariate statistical framework are governed by one crucial concept from biomathematics, the notion of *homology*. The ties between the morphometric and the biomathematical uses of this term are discussed in Section 1.2 of Bookstein et al. (1985). Morphometricians *qua* morphometricians have nothing much to say about "right" or "wrong" notions of homology, and the term will go undefined in these pages; but it is necessary to say a few words about the *semantics* of this construct.

In theoretical biology, homology is a matter of correspondence between parts; thus "the bones of the fish's jaw are homologous to the bones of the mammalian inner ear," or "the human arm is homologous to the chicken wing." This diction, unmodified, empowers only the most rudimentary sort of morphometrics, the invocation of variables that represent "extents" of homologous parts without any additional geometrical content. Morphometrics based on this primitive utilization of the notion of physical distance is generally called "multivariate morphometrics" (cf. Reyment et al., 1984). These variables usually are measured in cm (or cm^2 or cm^3), or log cm, or log ratios (differences of log cm), or various nonlinear transformations of these (such as degrees of angle). For instance, one common choice of variable in conventional morphometric analyses is the volume or weight of a well-delineated organ. For such variables, the physical notion of distance is present implicitly in the definition of volume as the integral of cross-sectional area, and area, in turn, as the integral of lengths of parallel transects – for lengths are physical distances as just described.

But the lengths and other elements that go into the integrals are not claimed separately to be homologous as extents upon the organism; they are simply conveniences in the computation of multiple integrals, which could be taken instead, according to Green's theorem, by surface integrals of position around the boundary. If, instead, the length of a linear structure, such as a long bone, is to be taken as a proper morphometric variable on its own, then the endpoints of the calipers that measure it must be themselves located upon homologous substructures: not, for instance, measured to the end of a bone spur on one form, a condyle on another. The primitive biological notion of homology gives us no further guidance regarding the precise measurement of "length" and, in particular, does not tell us what to do with structures that curve inconsistently between their "endpoints" over a sample of forms.

Beginning with D'Arcy Thompson, there has emerged an alternative extension of the notion of homology into biometrics, one in which the biological properties of the objects of study are considerably more richly articulated. In this replacement for extent-based morphometrics, the object of measurement is the relation per se between forms, not the single form. That is, what we are measuring is ultimately a matter not of shape but of homology. To pass from the biological to the biometrical context, homology must be considered as a *mapping function*, a correspondence relating *points to points* rather than parts to parts. That notion of homology can often be realized as a mathematical *deformation* (i.e., a smooth map), which can, in turn, often be described efficiently by way of its derivative (Bookstein, 1978). We shall not use this further mathematical development here, but only the reduction to a point-to-point mapping.

In this revised version of homology, the ordinary integral extents of organs – areas, in two dimensions; volumes, in three – carry over without change. But the lower-dimensional reductions of extended data, such as "lengths" of three-dimensional objects, in

57

general cease to be acceptable morphometric variables. They presume a prior knowledge of homology, that of the points at which the endpoints of the calipers are put down. If we would assert that prior correspondence directly, by recording sets of homologous locations of the same points over a sample of forms, then the higher-level concept ("length") is made quite unnecessary. We can found morphometrics purely upon a language of maps sampled by point correspondences, without any mention of homologously measured "variables" at all. The variables aid in interpretation and publication of findings, but are not required for computation. On the contrary, much of the intellectual task of morphometrics is the explicit computation of the variables that best summarize observed findings, or best suggest an interpretation in terms of biological process, a posteriori, after all specifically statistical computations are completed.

To proceed in this wise, we represent the data base of a morphometric inquiry by samples of discrete points that correspond among all the forms of a data set. These points are called **landmarks**. That they are to be considered biologically homologous is, as it was for parts and regions, a primitive concept, not the morphometrician's to argue for or against (although professional experience may be helpful). Our survey of morphometrics then becomes a survey of reasonable descriptors of covariance patterns involving corresponding sets of mathematical points *given that they have been previously assigned the same names*. In the notion of the naming ("bridge of the nose," "tip of the fin") is embodied the concept of biological homology represented by these maps. Different versions of homology lead to different computations of features. These do not necessarily share any common factor: In contradiction of the hopes of the early numerical taxonomists, there is no "true, underlying" morphometric distance between forms. We can hope, however, for factors underlying their covariance structure with other domains of measurement, such as the ecological or the biochemical (see Section 2.3.2).

A morphometric analysis of outline data is founded on the knowledge that to a particular curve in one form correspond particular curves on all other forms of a data set. For the analysis to be interpretable in terms of homology, it is required further that we know certain points that match from form to form upon those curves. The mathematical model of homology for curves must be founded on the correspondence of the labeled landmark points, and only then extended to the other points of a continuously curving form (and perhaps to the points inside the form as well) by one or another computational interpolation. When observed point landmarks make no appearance in the interpolation rule, it is impossible to consider the computed correspondence as embodying any aspect of biological homology; the problems caused by this hiatus of meaning have been explored in Section 2.4.1.

Section 2.3 reviewed the delicate relationship between conventional statistical methods and the distributed information of biological forms. Even when we actually mark particular bits of tissue over ontogeny, as by following natural variations of pigmentation, the resulting regression coefficients do not necessarily support any interpretation in terms of explanations of form (cf. Bookstein, 1978). In root tips, mammalian bone, and several other common examples, explanations "move" upon tissues: A process (e.g., a muscle insertion) applying at one place at one time applies at "another" place at a later moment in ontogeny. In fact, the relevance of biological explanations to line elements, or any other coordinate system applied to a form, is logically circular. No laws control our decisions about matching locations for the ends of the ruler separately prior to carrying out our regressions. Rather, it is the regression analysis itself, perhaps an exploration of allometry in one guise or another, that is to justify (however, retroactively) the comparisons of segments among these tentatively labeled endpoints. To the extent that the "lengths" covary with other measurable entities – weight, other lengths, fitness, habitat, histology, date – we assert these endpoints to be "landmarks." If the distances did not manifest interesting covariances, they would be useless as landmarks, no matter how clearly or objectively they had been observed.

Then *landmarks delimit our explanations of effects upon form*; their function is not to just *be* there but to encourage hints about the processes that *put* them there. Except in one dimension, the axial case treated by Huxley (1932), there is no easy way to automatically generate morphometric "variables," anyway (Bookstein, 1978). In two or three dimensions, the construction of a space in which to sift through covariances so as to uncover possible biological meaningfulness without any geometric bias requires algebraic tricks, for instance, the scheme of "shape coordinates" on which this volume relies. Yet most of the shape variables explicitly required for fair coverage of any set of landmarks will prove uninteresting. Even in one dimension, the set of possible objects of a subsequent biological explanation includes all of the distances between pairs of landmarks, and all ratios of those distances. These are all equally meaningless prior to a sophisticated study of their covariances among themselves and with exogenous factors, and all but a few will remain meaningless composites even after the study is completed.

Thus in all cases there are more morphometric variables than one can use in useful descriptions of particular effects upon form. The logic by which these alternatives are sifted is as crucially bound up with the *geometric* ordering of these variables as with their *statistical* ordering. Quantifications of organismic form lacking an appropriate morphometric discipline may be both accurate and taxonomically useful and still be indistinguishable, for our purposes, from meristics, colors, or variables of any other disorganized class. I do not include such quantifications among the morphometric methods. Although they appear to suit the etymology, they do not suit the context of biological explanation: One cannot interpret their covariances. For instance, a list of elliptic Fourier coefficients serves the biologist essentially as a list of ingredients serves the supermarket shopper. One can duplicate the outline (the product), but it remains wholly unclear why just those ingredients are there. In the absence of an epigenetic theory, we can have no expectations about the "causes" or "effects" of these ingredients. Analogously, certain sorts of "similarities" between evolutionary recipes might express some combination of common causes of the lists in question. The methods of systematic biology attempt to separate these causes into those that express common ancestry, case by case, versus those that do not. Whether or not that separation is even a well-posed problem (I believe it is not), *as evidence for establishing common ancestry* morphometric methods are not necessarily either better or worse than other methods. That is not their purpose at all.

The information we morphometricians are after is not the similarity due to common ancestry, but the other part, that due to the covariances with explanatory factors. There, at last, we can revert to a theoretical grounding stated first and most passionately by D'Arcy Thompson in 1917 in the well-known passage from *On Growth and Form* (1961:275–6) that I shall spare the reader the chore of rereading here. Thompson asserts that our descriptions of the processes that regulate form tend usefully to proceed in terms of the sizes and shapes of parts relative to others, and so will conduce to descriptions of relations among those forms in terms of geometric deformations. Conversely, deformations, as extended systems of distributed change, provide a likely mathematical scaffolding to support the search for evidence of explicable biological processes. It is one implication of this position that Huxley's basic model of "growth gradients" (Section 2.3), which came 15 years later, would get its geometry wrong: The issue is one of size, shape, and relative position, not merely of a scalar "length" along a conventional axis.

Many after Thompson attempted to discover methods for objectively seeking biologically meaningful descriptions within the mathematical space of deformations. As it happens, the algebra of landmark points provides the solution to that problem. That is, the statistics of the landmark locations are also the statistics of all models of deformation driven by the landmarks (cf. Section 6.6) – but that is not the issue here. Rather, the question at hand is the manner in which the model of deformation can usefully be applied to multiple sets of data, not just single pairs of forms. On this matter contemporary morphometricians are approaching a consensus. The methodology underlying landmark-based morpho-metrics currently runs somewhat as follows. We know that epigenetic processes regulate form as it unfolds and as it is arrived at in adulthood. We understand, too, certain influences on these processes. Some of the covariates of form are global, like net food intake; others are extremely local, as in the hypermorphosis resulting from muscular exertion or in the sequelae of particular mutations. Over this variety of causes and covariates of form, and in functional explanations throughout the huge diversity of taxa of which we have knowledge, it is found that the elements to which explanations point are often identifiable with specific organs or tissues, and, further, they usually can be represented by specific *boundary points* of those organs or tissues. By a "boundary point" is meant a location at which tissue types are juxtaposed with other tissues or with the surrounding medium. Then landmarks are the boundary points, between organ and organ or between organism and environment, at which our epigenetic explanations adhere.

This ideal type for landmarks will be searched for throughout the examples of this volume, just as they are devoutly sought throughout (the valid) part of contemporary morphometric literature. **Landmarks are the points at which one's explanations of biological processes are grounded.** They are signposts the organism conveniently erects to ease our task of being functional or evolutionary biologists while remaining biometricians.

I have claimed that landmarks are located to ease the task of biological explanation, and I seem to be justifying this claim by noting that many of the explanations of form we accept today as epigenetically valid seem to invoke deformations of the locations of landmarks. All this would seem to involve only the psychology of the biological profession. There is an additional advantage of landmark data, however, that in my view supersedes the preceding difficulty, by permitting us, at last, to transcend the context of classic biometry (Galton, Pearson, Wright) with its arbitrary separation of path coefficient from datum. In the appropriate multivariate context, such as the shape coordinates supply, landmarks permit the biologist to circumvent this distinction. (Though D'Arcy Thompson suspected it, it has been formally recognized only in the development of morphometrics in the last decade or so.) The space of "configurations" in which landmark locations are recorded is, at the same time, the space of possible depictions of effects upon form *and* the space of statistics of deformations relating those forms. Thus, *landmark-based morphometrics is the embodiment within biometrics of the functional form of biological explanation.* The statistical formalism that can be used to delineate *explanations* is the same formalism that was used to organize the individual instances subject to explanation. The landmarks link three separate scientific thrusts: (1) the geometry of data, (2) the mathematics of deformation, and (3) the explanations of biology. For example (Bookstein et al., 1985), any instance of (3) size allometry, computed in the appropriate multivariate way, can be immediately interpreted as (2) a deformation of the "mean," or can be equally effectively used to "grow" any single form (1) into others.

The importance of this formal property cannot be overstated. It applies to all the statistical manipulations of landmarks from Procrustes fits (which represent the no-deformation deformation) through my relative warps. By contrast, outline methods are incapable of leading to biological explanations. Landmark-based explanations can be localized, whereas those based on Fourier coefficients cannot be. The same objection applies to any other technique of integral measures, from eigenshapes to body weight: The language of *their* statistics is not a biometrical language, whereas the language of landmark statistics, the language of variables selected by virtue of their covariances with deformation models, *is*. In morphometrics, the same landmarks that we locate on the image are "put there," or, rather, put nearby (there is always a "residual," a composite of individual variation and measurement error), by the processes we use to explain their patterns. The name of a species does not account for differences among configurations of landmarks on a page, but the biomechanics of a jaw joint can. We draw the effect of that biomechanical explanation using vectors, or describe its effect on shapes using tensors; likewise, we draw the pattern of morphometric covariances with size using vectors, and then interpret it as a tensor field of allometric growth. But we cannot draw the change of a Fourier coefficient, or of an eigenshape, or of a net weight, using vectors: There is no place to put the arrowheads. For that matter, one cannot draw change in a single interlandmark distance (at which end does the arrowhead go?), or change in an angle or ratio among landmarks. The methods of conventional multivariate morphometrics (cf. Marcus, 1990; Reyment, 1990), like the other integral methods, are generally not supportive of subsequent biological explanations (Bookstein and Reyment, 1989).

In so radically empirical a context, the meaning of *homology* becomes far different from the usual. "Homology" is detectable only by its opposite, for which let me coin an abominable neologism, "heterology." If it were a word, "heterology" would mean an ineluctable interference, an intellectual jamming of the tie between morphometric pattern and epigenetic description: They would be "different words," as the etymology might imply. We do not draw any conclusions about the relation of shapes between the fish jaw and the human jaw, for instance, because they are heterologous. In other words, "homology" is a residual category (which is why it is so very difficult to talk about it). The term applies to similarities of form and covariation with exogenous variables for which arguments in favor of heterology are not considered definitive. In the absence of a continuous record of

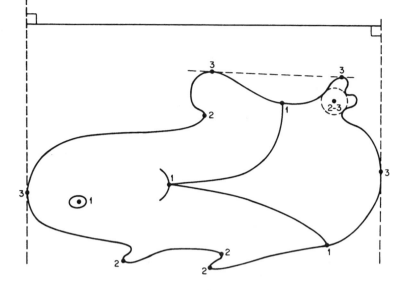

Figure 3.3.1. The three types of landmarks. Type 1: Juxtapositions of tissues. Type 2: Maxima of curvature. Type 3: Extremal points.

evolution or growth, then "homology" is just another name for effective morphometrics. My 1978 book argued that for statistical purposes, the classic notion of homology reduces to the applicability of the deformation model. I maintain the same position now.

From this point of view, the class of phenomena considered "homologous," and thus subject to morphometrically based evolutionary explanation (using landmarks or otherwise), will enlarge or contract over the years as phylogenies or disease states come and go in the journals. Morphometrics cannot settle these arguments, but it can supply pictures of the processes claimed to "explain" any such series of forms.

3.3. TYPES OF LANDMARKS

Three principal types of points that frequently are usable as landmarks correspond to three ways of grounding the epigenetic explanations that motivate these measurements in the first place (Figure 3.3.1).

3.3.1. Type 1: discrete juxtapositions of tissues

This category includes points in space at which three structures meet, such as the following: the bony sutures under the bridge of the nose in humans; branching points of tree structures of constant topology, such as larger-scale features of arterial or nervous systems, whether in two dimensions or three; centers or centroids of "sufficiently small" inclusions, preferably convex, such as the vertebrate eye or the nuclei of the brain; intersections of extended curves with planes of symmetry. Such points can be modeled as displayed in any (geometrical) direction by relative growth immediately adjacent or at a distance.

Landmarks of this first category can enter into many familiar sorts of biometrically valid functional explanations. Among the alternative accounts for deformation, for instance, is the conservation or optimization of biomechanical strength or stiffness under systematic changes of load; another is the biomathematical efficiency of sensory systems; yet another, the bioenergetics of propulsive systems. In particular, the statistics of landmarks are the same as the statistics of descriptive finite-element schemes, which rely on landmarks to quantify strains in a manner comparable from form to form. Another common suggestion is the conservatism of enclosing structures under changes of their contents (the "functional-matrix hypothesis" of Melvin Moss). When a lobe of a brain expands in ontogeny, for instance, there is induced a deformation of the surrounding bone. Although the brain behaves approximately like a fluid, expanding directionlessly, the enclosing bone must adjust to several considerations other than mere hydrostatic pressure and generally will respond by a shape change that is not isotropic (cf. the example for rat calvarial growth in Section 7.2). In other examples (cf. Bookstein, 1985*a*), localized changes of function near the margin of an organ are propagated only a short ways across it, leading to equally localized changes of position among landmarks exactly upon the margin. All such explanations are most persuasive within single ontogenies or functional cycles; their extension to comparisons across organisms involves inferences about fitness gradients, inferences that rely on faith to a greater or lesser extent.

3.3.2. Type 2: maxima of curvature or other local morphogenetic processes

These include tips of extrusions and valleys of invaginations. Landmarks of this second sort often serve as points of application of real biomechanical forces, pushes and pulls. Included are tips of predatory structures – claws and teeth, for instance – and tips of bony processes where muscle attachments may be centered. Landmarks of this sort may also signify a response to a bulge or other radial phenomenon at some distance from the geometrical boundary under study. As reviewed in Bookstein et al. (1985), one cannot, in principle, discriminate displacements of such landmarks lateral to the boundary direction from combinations of normal displacements outward to one side of the landmark, inward to the other. The more complex explanations of the latter category are less credible in general, but may be more valid in particular cases. Landmarks of the first category may enter into explanations of this second sort as well: for instance, tips of incisors.

For three-dimensional data (the case of surfaces rather than curves), gathering the raw information about a shape is a problem all its own. Direct observation of surfaces by one or another optical method is the concern of the field called *biostereometrics*, the subject of occasional SPIE proceedings volumes. An example currently of medical importance is tracking the vertex of the "hump" in cases of scoliosis (curvature) of the human spine (Frobin and Hierholzer, 1982). In three dimensions, extrema of curvature can be bulges, dips, or the "mixed" case of a saddle point. Another hybrid applying to surfaces (Bookstein and Cutting, 1988) first extracts a curve of points that are locally "curvature-landmark-like" in planes perpendicular to the curve, and then scans the curve itself for points that appear to be landmarks, again of the curvature-characterized type. The "corner" of the jaw and the "corners" of the orbital rim can be located in three dimensions by this approach.

3.3.3. Type 3: extremal points

Extremal points are points the definitions of which refer to information at diverse, finitely separated locations. This category, commonest in multivariate morphometrics, incorporates endpoints of diameters, centroids, intersections of interlandmark segments, points farthest from such segments, constructions involving perpendiculars or evenly spaced radial intercepts, and the like. Points taken as "farthest" from other points, or as "endpoints" of a diameter of the form (i.e., as farthest from a point that is farthest from them), are rarely meaningful as landmarks. Although the statistical methods to be discussed later attach vectors to them just as if they had two or three real coordinates, their displacement is meaningful principally in a single direction representing the length ("size") of the defining segment; other directions are confounded by unmeasured aspects of local shape. We often refer to these as **deficient** by virtue of the coordinates they are missing. For an example that supports an appropriate explanation nevertheless, see Section 4.3.2. Similar difficulties apply in the case of points computed as intersections of a contour with perpendiculars to a chord: Series of such points represent functions, not landmark configurations, and their statistics must be reinterpreted appropriately.

Landmarks upon the medial axis of an outline (Bookstein et al., 1985; Straney, 1990) are hybrids of the second and third types here. Endpoints (centers of curvature of boundary segments having locally extreme values of curvature) are at a distance from the boundary equal to that minimum radius of curvature along a vector aligned with the boundary normal. If the morphogenetic process regulating the form in this region is boundary-driven, as it may be for relatively small, heavily sculpted forms like teeth, the displaced point is less useful than the boundary point that it represents; if the process is driven from an interior center, like a bulge, the better point for explanations is the medial point. In contrast, triple points of the medial axis necessarily represent organizations of three or more boundary arcs at considerable separation. When these stand for biochemical integration, as in the human mandible (Bookstein et al., 1985), they are likely more informative than the boundary points they summarize; otherwise, they are not likely to be useful (see also Figure 3.4.12 and Section 3.5).

Some other landmarks of the third type are associated with the convenience of extracting data from plane representations of solid form. The plane involved may be a homologously oriented plane of section of the form, typically a plane of symmetry, or instead the apparent "plane" of a photograph or drawing. In space, certain structures *are* curves, and other structures, such as pairs of surfaces, may abut along curves. The points where curves begin and end in space are fine landmarks; but in plane descriptions, additional apparent landmarks arise where these curves appear to touch the apparent boundary of the organism. In reality, such a "landmark" is merely a point at which the plane normal to the surface, which includes the tangent to the curve, passes through the point of view of the pictorial representation. This is obviously not a local characterization of the "landmark" unless the view is normal to a plane of symmetry. Even less landmark-like is the bulge point of a surface (the point farthest from a chord at some distance) in such a view; it corresponds to no recognizable location on the actual surface material.

When data are derived from radiographs of surfaces, the value of a two-dimensional representation is somewhat enhanced. Landmarks digitized in two dimensions from projection images typically have at least two-thirds of the information available in three dimensions. This compromise is not necessary. Landmarks can be digitized directly in three dimensions or reconstructed there from multiple projections (cf. Grayson et al., 1988, Metz and Fencil, 1989). Any explanation of a two-dimensional analysis of a three-dimensional configuration must acknowledge, of course, the absence of information normal to the plane of the representation.

3.4. EXAMPLES OF LANDMARK CONFIGURATIONS

This section includes descriptions of the main data sets used for examples of the morphometric computations in the remaining four chapters, along with some alternatives and extensions. I indicate the geometry of the landmarks available, assort them by the typology of the preceding section, and justify some choices that might otherwise appear more arbitrary than they actually are. Additional annotated examples may be found in Bookstein (1990*d*).

3.4.1. Rat calvarial growth

This simple data set, Table 3.4.1, appears in many demonstrations: factor models for interlandmark distances (Section 4.3), uniform components of growth (Section 7.2), growth gradients (Section 7.4), relative warps (Section 7.6), and their covariances. The data, listed in Appendix A.4.5, are eight landmark locations for 21 male laboratory rats observed at eight ages. The data base is a nearly complete three-way array: Locations were missing for only 4 of the 1,344 combinations of landmark, animal, and age. The original roentgenograms were collected by Henning Vilmann of the Royal Dental College, Copenhagen. The coordinates of the landmarks were digitized by Melvin Moss at Columbia University. These 8 landmarks are selected from a set of 20 covering the face as well as the calva. Their locations have been used previously in his articles on the finite-element method (Moss et al., 1985, 1987) and in Goodall's approach to the same coverage of shape space by a different algebraic formalism (Goodall and Bose, 1987; Goodall, 1991), as well as in my earlier publications of the examples in which they appear here (Bookstein, 1983, 1987*a*, 1989*b*).

Table 3.4.1. *Rat calvarial landmarks, Figure 3.4.1*

Name	Number	Type	Description
Basion	1	2	Ventral extreme of foramen magnum (tip of basioccipital bone in midplane)
Opisthion	2	2	Dorsal extreme of foramen magnum (tip of supraoccipital bone in midplane)
Interparietal suture	3	1	Interparietal-supraoccipital suture where it crosses the midplane
Lambda	4	1	Parietal-interparietal suture where it crosses the midplane
Bregma	5	1	Frontoparietal (coronal) suture where it crosses the midplane
Spheno-ethmoid synchondrosis	6	3	"Middle" of gap between cribriform plate of ethmoid bone and presphenoid bone along axis of presphenoid
Intersphenoidal suture	7	2	"Middle" of the presphenoid-basisphenoid synchondrosis in the midplane
Spheno-occipital synchondrosis	8	2	"Middle" of the basisphenoid-basioccipital synchondrosis in the midplane

3.4. Examples

Figure 3.4.1 is a hybrid drawing, showing the actual midsagittal plane of a typical 15-day-old rat skull (Baer, Bosma, and Ackerman, 1983:395), soft contents deleted, fitted to the mean landmark configuration observed in our 7-day-old specimens. The landmarks are quite easy to visualize in conventional lateral cephalograms. Places where sutures cross the midplane are visible at the horizon of the cranial form; synchondroses are equally visible as gaps between bony shadows. Figure 3.4.2 shows two typical effects of age upon this configuration.

3.4.2. The University School Study subsample

Figure 3.4.3 shows the scheme of landmarks for the University of Michigan University School Study, a major archive of 45 points in lateral view for 1,296 lateral cephalograms of about 200 children at the University of Michigan laboratory school in the 1950s and 1960s. Not all these points are used in the examples in this book, but in their variety of definitions they provide a most instructive example of the fruits (and pitfalls) of hard work at landmark definition (Moyers, Bookstein, and Hunter, 1988).

As Table 3.4.2 indicates, all three types of landmarks crop up in this typical practical investigation. The 35 landmarks not on the molars include 7 of Type 1 (anatomical), 1 (#35, Sella) unclassifiable between Types 1 and 2, 8 of Type 2 (processual), and 18 of Type 3 (extremal). The coordinate system referenced in these

Figure 3.4.1. Representation of midsagittal section, rat calvaria. Landmarks are as in Table 3.4.1.

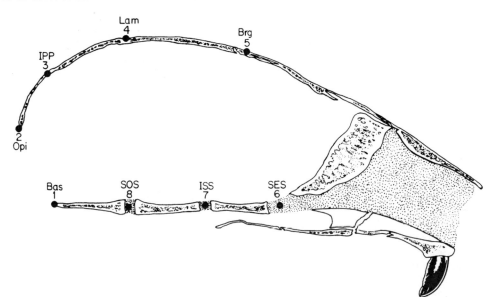

(a)

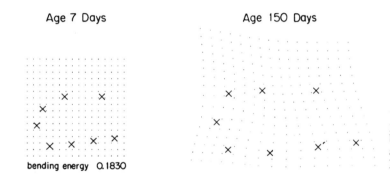

Age 7 Days   Age 14 Days

bending energy 0.0036

(b)

Age 7 Days   Age 150 Days

bending energy 0.1830

Figure 3.4.2. Change of mean landmark configuration, calvaria of 21 male rats, from age 7 days to age 14 days and age 150 days. The representation in this and similar figures to follow in this section is the interpolant via the thin-plate spline reviewed in Section 2.2. Mean forms are computed as explained in Section 5.4 by averaging shape coordinates to a convenient baseline. Compare Bookstein (1983).

definitions by such words as "anterior," "anterior-inferior," and the like is *not* the system in which the diagram is printed, but instead the conventional "Frankfurt orientation." This sets to horizontal a line from point #40, Orbitale (bottom of the eye socket), to Porion, "top of the auditory meatus (earhole)," a point not included in this data base even though it is clearly visible in the films.

Landmarks 1 through 3 are statistically equivalent deficient landmarks clustered at the chin. One is taken where the outline shows a tangent that is horizontal, one where the tangent is at 45° to the horizontal, and one where it is vertical. These are clearly meant to be not homologous points but merely termini for length measurements (height of face, protrusion of teeth beyond chin, length of mandible); the "center" of the chin as supplied by the

3.4. Examples

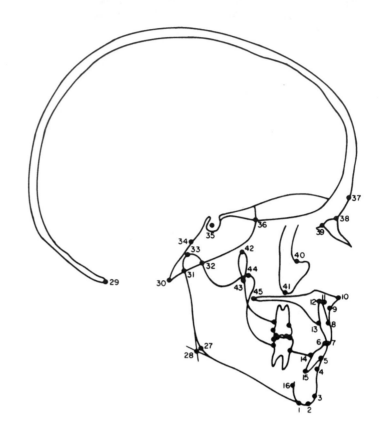

Figure 3.4.3. Forty-five landmarks (Table 3.4.2) from the University of Michigan University School Study (Riolo et al., 1974).

medial axis (i.e., the center of the circle of curvature at the outline point of smallest radius of curvature; see Section 3.5.2) would be a better landmark than any of these three for most explanatory purposes. Point 11, "L" (for "van der Linden") is a wonderful example of the heterologous "landmark" that can be located by only one practitioner. I extract its definition, in full, from Riolo et al. (1974:14–16):

L Point represents a point on the anterior surface on the image of the labial lamella at the apex region of the maxillary central incisor. When the permanent incisors (before eruption) are positioned within bone with their crown in the apical base region, L Point is taken 1–2 millimeters anterior to the height of contour of the crown relative to and on a line drawn through supradentale and parallel to the axis of the central incisor. When the permanent incisors are erupted and their roots are not fully formed, L Point is located at the root end along an axially placed line through supradentale. When the root is completed, L Point is located along the same axial line at the root tip.

If a definition of one of your landmarks sounds like that, rewrite it immediately!

70

Table 3.4.2. *Landmarks of the Michigan set, Figure 3.4.3*

Name	Number	Type	Description
Menton	1	3	Most inferior point of mandible
Gnathion	2	3	Most anterior-inferior point of mandible
Pogonion	3	3	Most anterior point of mandible
B	4	3	Most posterior point between lower incisor and chin
Infradentale supradentale	5, 8	1	Labial contact of alveolar ridge and mandibular/maxillary central incisor
Lower/upper incisal edge	6, 7	2	Tip of lower/upper incisor
A	9	3	Most posterior point between upper incisor and point 10
Anterior nasal spine	10	2	Tip of the median bony process of the maxilla
L	11		See text
Upper/lower incisal apex	12, 15	2	Root tip of maxillary/mandibular incisor
Upper/lower incisor lingual	13, 14	1	Lingual contact of alveolar ridge and maxillary/mandibula central incisor
Symphyseal point	16	3	Intersection of line through point 3 parallel to mandibula "plane"
Molar points	17–26		Not referenced in this book
Gonion	27	3	Intersection with mandibular border of bisector of angl between mandibular "plane" and ramal "plane"
Gonial intersect	28	3	Intersection of mandibular "plane" and ramal "plane"
Opisthion	29	2	Posteriormost point of foramen magnum
Basion	30	2	Posteriormost point on clivus
Articulare	31	3	Overlap of shadows of posterior condylar border and clivus
Anterior articulare	32	3	Overlap of shadows of anterior condylar border and clivus
Condylion	33	3	Most superior axial point of condylar head
Spheno-occipital synchondrosis	34	1	Midpoint of the synchondrosis
Sella turcica	35	1–2	Center of the pituitary fossa
Ethmoid registration	36	3	Overlap of shadows of anterior wing of sphenoid an(sphenoidal "plane"
Glabella	37	3	Bulge point of eyebrows
Nasion	38	1	Junction of frontonasal sutures
Frontomaxillonasal suture	39	1	Junction of the three bones specified
Orbitale	40	3	Lowest point on the bony orbit
Inferior zygoma	41	3	Lowest point on the zygoma
Superior pterygo-maxillary fissure	42	3	Most superior point of the outline of the fissure
Inferior pterygo-maxillary fissure	43	3	Locus of "disappearance" of outline as sketched
Coronoidale	44	3	Most superior point of coronoid process
Posterior nasal spine	45	2	Posterior tip of midsagittal bony palate

Source: Adapted from Riolo et al. (1974).

Points #31 and #32 are explicit overlays of silhouttes of spatially separated bones (the condylar head and the clivus of the cranial base). They appear to enter into no valid biological explanations (but compare #36). The definition of point #33, Condylion, is one of a variety of alternatives that try to find the "tip" of this mushroom-like structure. The effort is worthwhile, because the shape of the tip is functionally highly regulated (it has to be able to shift smoothly in its fossa), and because its shape reflects the underlying local chondrogenic processes that formed it.

Landmark #35, Sella, is taken in "empty space." Yet it is very reliably locatable in humans, as the pituitary fossa is nearly circular in this cephalometric projection. The point defined so, however, is nearly useless for comparisons involving the majority of species, in which the fossa is not cylindrical. Primatologists might use the tip of the process called dorsum sellae, just posterior to Sella, or the posterior clinoid process just lateral to the midline at the chiasmatic groove anterior to Sella. Landmark #36, in contrast to #31, is an intersection of shadows that *does* appear to enter into biological explanations, as each of its coordinates has a well-defined meaning even if they are not linked at the tissue level (see the example in Section 7.3.3). Landmark #40, Orbitale, is clearly an inappropriate way of recording the "position" of the eyes. In the frontal cephalogram, in which the eye sockets appear as slightly squared circles, it is clear that the "corners" of the eye are not its north, south, east, and west compass points, but rather its northeast, northwest, southeast, and southwest points, where the circumorbital sutures often can be found. Landmarks #42 and #43 both lie on a "structure" that does not properly exist – a "fissure" that is an artifact of the angle at which the posterior part of the maxilla is viewed. Point #43 is particularly badly behaved, as it is the place where a shadow "disappears." Point #44, the "top" of the coronoid process, proves quite difficult to see, in view of the maxillary structures superimposed upon it. We shall substitute a better alternative, the "tip" of this process (point farthest from the middle of the ramus), in Section 3.5.

Landmarks are drawn from this set or studies of normal craniofacial growth and Apert and Crouzon syndromes. A selection for the normal-growth study is presented in Appendix A.4.1, and for Apert syndrome, in Appendix A.4.2. A subset of five from the mandible is extended to three dimensions for the example of Sections 5.4.4 and 6.5.4. Figure 3.4.4 suggests the subtlety of the effects of growth upon this landmark configuration.

3.4.3. Assorted small creatures

In three papers published in the late 1980s, Richard Reyment and I and some colleagues applied landmark-based morphometrics to

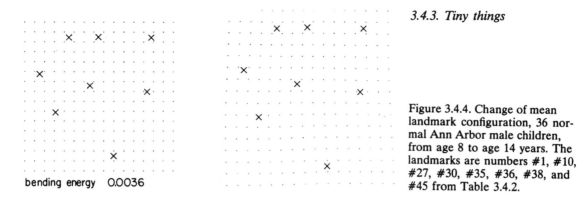

bending energy   0.0036

Figure 3.4.4. Change of mean landmark configuration, 36 normal Ann Arbor male children, from age 8 to age 14 years. The landmarks are numbers #1, #10, #27, #30, #35, #36, #38, and #45 from Table 3.4.2.

some problems in quantitative paleontology that previously had been explored principally by the methods of multivariate morphometrics and the ordinations that ensue (Reyment, 1991). Some of those analyses appear in this volume as exemplifying one sort or another of landmark finding. Also included here are two schemes of landmarks for *Globorotalia*: one developed in Bookstein (1986*a*), and another, much richer, developed by Elena Tabachnick in the course of her dissertation (Tabachnick, 1988); see also Tabachnick and Bookstein (1990*a*, *b*).

3.4.3.1. Brizalina.—

Figure 3.4.5 shows six landmarks for a Miocene foraminiferan; the landmarks are defined in Table 3.4.3. The locations of these

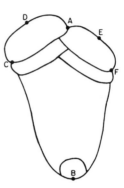

Figure 3.4.5. Landmarks for the Miocene foraminiferan *Brizalina*, Table 3.4.3.

Table 3.4.3. *Landmark definitions for Brizalina, Figure 3.4.5*

Name	Letter	Type	Definition
Aperture	*A*	1	Point at which the convexity of the final chamber appears to spring from that of the penultimate chamber
Proloculus	*B*	2	Sharpest curvature of this structure, which is the first part of the organism to be laid down
Final chamber proximal	*C*	1	Point where the convexity of the final chamber appears to spring from the earlier body wall
Final chamber bulge	*D*	3	Point on the margin of the final chamber farthest from the chord from *A* to *C*
Penultimate chamber bulge	*E*	3	Point on the margin of the penultimate chamber farthest from the chord from *A* to *F*
Penultimate chamber proximal	*F*	1	Point where the convexity of the penultimate chamber appears to spring from the earlier body wall

landmarks for 10 specimens each from five levels of a Cameroun borehole are listed in Appendix A.4.4. I digitized these locations from a series of photomicrographs executed by Eva Reyment. All landmarks are defined in reference to the image in a particular view, that "across" the plane of the organism (which is assembled in an alternating, not a spiraling, fashion).

Landmarks *A*, *C*, and *F* are quite well defined in the specified view. (*C* and *F* are sometimes the intersection of two curves both visible in the image and sometimes the terminus of one suture that is plainly visible. When all three features can be seen, their locations are concordant.) Landmark *B*, originally suggested as the endpoint of a length measure (Bookstein and Reyment, 1989), is nevertheless localizable fairly well; the analysis in Section 4.3 exploits it as one end of a baseline. Landmarks *D* and *E* are wholly deficient in the coordinate parallel to the chord *AC* or *AF* that is entailed in their definitions; this deficiency is apparent in the ensuing statistical analysis (Bookstein and Reyment, 1989). Figure 3.4.6 displays a typical effect upon this configuration of landmarks.

3.4.3.2. Veenia. —

Abe et al. (1988) analyzed nine levels of specimens of two species of ostracods from the Santonian (Cretaceous) in Israel. The landmarks are sketched in Figure 3.4.7 and defined in Table 3.4.4. I shall use one of these sequences to exemplify a higher-order growth gradient in Section 7.4.4. Specimens were positioned in the apertural plane and were digitized from scanning electron micrographs. Effects on these landmarks (Figure 3.4.8) typically do not alter the general outline.

3.4.3.3. Mutilus. —

Another ostracod, *Mutilus*, is a living form found along the southern coast of Australia. The scheme in Figure 3.4.9 was previously published (Reyment et al., 1988). These landmarks

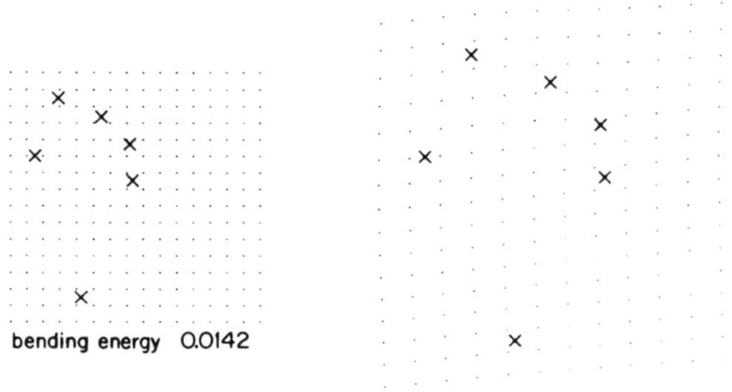

bending energy 0.0142

Figure 3.4.6. Change of mean configuration, six landmarks, between stratum 2 and stratum 4 of Reyment's *Brizalina* data.

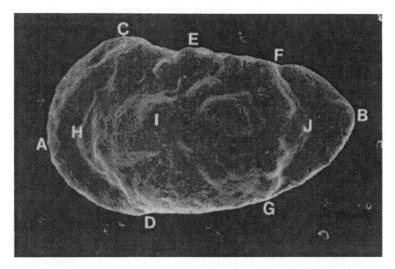

Figure 3.4.7. Ten landmarks for an ostracod, *Veenia*, Table 3.4.4.

were not named, but only depicted, and so we do not tabulate them here. All are of Type 2, the "centers" of fairly small regions at which homologous structures intersect. A typical group difference is depicted in Figure 3.4.10.

The measurement of ostracods is quite difficult in general, and the species shown here are unusually landmark-rich; analysis of other data sets may find none of these landmarks, or, indeed, no usable landmarks at all.

3.4.3.4. *Globorotalia.* —

Section 6.5.2 exemplifies the study of ecophenotypy using the landmarks from Figure 3.4.11, and Section 7.3.3 pursues the example further. I digitized the landmarks here from computer listings of *eigenshapes* (see Section 2.4.1), Lohmann's method of sample ordination, which preserved these as landmarks even while

Table 3.4.4. *Ten landmarks for Veenia, an ostracod, Figure 3.4.7*

Name	Letter	Type	Description
Anterior pole	*A*	3	Midpoint of anterior margin
Posterior pole	*B*	3	Midpoint of posterior margin
Eye tubercle	*C*	1–2	Center of the bulge
Anterior rib ventral	*D*	1	Intersection of anterior rib with anteroventral margin
Anterior rib dorsal	*E*	1	Intersection of anterior rib with centrodorsal margin
Posterior rib dorsal	*F*	1	Intersection of posterior rib with posterodorsal margin
Posterior rib ventral	*G*	1	Intersection of posterior rib with posteroventral margin
Anterior furrow	*H*	3	"Tip" of anterior furrow (near *A*)
Adductor tubercle	*I*	1–2	Bulge of adductor muscle tubercle
Posterior ridge	*J*	3	"Tip" of posterior ridge (near *B*)

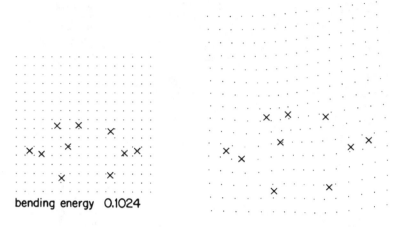

Figure 3.4.8. Change of mean configuration, 10 landmarks, from strata 1–5 to strata 6–9 for Abe's *Veenia* data. The difference is extrapolated fivefold.

bending energy 0.1024

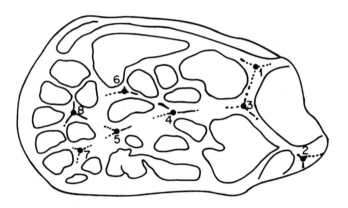

Figure 3.4.9. Eight landmarks for *Mutilus*, located upon the median rib and associated ornamental features.

Figure 3.4.10. Change of mean configuration, eight landmarks upon *Mutilus*, between the Seaholme and the Kingston samples (Reyment et al., 1988, Fig. 1). The difference is extrapolated threefold.

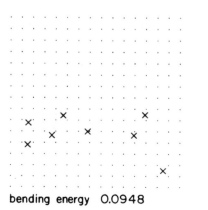

bending energy 0.0948

paying no attention to them. Lohmann described these shapes as follows (1983:664–5):

> Between 15 and 30 specimens of left-coiling. *G. truncatulinoides* larger than 0.25 mm in diameter were randomly drawn from each of 16 [later, 20] seafloor sediment samples [from 16° to 51° S in the Indian Ocean]. The outline of each specimen (oriented in edge view) was digitized, interpolated to the same number of equal segments around its perimeter, ... and represented by a Zahn and Roskies $\phi^*(l)$ shape function. These shapes were then rotated to mutually homologous positions.

Eigenshapes were then computed by singular-value decompositions of cross-products between these functions sample by sample. The function ϕ^* is $\phi(l) - l$, where ϕ is the tangent angle (cf. Bookstein, 1978) at the point a fraction l of the way around the form (from a presumably homologous starting location). The landmarks are the "corners" of the form, numbered #1 through #3 in the figure. These were operationalized as the points of greatest net curvature (change of tangent angle) of the sample-specific first eigenshape ("mean form") over runs of six points spaced at intervals of $1/128$ of the net perimeter of the form of this view. Additional deficient landmarks #12, #23, and #31 were chosen halfway between these landmarks, in pairs, along the "eigenshape" curves joining them.

3.4.3.5. *Another scheme for Globorotalia.* —

In her 1988 dissertation, Elena Tabachnick digitized a different group of globorotaliids in a great deal more detail. As Figure 3.4.12 shows, there are two schemes of proper landmarks here, corresponding to two views of the same organisms at approximately 90°. No attempt is made here to correlate landmarks between the views. In the spiral view, the landmarks lie on well-defined space curves (juxtapositions of successive chambers)

3.4.3. *Tiny things*

Figure 3.4.11. Form of *Globorotalia truncatulinoides*. Left: Drawing of a single specimen. Right: Outline after the smoothing and averaging that is Lohmann's eigenshape analysis, with six landmarks, three of which are deficient.

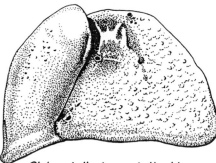

Globorotalia truncatulinoides

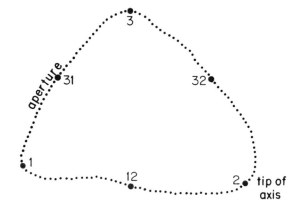

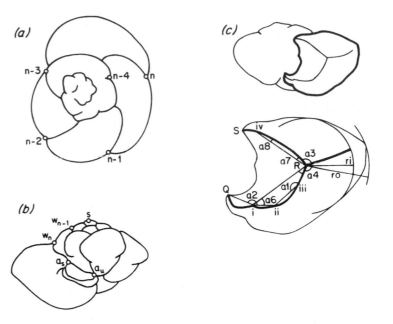

Figure 3.4.12. Three schemes for representing globorotaliid form, from Tabachnick (1988). (*a*) Landmarks in spiral view. (*b*) Landmarks in apertural view. (*c*) Angles and ratio chosen to measure medial axis of chamber shape, apertural view.

where those curves intersect the edge of the regression of the form in the chosen view. In the apertural view, landmarks on the aperture itself appear to be of Type 1, juxtapositions of structures. The spiral point *s* is likewise of Type 1, as the earliest recognizable point of the organism. Landmarks labeled *w* are loci at which well-defined curves have tangents passing behind the surface according to the chosen plane of view. The selection of features of the medial axis (see Section 3.5.2) consists of eight angles and one log ratio of radii as shown.

3.4.4. Lateral photographs of seven-year-olds

Sections 5.4.3, 7.2.5, and 7.3.3 exploit data from lateral photographs of the faces of normal and nearly normal human seven-year-olds. (The analysis of the frontal photograph has already been exemplified in Chapter 1.) Analyses of these data were first published in Clarren et al. (1987) and also supported the earlier publication of the method of quadratic growth gradients in Bookstein and Sampson (1987, 1990). The 36 photographs represent the morphometrically usable pairs from a slightly larger study of perception involving 21 seven-year-olds prenatally exposed to substantial amounts of alcohol, and 21 others not so substantially exposed, from the Seattle Longitudinal Prospective Study of Alcohol and Pregnancy. The original 42 were matched on sex, race, and a "waif factor" (hair care, holes in T-shirts, etc.); the original design involved only subjective classification of the images by dysmorphologists, not actual morphometrics. When we augmented the psychological study by a quantitative analysis, considerations of data quality in both lateral and frontal views reduced the data set to 36 cases, which proved best analyzed as the 8 most highly exposed versus the 28 others. Landmarks were marked directly on the photographs with pinholes, the locations of which were subsequently digitized at a digitizing tablet.

The protocol of Table 3.4.5 embodies a fairly interesting set of compromises. Many of these points are difficult to locate, at least in comparison with their cephalometric equivalents (cf. Table 3.4.2); but, of course, the whole point of anthropometry from photographs is to avoid the cost and the radiation dose associated with roentgencephalometry for population studies. All the landmarks described as "maxima of curvature" in Table 3.4.5 actually correspond to quite gentle maxima; that is why the table declares them intermediate between Types 2 and 3. Point #18, in particular, while useful, has no good name; it is the place at which uncles pinch their nephews and nieces after not having seen them for some months. The effect of alcohol exposure upon this landmark configuration (Figure 3.4.14) will be reduced to three features in Section 7.3.

3.4.4.1. Landmarks of Figure 1.2.1. —

At the time that the landmarks of the frontal view were introduced (Figure 1.2.1 and Table 1.2.1), our terminology of landmark types was not yet in place. It is appropriate to review those landmarks now. Points #5, #6, #8, #9, #11, #13, and #14 seem to be good Type-1 landmarks, referring to the juxtaposition of explicitly distinct anatomical structures. All the points on the eyebrows (#1, #2, #3, #4) are of Type 3, intersections at a distance, as they are defined by lines crossing the eyebrows that have sprung from various features of the eyes. Points #1 and #4, in particular, were included mainly to corroborate a clinical hunch

3.4.4. Photographs

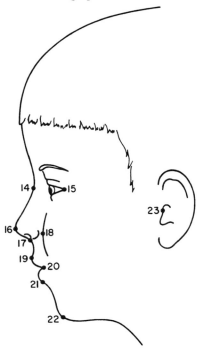

Figure 3.4.13. Ten lateral landmarks (Table 3.4.5) for human facial photographs, from Clarren et al. (1987).

Table 3.4.5. *Lateral landmarks for the human face, Figure 3.4.13*

Name	Number	Type	Description
Nasion	14	2–3	Point of maximum curvature over nasal bridge
Exocanthion	15	1	Lateral intersection of upper and lower eyelids
Pronasale	16	2–3	Point of maximum curvature over nasal tip
Subnasale	17	2	"Intersection" of columella and philtrum
"Pinch point"	18	2–3	Point of maximum curvature of soft-tissue fold from zygoma
Vermilion upper	19	1	Boundary of upper vermilion border at midline
Cheilon	20	1	Lateral intersection of upper and lower vermilion borders
Vermilion lower	21	1	Boundary of lower vermilion border at midline
Gnathion	22	2–3	Point of maximum curvature of chin
Meatus	23	2	"Center" of external auditory opening

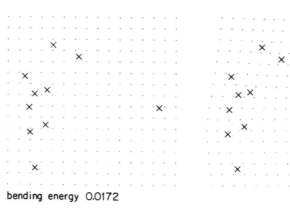

bending energy 0.0172

Figure 3.4.14. Effect of prenatal exposure to alcohol upon configuration of 10 lateral landmarks.

about "Harlequin eyebrow," a redirection of the lateral part of the eyebrows quite a bit higher on the face in certain syndromes. Landmark #7, Nasal bridge, is probably of Type 3, the digitizer's best guess at the "deepest" point of that structure as viewed from shading, shadow, or the corresponding lateral photo. This landmark is clearly *not* the same as the point halfway between the eyes (average of #6 and #8), as that average moves vertically as well as horizontally with respect to point #7. Landmarks #10 and #12, Nasal alae, are of Type 3, as each is "most lateral" either with respect to the plane of symmetry or with respect to the other ala. Point #16, Chin, is of Type 3 (the "bottom" of a structure). It is surprisingly clear in this view, as the skin of the throat behind it is ordinarily out of focus.

3.5. THE MEDIAL AXIS AND THE LIMITS OF LANDMARKS

My introductory material frequently mentioned the difficulties of incorporating information about curving form within the landmark formalism. Forms to which this objection often applies are those that are assembled out of more or less blobby "parts" whose junctions cannot be observed in the adult form being measured. I shall explore this point in the context of a small study carried out jointly with Drs. Barry Grayson and Joseph McCarthy of New York University: the discrimination of mandibular shape between the normal condition and that found in the heads of patients with Apert syndrome or Crouzon syndrome (see Section 6.5.3). The study is part of a larger investigation into new techniques of surgical planning for these corrections. The sample for this part of the study included 24 normal 7-year-old subjects from the Michigan series and 12 subjects each with Apert and Crouzon syndromes in the age range of six to eight years, from the files of the Institute for Reconstructive Plastic Surgery, New York University (Grayson et al., 1990).

3.5.1. Six mandibular landmarks

From the public archival file of the University of Michigan University School Study (Section 3.4.2) were extracted the locations of six landmarks characterized in Figure 3.4.3: Condylion, Gonion, Menton, Pogonion, Lower incisal edge (LIE), and Infradentale (ID). The same points were located in the 24 films of the two syndromal populations. A seventh landmark, Coronoidale, *sensu* Riolo et al. (1974), apparently had been quite difficult to locate accurately in these films; it was missing from too many of the archived cases to be of use in that form. A point defined slightly differently will prove quite useful, as we shall see in a moment.

Multivariate analysis of the shapes of these 48 configurations of six landmarks is by the method of shape coordinates (Section 1.1.2) to a baseline from Condylion to Menton. The shape of the configuration reduces to four pairs of shape coordinates: the positions of Gonion, Pogonion, LIE, and ID in a coordinate system for which Condylion is fixed at $(0, 0)$, and Menton at $(1, 0)$. Means of these coordinate pairs – the mean shapes of the landmark configurations for our three samples – are displayed in Figure 3.5.1.

It is possible to augment a landmark data set by incorporating additional information on the curving of outline form between landmarks (Bookstein, 1988a; or see Appendix A.1). Because the mandibular outline is so poorly sampled by landmark locations to begin with, we chose instead to represent it wholly independently of these landmarks by a measurement scheme following entirely different principles.

Figure 3.5.1. Mean coordinates of four mandibular landmarks to a baseline from Condylion to Menton. Michigan group, 24 normal University of Michigan University School Study 7-year-olds. Apert group, 12 cases of Apert syndrome, aged 6 to 8 years. Crouzon group, 12 cases of Crouzon syndrome, aged 6 to 8 years.

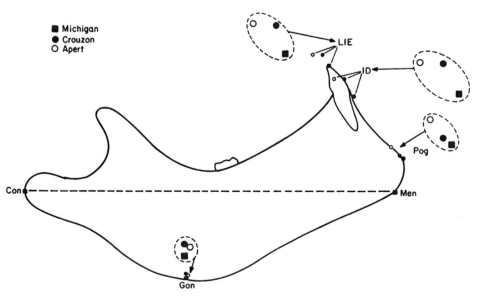

■ Michigan
● Crouzon
○ Apert

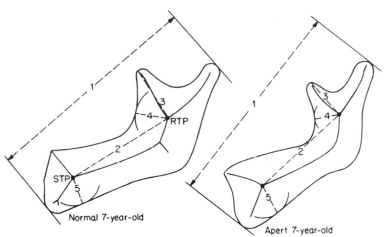

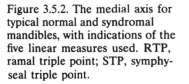

Figure 3.5.2. The medial axis for typical normal and syndromal mandibles, with indications of the five linear measures used. RTP, ramal triple point; STP, symphyseal triple point.

3.5.2. The mandibular medial axis and its measurement

The **medial axis** of an irregular plane curve is the collection of centers of circles that touch the curve at at least two separate points. The idea of representing a biological outline by centers of circles in this fashion was introduced by Harry Blum (1973). Straney (1990) reviews several algorithms for the automatic computation of this structure. Its application to the particular form of the human mandible has been the subject of several earlier experiments (Blum and Nagel, 1978; Bookstein, 1979, 1981*a*; Bookstein et al., 1985; Grayson, Bookstein, and McCarthy, 1986). The typical mandibular medial axis (Figure 3.5.2) has two *triple points* at which inscribed circles touch the form upon *three* separate arcs of the outline. At such points the medial axis branches to penetrate between each pair of boundary arcs separately. It is common for mandibular forms in older children and adults to manifest a third triple point as well, where the medial axes of the corpus and the ramus fork to generate a branch that penetrates somewhat into the gonial angle. The gonial triple point is not reliably present in the forms of this series.

Complete mandibular outlines were traced by Mr. H. C. Kim of New York University for the subsample of 24 syndromals, and the same traces were retrieved from the unpublished University School Study archives for the 24 normal subjects. Medial axes for these 48 mandibular outlines were computed by the algorithm of Bookstein (1979).

There is no standardized way of "measuring" the medial axis. Indeed, when it is augmented by the record of radii of those doubly tangent circles, it contains precisely as much information as the original outline tracing. It is a transformation, not a summary, of the outline form (Blum, 1973). Judicious scrutiny of these 48 examples suggested the recording of the five distances shown in the figure. The analysis incorporates the locations of the Ramal triple point (RTP) and the Symphyseal triple point (STP) and a modified version of Coronoidale: not the elusive "most superior point" of the process, but instead the more reliably locatable point farthest from RTP upon the process. The "mandibular diameter" measured here is simply the longest distance across the traced outline. It approximates the distance from conventional Condylion to conventional Gnathion, but those landmarks are not in fact referenced. Thus the five-distance record of the medial axis shares no loci with the set of all readily available conventional landmarks for the same images. In fact, the radii at RTP and STP cannot be construed as distances between pairs of landmarks at all. Still, because ratios to overall mandibular diameter serve the same conceptual function as ratios to the length Condylion–Menton in the landmark analysis, we believe that the comparison of the two measurement schemes is quite fair to both. The medial axis also supports various angle measurements (Blum and Nagel, 1978; Bookstein, 1981*a*). All these proved uninformative in the current application, though they were quite effective in the analysis of Tabachnick's *Globorotalia* (Section 3.4.3.5; Tabachnick and Bookstein, 1990*a*).

3.5.3. Findings

In Figure 3.5.1, the mandibular form typical of synostosis is most clearly differentiated by the triangle involving the anterior dental landmark ID. With respect to the Condylion–Menton (Con–Men) baseline, in Apert syndrome the point ID is displaced from the normal position by about 7% of baseline length anatomically upward (i.e., both relatively away from the baseline and relatively backward along it). By the methods of Chapter 6, this can be described as an increase over normal of some 25% in the ratio of distances ID–Men : ID–Con. The backward, but not the upward, component of this displacement is halved in the typical Crouzon mandibular shape. The extent of displacement from the normative position away from the baseline is somewhat lower for the point LIE, perhaps because some of the incisors in this sample are still erupting. The scatters of this pair of shape coordinates for the three groups are shown in Figure 3.5.3; an optimal linear discrimination using all eight shape coordinates is based on a score very similar to that obtained by projection upon the northwest–southeast diagonal here. The net separation of the Michigan normals from the syndromals is clear, the overlap modest.

We turn now to the alternate set of measures of the same 48 mandibles, the five distances (Figure 3.5.2) selected to represent features of the medial axis. In order to restrict the analysis to shape information, we considered these variables in terms of their ratios. Table 3.5.1 presents the statistics of all the simple ratios (or their inverses).

The ratios having the best *F*-statistics all involve either the distance from RTP to Coronoidale or the radius of the touching

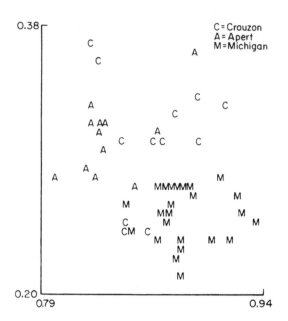

Figure 3.5.3. Shape coordinates of Infradentale to a Condylion–Menton baseline.

circle at STP; the best simple ratio, indeed, is the ratio of these two quantities. As Figure 3.5.4 shows, all by itself it discriminates the 24 syndromals from the 24 Michigan normals with only two misclassifications. The average of this ratio is nearly 25% lower in the syndromals than in the normals, as typified in Figure 3.5.2. Notice that there is one modest outlier in each syndromal group.

Following the logic of Section 2.3.1, or Crespi and Bookstein (1989), we can compute a discriminatory factor without reference to the correlations among our ratios (correlations built in by virtue

Table 3.5.1. *Elementary ratios of distances measured on the medial axis*

Ratio[a]		Crouzon sample		Apert sample		Michigan sample		Net F for ANOVA by group
Numerator	Denominator	Mean	S.D.	Mean	S.D.	Mean	S.D.	
Rad. RTP	Diam.	0.137	0.014	0.138	0.019	0.142	0.008	0.505
Rad. STP	Diam.	0.144	0.013	0.149	0.006	0.128	0.006	31.710
RTP–Cor	Diam.	0.228	0.025	0.242	0.041	0.273	0.015	13.252
RTP–STP	Diam.	0.493	0.021	0.475	0.029	0.492	0.023	2.412
Rad. STP	Rad. RTP	1.052	0.104	1.095	0.141	0.910	0.064	17.210
RTP–Cor	Rad. RTP	1.664	0.124	1.747	0.101	1.930	0.130	21.766
RTP–STP	Rad. RTP	3.629	0.461	3.520	0.717	3.491	0.313	0.340
RTP–Cor	Rad. STP	1.595	0.180	1.623	0.245	2.126	0.147	47.916
RTP–STP	Rad. STP	3.458	0.382	3.190	0.264	3.839	0.281	19.447
RTP–STP	RTP–Cor	2.187	0.283	2.031	0.491	1.811	0.150	0.674

[a]RTP, Ramal triple point; STP, Symphyseal triple point; Diam., mandibular diameter; Rad., radius of triply tangent circle; RTP–Cor, distance from RTP to the farthest point on the coronoid process.

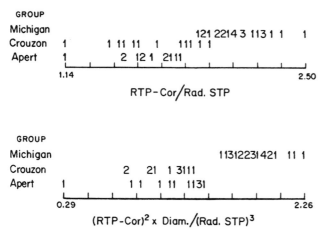

GROUP

Michigan   121 2214 3 113 1 1   1

Crouzon   1   1 11 11   1   111 1 1

Apert   1   2 12 1 21 11

1.14   2.50

RTP–Cor/Rad. STP

GROUP

Michigan   11312231421 11 1

Crouzon   2   21   1 3111

Apert   1   1 1   1 11 1131

0.29   2.26

$(RTP–Cor)^2 \times$ Diam./(Rad. STP)^3

3.5.3. Findings

Figure 3.5.4. Separations of samples by ratios of distances among medial-axis "landmarks." Top: Best single ratio, (RTP–Cor)/(Rad. STP). Bottom: A partial-least-squares composite: log of the ratio (3.5.1).

of their sharing a denominator, of course) if we combine their logarithms with weights equal to their separate covariances with group. (Compare the approach in Mosimann and James, 1979, or Darroch and Mosimann, 1985.) These covariances are just the logarithms of the ratios of Michigan and syndromal means in Table 3.5.1. The two largest F-ratios correspond to the ratios of Rad. STP to Diam. and to the distance RTP–Cor. The mean differences of the logs of these ratios between the syndromal and normal groups [approximately $\log(0.128/0.1465)$ and $\log(2.126/1.609)$] are -0.138 and 0.279, in a ratio of almost exactly $-1:2$. This suggests a discriminatory factor of the form $(\text{Rad. STP/Diam.})^{-1} \times (\text{RTP–Cor/Rad. STP})^2$, or

$$\frac{(\text{RTP–Cor})^2 \times \text{Diam.}}{(\text{Rad. STP})^3}. \tag{3.5.1}$$

By comparison, an optimal linear discriminant analysis using as basis of the log contrasts the first four variables in the table (ratios to mandibular diameter) generates coefficients proportional to -0.95, -3.34, 2.09, and 0.30 for the logs of these ratios. The discrimination afforded by these is indistinguishable from that given by the ratio (3.5.1), which is equivalent to using coefficients $(0, -3, 2, 0)$, as shown in the second panel of Figure 3.5.4.

The expression (3.5.1) might be summarized as something like a ratio of ramal *volume* to corporeal width cubed. The syndromal cases have small values of these ratios – their symphyseal regions are quite a bit larger than normal in relation to ramal width and length. The change of ratio owes to diminution of the ramal measures, and also mandibular diameter, in both of the syndromal groups, in comparison to a symphyseal width Rad. STP that is not distinguishable from the corresponding normal mean.

85

3.5.4. Implications of the example for landmark selection

In these synostoses, the analysis of the mandibular deformity by measures of the medial axis results in a much clearer characterization of the underlying deformity than does the analysis of the same samples by a larger number of landmark-based shape measures. One particular ratio of medial-axis measures, RTP–Cor/Rad. STP, separates the normals from the pooled syndromals better than could an optimal linear combination of all the shape information available in the configuration of six conventional landmarks.

In hindsight it is easy to see why this should be so. The effect of the synostosis is to generate a relatively gracile mandibular ramus. But, in view of the difficulty in locating Coronoidale according to the Michigan definition, there are *no* conventional landmarks to support a point-to-point measurement of this width. The medial-axis analysis permits the substitution of a somewhat more visible alternative to Coronoidale, and includes, as well, an alternate measure of ramal width (Rad. RTP) making no reference to landmarks at all. Likewise, the measure Rad. STP of symphyseal width available from the medial axis seems more stable than the most straightforwardly corresponding landmark measure, the distance Menton–Infradentale, which proved the most significant in the landmark analysis. Its ratio to the distance Condylion–Menton lies along the line 26° to the left of vertical in Figure 3.5.1, the direction along which the groups most clearly separated in the tensor computations. The shape-coordinate finding is thus equivalent to the *minor* component Diam./Rad. STP of the expression (3.5.1).

The manner in which the ramus and the corpus articulate with one another – as assessed by the largest mensural structure that one can place upon the form, the triangle Condylion–Gonion–Menton – shows *no* effect of the synostosis: The mandibular deformity is entirely "above" that triangle, precisely in the region where conventional landmarks seem unobtainable. For instance, there seems to be no possibility of locating a homologous landmark in the upper curve of the alveolar ridge as it blends into the anterior border of the ramus; but *both* of the triple-point constructions sample aspects of this anterior-superior curve as it springs from Coronoidale or from Infradentale.

As I have argued before (Bookstein, 1978, 1988*a*), there is substantially more information available in the record of curving form than can be associated with the positions of discrete, recognizable landmarks alone. For two-dimensional data, such as we explored in Grayson et al. (1986) and have been exploring here, that additional information includes, at the least, tangent direction and outline curvature at each landmark. These involve two additional parameters at each point, the same number as are incorporated in the Cartesian coordinates of the landmark itself.

For three-dimensional data (Bookstein, 1980b; Bookstein and Cutting, 1988), the missing information is even more extensive; there are six parameters of normal direction and surface curvature at every point, in addition to the three Cartesian coordinates.

It is not surprising, then, that under certain circumstances the landmark-based characterization of processes affecting form might be expected to be weak. Such failures might be expected, for instance, in most landmark-poor regions of the human head – the mandible, but also the bony orbits, the wings of the sphenoid, and the forehead. The mensural parameters afforded by the medial-axis construction might often provide precisely the information unavailable from landmarks – "widths" of structures whose outlines, by their irritatingly gentle tapering, afford no place to "take hold" of a specific outline position. The medial axis offers two sorts of these homology-free landmark substitutes: triple points, such as those shown here, and endpoints, extrema of outline curvature, similar to our modified Coronoidale.

Together these two types of measures compensate for two of the greatest lapses of the landmark formalism. Had there been some anterior-superior mandibular landmarks, we might have been able to treat the curving information as modifying a landmark-based analysis. That possibility is not available in this instance, whereas in the sense of Blum's "transformation" theorem (1973) there can be no parameters of the curving outline that are *not* measurable upon the medial axis. In its diversity of features – radii, locations, angles at which lobes articulate – is a much-needed extension of the landmark technology.

3.5.4. Implications

4

Distance measures

For a data set comprising locations of homologous landmarks in a sample of forms, the simplest size variable is the distance between a pair of landmarks. This chapter considers, in addition to the discrete landmarks presented by the data, the **constructed landmarks**, arbitrarily weighted centroids of sets of landmarks, and the set of all distances measured between pairs of these. For shapes constrained to a sufficiently modest range, this set of distances behaves like a linear vector space. Of special interest is the size variable S that is the summed-squared distance between pairs of landmarks. S is a multiple of the spatial variance of the landmarks of a single form about their common centroid.

The construction of this space of distance measures is necessary mainly so that the next chapter can introduce a statistical structure for the collection of all their ratios. This chapter introduces one specific class of multivariate models that can be handled by linear combinations of distances alone, without the passage to ratios: the path modeling of lists of distances by multiple morphological explanations (factors), including General Size. These models, implemented via factor analysis and analysis of covariance, apply as well to size data that are not distances between homologous landmarks. We shall see how questions about ratios arise naturally by inspection of residuals from certain path models applying to data in the form of distances. Although rearrangement of the analyses of covariance suggests that explanations might proceed further in terms of shape measurements like these ratios, those extensions require that we exploit the geometry of landmark data more extensively than by studying only covariances of distances. The ground is thus prepared for the direct construction of shape variables without reference to size variables, the concern of Chapter 5.

Much of this material was first published in Bookstein (1986*a*).

4.1.1. Constructed distances

Suppose we have a data set of configurations of K landmarks $Z_1, \ldots, Z_K$. The simplest sort of size variable is the distance $|Z_i - Z_j|$ between two of these landmarks, as measured in each landmark configuration of the sample. In this chapter, the arithmetic is that of vectors. (In Chapter 5 the same symbols will be treated as complex numbers.)

Consider now a weighted average of landmark locations: a new point $\Sigma a_i Z_i$ for which all a_i are positive and $\Sigma a_i = 1$. Because, for vectors Z and rotation matrices A,

$$\Sigma a_i(Z_i + Z) = \Sigma a_i Z_i + \Sigma a_i Z = \Sigma a_i Z_i + Z,$$

and

$$\Sigma a_i(AZ_i) = A\Sigma a_i Z_i,$$

the quantity $\Sigma a_i Z_i$ moves precisely in accordance with similarity transformations (such as rigid motions) of the landmarks used to compute it, so that it may fairly be called a **constructed landmark**. (In fact, the invariance holds for any 2×2 matrix A: The linearity is an affine, not a Euclidean, property; but if A is not skew-symmetric with diagonals identical, it changes length ratios.) For instance, the midpoint of the segment between two landmarks Z_j and Z_k is $\Sigma a_i Z_i$, with $a_j = a_k = \frac{1}{2}$ and all other a_i equal to zero. The distance between two constructed landmarks, which will become our most general landmark-based measure of size, is $|\Sigma a_i Z_i - \Sigma b_i Z_i| = |\Sigma c_i Z_i|$, with $\Sigma c_i = \Sigma a_i - \Sigma b_i = 0$. For instance, the length of the median line from vertex Z_i to the point $(Z_j + Z_k)/2$ is $|Z_i - \frac{1}{2}Z_j - \frac{1}{2}Z_k|$, having coefficients c_i of $1, -\frac{1}{2}, -\frac{1}{2}$, totaling zero. That length is half of $|2Z_i - Z_j - Z_k|$ $= |(Z_k - Z_i) - (Z_j - Z_i)|$, the diagonal of the parallelogram with $Z_k - Z_i$ and $Z_j - Z_i$ as edges. That the coefficients of these forms total zero makes their values independent of the origin of coordinates; and independence of orientation is a property of the length operation $|\cdot|$ itself. If your algebra is rusty for this sort of thing, review tactics in Chapter I of Pedoe (1970).

Every size variable $|\Sigma c_i Z_i|$, $\Sigma c_i = 0$, is a multiple of an actual observable distance between two constructed landmarks. Renumber the landmarks into a run of the positive terms followed by a run of the negative terms:

$$\Sigma c_i Z_i = \Sigma_{c_i > 0}(c_i Z_i) - \Sigma_{c_i < 0}(-c_i Z_i).$$

4.1. The vector space

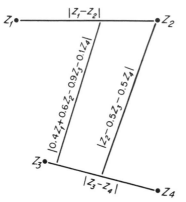

Figure 4.1.1. Some distance measures between constructed landmarks.

By rescaling, we can arrange that coefficients of each sum separately total 1. Then each term is a constructed landmark, the weighted average location of the landmarks in its run. Figure 4.1.1 shows several examples.

This class of size variables, though algebraically very tractable, includes a subset that proves to be of no morphometric use. The two components $\Sigma_{c_i > 0}(c_i Z_i)$ and $\Sigma_{c_i < 0}(-c_i Z_i)$ may have the same expected location in the plane specimen by specimen: For instance, they may be the midpoints of the two diagonals for four landmarks arranged approximately in a square. This circumstance leads to the vanishing of denominators that underlie certain approximations in the space of shape coordinates to be introduced in the next chapter. In practice, attention should be restricted to those size measures $|\Sigma c_i Z_i|$ for which the landmarks involved in the two partial sums have nonoverlapping convex hulls. In the case of the square, this class includes (but is not limited to) distances between constructed landmarks defined on opposite edges, but excludes those that are distances between points on different internal diagonals.

4.1.2. The interlandmark distances span the constructed distances

One might reasonably be interested in the behavior of many of these distances $|\Sigma c_i Z_i|$, $\Sigma c_i = 0$, among constructed landmarks; indeed, it would be useful to be able to talk about all of them at the same time. For studies of changes that are not too large, it will prove possible to be guaranteed of this by a consideration of the simple interlandmark distances only, as they span a vector space of their own linear combinations. These combinations appear, for the most part, strange analytic creatures like $5|AC| + 3|CD| - 2|EF|$ – an algebraic chaos of unrelated linear quantities. The truth is otherwise. *In the vicinity of a mean form*, the change in any distance between constructed landmarks can be considered to be some linear combination of changes in the interlandmark distances alone. In more technical language, the interlandmark distances form a **basis** for the set of (linearized) distances between constructed landmarks. This construction is by way of prologue to one in Chapter 5, where the space of *ratios* of these distance measures is shown likewise to have a straightforward statistical structure based on triangles.

The structure of a general proof of this proposition may be glimpsed in the detailed consideration of our running example: the median line of a triangle, the line from one vertex A to the midpoint $(B + C)/2$ of the side opposite. Let us show how small changes in its length can be expressed in terms of concomitant changes in only the sides of the triangle ABC. For small changes, we may as well work with the length of this line in terms of its square. In this section we shall use the notation $|A|^2$ for the squared length of a vector A, the dot product $A \cdot A$, and we shall frequently exploit the differential approximation

$$\Delta |A|^2 \sim 2|A|\Delta|A|.$$

A theorem about parallelograms sets us in the right direction. For parallelograms, the sum of the squares of the two diagonals equals the sum of the squares of the four sides. In the present notation, for a parallelogram with vertices at $(0,0)$, B, C, and $B + C$, the assertion is the identity

$$|B + C|^2 + |B - C|^2 = 2|B|^2 + 2|C|^2.$$

(The mixed terms $\pm 2B \cdot C$ cancel.) Now [with A at $(0,0)$] the median line of the triangle ABC is the vector $(B + C)/2$, and the side of the triangle to which it is erected is the vector $B - C$; hence, rearranging the identity, the squared length of the median line, $\frac{1}{4}|B + C|^2$, is $\frac{1}{2}(|B|^2 + |C|^2 - \frac{1}{2}|B - C|^2)$. Small changes in the median length are thus easily expressed in terms of small changes in the lengths $|B|$, $|C|$, and $|B - C|$ of the sides of the triangle by the differential approximation introduced earlier.

The generalization to K landmarks is easy. In considering the distance measure $|\Sigma c_i Z_i|$ we can always arrange for one of the coefficients c to equal -1, so that we measure distance from one landmark – call it landmark 1 – to a combination of all the others; and we can always assign Cartesian coordinates so that that landmark remains at location $(0,0)$. Then the squared distance in question is

$$|\Sigma c_i Z_i|^2 = \Sigma c_i^2 |Z_i|^2 + \Sigma\Sigma c_i c_j (Z_i \cdot Z_j)$$
$$= \Sigma c_i^2 |Z_i|^2 + \tfrac{1}{4}\Sigma\Sigma c_i c_j \big(|Z_i|^2 + |Z_j|^2 - |Z_i - Z_j|^2\big),$$

where all sums now run from 2 to K. Changes in the square of this length, and hence changes in the length itself, are thereby expressed as a linear combination of changes in the distances $|Z_i|$ of the other landmarks from landmark 1 and the distances $|Z_i - Z_j|$ of the other landmarks from each other. The coefficients of the combination combine the coefficients c_i of the formula with the means $|Z_i|$, $|Z_i - Z_j|$ of the interlandmark distances. This proof is valid in any number of Cartesian dimensions.

A sort of "converse" to this construction is *not* true. An arbitrary combination of interlandmark distances usually cannot be written as a single distance between constructed landmarks. The space of distances between constructed landmarks has dimension $K - 1$ only (the dimensionality of the coefficient vectors $\{c_i\}$ subject to the constraint of adding to zero). This is not enough to cover the $2K - 3$ independent geometric degrees of freedom of the landmark configuration ($2K$ coordinates, minus two for arbitrariness of the centroid and one more for arbitrary orientation). One might conjecture that for planar data *two* constructed distances are usually sufficient – indeed, there should be some redundancy there, as together they have one geometric degree of freedom too many. William D. K. Green has pointed out to me that for planar data, two constructed distances are sufficient precisely when the deformation dual to the diagram of forces specified by the system of arbitrarily many distances is not purely inhomogeneous (Section 7.3). In other words, the reduction to a pair of constructed distances can proceed if and only if the constraint specifying constancy of the given combination of arbitrarily many distances entails a nontrivial (linearized) constraint upon the affine subspace (Section 7.2) of the general shape change. This criterion is a function of the mean locations of the landmarks as well as of the list of constructed distances involved.

We have shown that the set of changes of interlandmark lengths spans the set of small changes in all homologously defined size measures $|\Sigma c_i Z_i|$ with $\Sigma c_i = 0$ – *all* the homologous distance measurements that might be made upon our configuration of landmarks. This will be our space of size variables: the linear parts of variation in distances between landmarks, and all of their linear combinations, some of which are sketched in Figure 4.1.1.

For configurations of more than three landmarks, this basis is redundant: It contains $K(K - 1)/2$ distance measures, whereas the set of configurations of K landmark points has only $2K - 3$ geometric degrees of freedom. The full set of distances is subject to a series of constraints that impose flatness upon all quadrilaterals of landmarks (in three dimensions, all pentahedra). This constraint itself is somewhat nonlinear, as is clear from Salmon's formula (1914:47)

$$\begin{vmatrix} 0 & 1 & 1 & 1 & 1 \\ 1 & 0 & d_{12}^2 & d_{13}^2 & d_{14}^2 \\ 1 & d_{12}^2 & 0 & d_{23}^2 & d_{24}^2 \\ 1 & d_{13}^2 & d_{23}^2 & 0 & d_{34}^2 \\ 1 & d_{14}^2 & d_{24}^2 & d_{34}^2 & 0 \end{vmatrix} = 288 \, V^2$$

for the volume of the tetrahedron having the six distances d_{ij} among four points for its edge lengths. Here we require $V = 0$. Of course, this formula, like all the others we borrow from analytic geometry, may itself be linearized.

It is not just explicitly measured distances that can be approximated in this space; equivalents of most familiar size measures may be located here as well. For instance, the area of a triangle of landmarks is spanned by this basis. By a formula from antiquity [high-school textbooks call it the formula of Heron, but Coolidge (1940:59) attributes it to Archimedes], the area of a triangle with edge lengths a, b, c is

$$A = [s(s - a)(s - b)(s - c)]^{1/2},$$

where $s = (a + b + c)/2$. Small changes ΔA of area may thereby be expanded as a sum of products of small changes $\Delta a, \Delta b, \Delta c$ by real coefficients $\partial A / \partial a$, and so forth, that may be treated as formulas in $\bar{a}, \bar{b}, \bar{c}$, the means of these distances in the sample under study; but $\Delta a, \Delta b, \Delta c$ are themselves basis elements of this size-variable space. The area of any polygon may be broken up into triangles and expressed using the interlandmark distances in the same way. A quite different approximation of area will be introduced in Section 5.5.1. Throughout the sequel I shall refer to variables as "statistically equivalent" if, regardless of mean values or higher-order terms, their differentials under small changes of shape can be expressed in the same ratios of the coefficients multiplying changes of interlandmark distances like Δa.

4.1.2.1. Cartesian coordinates are not homologous size variables. —

Cartesian coordinates locating one landmark in a system registered upon some other landmarks are not members of the size-variable space introduced here. One Cartesian coordinate of Z_3, for instance, might be the distance of Z_3 from the line connecting Z_1 and Z_3 (or from the line through Z_1 perpendicular to the segment $Z_1 Z_2$). Being the distance from a point to a line, the coordinate is properly the distance from Z_3 to the foot of the perpendicular from Z_3 dropped onto the line $Z_1 Z_2$. But the location of the foot of this perpendicular is not homologous from configuration to configuration in a sample – it will divide the segment between Z_1 and Z_2 in varying proportion. Thus the x-coordinate of Z_3 is not expressible as the distance between Z_3 and any constructed landmark $a_1 Z_1 + a_2 Z_2$; neither is the y-coordinate. That is, they are not members of the space of size variables. (This is good, as the next chapter will be mainly concerned with a space of approximations to *ratios* of size variables; Cartesian coordinates, which pass through zero, cannot serve as denominators of such ratios.)

4.1.3. Centroid Size

One particular linear combination of these size measures will be of considerable use to us later on. Consider the function S that is

4.1. The vector space

the sum of all $K(K-1)/2$ squared interlandmark distances of the configuration:

$$S(Z_1, \ldots, Z_K) = \Sigma\Sigma_{i<j}|Z_i - Z_j|^2.$$

(The letter S stands for "size.") By the usual approximation for change in squared distance, $(x + \varepsilon)^2 \sim x^2 + 2x\varepsilon$, S is certainly a member of our space of size variables – its changes are very nearly identical with changes in $\Sigma\Sigma\mu_{ij}|Z_i - Z_j|$ if each μ_{ij} is taken equal to twice the mean of $|Z_i - Z_j|$. S can thus be approximated as a weighted sum of the interlandmark distances (rather than their squares) in which each distance is weighted by its own mean value.

In addition, two other simple interpretations apply. Let us consider the formula for S with each distance taken twice, once "measured from one landmark," once "from the other." Recall from elementary algebra that the sum of squared distances between one number x and a collection of $K - 1$ others y_i is equal to $K - 1$ times the squared distance of x from the mean of the y's plus the sum of the squares of the y's around their own mean. [This is the formula $\Sigma_1^L(y_i - x)^2 = \Sigma_1^L(y_i - \bar{y})^2 + L(\bar{y} - x)^2$ for $L = K - 1$. You may recognize this as the formula for computing the variance beginning with the raw sum of squares; actually, its origin is in the classical mechanics of moments about centroids and other points.] This identity applies to each Cartesian coordinate of each landmark Z_i in relation to the same coordinate of all the other landmarks. As the distance of a point from itself, 0, may be freely added in, the contribution of any point to the sum that is $2S$ is thus proportional to the squared distance of that point from the centroid of all, together with a term for the variance of the points about that centroid. But in the assembly of S taken twice, there is one such squared distance from the centroid to each landmark. Applying the identity at a second level, we see that S reduces to one extended multiple of the mean squared distance of points from their centroid. Hence S is equivalent to a simpler size variable, the sum of squared distances of each landmark from their centroid case by case, as shown in Figure 4.1.2.

When we consider the landmark coordinates of a single case to form one sample of K bivariate observations, the principal axes of their variance-covariance ellipse, squared, add to the sum of variances of the x- and y-coordinates separately. This sum, by a simple rearrangement, is proportional to the sum of squares of the Euclidean distances of the landmarks as points distributed about their centroid, proportional to the sum of squares S we are already discussing. Hence the variable S, Centroid Size, is also equivalent to the mean square of the axes of the scatter ellipse for the set of landmark coordinates case by case.

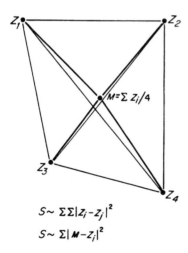

$$S \sim \Sigma\Sigma|Z_i - Z_j|^2$$
$$S \sim \Sigma|M - Z_i|^2$$

Figure 4.1.2. Centroid Size: the sum of all the squared interlandmark distances; equivalently (see text), the summed-squared distance of all the landmarks about their centroid case by case, or the sum of the variances of the two Cartesian coordinates for the landmarks of that case.

94

Centroid Size typically is not equivalent to any distance between constructed landmarks, but instead is irreducibly composite in terms of the basis reviewed in the preceding subsection. The linear combinations of landmarks of which it is the sum of the lengths may be taken as component scores on the two principal axes of the scatter ellipse case by case (or of any orthogonal rotation of these). If we want to represent S as a weighted sum of only a few interlandmark distances, rather than of all $K(K - 1)$, it is approximately a sum of two distances at 90° between weighted combinations of landmarks. One of these is the distance between a weighted sum of the landmarks to the left of the centroid and a weighted sum of the landmarks to the right, with weighting factors the mean displacements from the centroid, left or right, in the x-direction; the other of these is the distance between similarly weighted sums of landmarks above and below the centroid, with weights proportional to the displacements from the centroid in the y-direction. For a square of landmarks, for instance, S is statistically equivalent to the sum of the diagonals of the square, or the sum of the lengths of lines joining midpoints of opposite sides. The choice exemplifies the redundancy with which the combinations of two constructed distances redundantly span most combinations of more than two. We shall see other examples of this redundancy in Section 7.3.1.

4.1.4. A comment on the "truss"

An early attempt by the Michigan group at tying physical geometry to multivariate geometry was the *truss method* (Strauss and Bookstein, 1982; Bookstein et al., 1985). In that approach, a set of landmark locations was divided into neighborhoods of four points each, and each neighborhood was measured exhaustively by all six interpoint distances. The resulting assortment of segments was a reasonable list of features for studies of allometry as referred to a first-principal-component version of "size," and it also permitted estimation of landmark locations for diagramming (not for statistical analysis) by the classic technique of network relaxation.

But trusses are not appropriate substitutes for landmark locations in other multivariate morphometric maneuvers. For small size variation, the ordinary multivariate distance measure $\Sigma_i(X_i - Y_i)^2$ based on truss data is an oddly weighted approximation to the Procrustes distance $\Sigma_i|P_i - Q_i|^2$ relating the same set of forms. For larger size ranges, the conventional multivariate distance $\Sigma_i(X_i - Y_i)^2$ applied to the *logarithms* of the truss length measurements approximates a standardization of Procrustes distance to forms of varying scale. But this distance may be computed more expeditiously by the formula (5.6.1) making no reference at all to trusses. Except as a device for collection of data when landmark locations cannot be digitized (cf. Bookstein et al.,

1991), the truss analysis gains one nothing in a multivariate context, and it should be superseded by the scheme of Centroid Size and the shape coordinates. In particular, it makes no sense to apply it to data that are not landmarks, as the resulting distances are no longer homologous as scalars.

4.2. GENERAL SIZE AND SIZE ALLOMETRY

4.2.1. Size as an explanation

Over a period of growth of an organism, or over a sample having diverse weights or ages, the correlation coefficients among ostensibly distinct linear dimensions usually will be very high. Most such distances increase over time, and the covariance observed between pairs of such variables is due in large part to that joint "dependence." Only a small part of the covariance expresses functional regulation, morphological integration, shape differences between subgroups at constant size, or other specifically biological processes or constraints.

If that sort of functional explanation is one's goal, the best procedure might be thought to be removing the effects of time or size from each distance variable. If the data are sampled at fixed ages, for instance, this would be equivalent to centering the observed scores at each age. If residual variations about the age means are correlated, one might be tempted to infer biological "pattern." However, organisms sampled at constant chronological age will still vary in size, and, to that extent, residuals from age-corrected values will continue to show size-confounded correlations or covariances. Standardization by *any* variable explicitly measured, whether in units of days or grams or centimeters, confounds variation of that unit with covariation among the standardized quantities (Bookstein et al., 1985:114*n*). More seriously, any "size correction" (cf. Rohlf and Bookstein, 1987) destroys the possibility of detecting nonlinearities of size dependence, such as those in the example of Section 4.2.3, and makes more difficult the consideration of differences in the nature of size dependence between groups, which may be as important for biological explanation as is the description of the "size-free" effects that remain.

The notion of "size" here is somewhat "stylized" (that *mot juste* is Richard Reyment's). We have no guarantee that the data before us have a size range, that everything we may have cared to measure becomes larger with age, that all bivariate correlations are positive, and the like. Failure of any of these presumptions naturally invalidates the "explanation" implied by the analysis to follow. That is because such analyses, when numerically satisfactory, *represent* a certain form of explanation. That interpretation is much clearer for factors than for the principal components that often approximate them, and so the following discussion is set in factor terms.

When we have measured more than two variables we are faced with an entire matrix of covariances σ_{ij}. Supposing that they are all large and positive, it is tempting to explain the whole collection at once by "joint dependence on size," but now a bit of sophistication is needed. For instance, the covariances might not be all the same, or the correlations; those for one variable, or one block of variables, might tend to be higher than those for others.

Techniques of **factor analysis**, when applied in morphometrics, identify size by its explanatory property. They compute a **latent (unmeasured) variable** in relation to which the observed covariances are most plausibly or most completely explained. The operationalization of "most complete" by least-squares fitting to the covariance matrix was sketched in Section 2.3; here I show how it leads to biological explanations superior to those that are least squares in regard to the raw data. In these applications, the explanatory score, **General Size**, is constructed from the linear measures themselves, with no reference to any external standard of age, length, or mass. The factor model states that the regression of observed measurements (here, interlandmark distances) on this score is to be linear, with all prediction errors independent of one another. Inspection of the residuals from these regressions may indicate nonlinearities; scrutiny of the regression coefficients may indicate the spatial ordering of shape regulation; and study of the residual covariances may disclose additional systematic patterns of shape variation. In this section I shall exemplify only the first of these capabilities. Consideration of the second is delayed until the introduction of more powerful methods of reporting effects on shape. In the context of factor analysis, the third is elaborated in Section 4.2 of Bookstein et al. (1985), a presentation that it is unnecessary to duplicate. This book emphasizes a simpler case than the primary-secondary factor model, indeed, the simplest nontrivial case: "residual covariance" with a grouping variable that is explicitly measured. We shall see how a straightforward path model, very simple to estimate, keeps separate the two processes (size allometry and group mean shape difference) that can account jointly for differences between the forms typical of two groups. A conventional discriminatory analysis "separates" the groups more efficiently, but explicitly confounds these two distinct explanations, and so leads to no sort of understanding at all.

The Centroid Size introduced in the preceding section is the "opposite" of General Size in a sense to be clarified in Section 5.5. Under a certain model of error in the original landmark data, Centroid Size is *uncorrelated* with the entire space of shape variation: In the absence of allometry, it "explains" precisely nothing about shape. General Size, by contrast, is computed to

4.2.1. As explanation

97

explain as much as possible of shape variation, albeit under somewhat different circumstances.

4.2.2. Factors and covariances

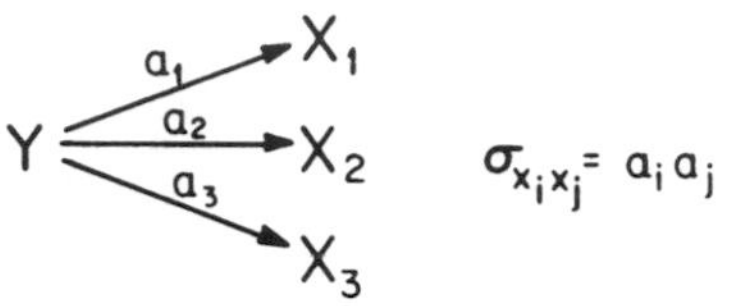

Figure 4.2.1. The single-factor model for three variables. This model has an exact solution.

Section 2.3 explained the grand strategy of least-squares fits to covariance matrices or their pieces, but supplied no details. In this section we review Wright's algorithm (1932, 1954, 1968) for the "best rank-1 fit" to a matrix of covariances, or, rather, to its off-diagonal part, and explain the meaning of the "factor score" corresponding to the formula that is computed.

A factor model is a list of related regressions (Figure 4.2.1). Suppose two variables X_i and X_j, of variances σ_i^2 and σ_j^2, manifest a covariance σ_{ij} that we wish to attribute to their joint regression upon a third variable, a *factor Y*. We mean by this to assert that for each subscript k,

$$X_k = a_k Y + e_k,$$

where each e_k is pure random noise uncorrelated with the other e's and with Y. To identify the scale of the a's, set the variance of the factor Y to 1.0.

Under these assumptions, the variance of each e_k is $\sigma_k^2 - a_k^2$, and the covariance of X_i and X_j ought to be $a_i a_j$ (Mulaik, 1972). If their covariance is observed to be something other than this product of the separate regression coefficients on a third variable, e_i and e_j must be correlated. If Y is the common cause of these variables, and we wish to remove its contribution to their covariance, then on this model we subtract $a_i a_j$. The residual covariance $\sigma_{ij} - a_i a_j$ measures the strength of functional constraint, size-free group differences, or the like. Note that this inference proceeds from residuals of *covariances*, not variables.

If there are three variables X_1, X_2, X_3 having sample variances $\sigma_1^2, \sigma_2^2, \sigma_3^2$ and covariances $\sigma_{12}, \sigma_{13}, \sigma_{23}$, the number of regression coefficients to be estimated (three: a_1, a_2, a_3) equals the number of covariances supplied, and the model

$$X_1 = a_1 Y + e_1, \qquad X_2 = a_2 Y + e_2, \qquad X_3 = a_3 Y + e_3$$

has a unique solution:

$$a_1 = \left(\sigma_{12}\sigma_{13}/\sigma_{23}\right)^{1/2}, \qquad a_2 = \left(\sigma_{21}\sigma_{23}/\sigma_{13}\right)^{1/2},$$

$$a_3 = \left(\sigma_{13}\sigma_{23}/\sigma_{12}\right)^{1/2}$$

because, by cancellation, $a_1 a_2 = \sigma_{12}$, $a_1 a_3 = \sigma_{13}$, and $a_2 a_3 = \sigma_{23}$.

The model fails (i.e., the error terms e_k must be correlated) if any of the a_k are greater than the corresponding σ_k or if just one of the observed σ_{ij} is negative. In the former case, some e_k would have negative variance; in the latter case, all the a_k would be imaginary.

98

On the factor model, each X_k is measured with noise e_k. Of the observed covariance of σ_k^2 between X_k and itself, only a_k^2 ($= a_i a_j$ for $i = j = k$) is due to the dependence of X_k on Size; the remainder is merely the covariance of the noise in X_k with itself. In the absence of a great many more measures like X_k, we cannot actually observe this noise term separately; but we can imagine being able to measure it less indirectly (by analysis of cloned replicates, left–right symmetry, and the like), and so we can imagine the explained part $\hat{X}_k$ of each variable X_k. For the example using three variables, the covariance matrix of the $\hat{X}_k$ is not

$$\begin{bmatrix} \sigma_1^2 & \sigma_{12} & \sigma_{13} \\ \sigma_{12} & \sigma_2^2 & \sigma_{23} \\ \sigma_{13} & \sigma_{23} & \sigma_3^2 \end{bmatrix}$$

but

$$\begin{bmatrix} a_1^2 & \sigma_{12} & \sigma_{13} \\ \sigma_{12} & a_2^2 & \sigma_{23} \\ \sigma_{13} & \sigma_{23} & a_3^2 \end{bmatrix},$$

wherein each diagonal term is diminished by the variance of its error term.

We can define Y, General Size, by formula:

$$Y = \frac{a_1 \hat{X}_1 + a_2 \hat{X}_2 + a_3 \hat{X}_3}{a_1^2 + a_2^2 + a_3^2}.$$

We cannot determine its value exactly, case by case, because the error components of the X_k, which we must subtract to arrive at the $\hat{X}_k$, are unknown (Mulaik, 1972:327). But it can be verified algebraically that this unmeasurable Y has variance 1 and has covariances a_1, a_2, a_3 with $\hat{X}_1, \hat{X}_2, \hat{X}_3$. This quantity therefore is General Size for three variables. We might estimate it by a multiple of $\Sigma a_i X_i$ having variance 1.

This formula is not quite the most precise possible estimate of the value of Y. Under the assumption that the single-factor model is true, one can "regress" the value of Y upon the X's by using the reconstructed covariance matrix in place of that given by the data. There results a predicted value of Y that is a differently weighted average of the X's:

$$Y \propto \Sigma a_i X_i / (\sigma_i^2 - a_i^2).$$

Each observed variable X is weighted inversely to the error variance of its prediction of Y. The formula takes this form because, by hypothesis, those prediction errors are independent.

Ignoring the denominator in applications of this formula is of no consequence when either (1) the denominators $\sigma_i^2 - a_i^2$ are nearly equal, as when the formula is applied to standardized variables with a relatively weak factor structure, or (2) the correlations among the X's are fairly high. This latter condition is almost always the case in applications to single-factor morphometric models, and the former almost always applies to standarized analyses of factors of residuals.

In the three-variable case, the products of the a_k exactly reproduce the off-diagonal σ_{ij} of the covariance matrix among the X_k. (There is no analogous set of a's for the two-variable case – their values are indeterminate, two parameters constrained by only a single equation. The consequences of this ambiguity will be noted in connection with a simulated example in Section 4.3.1.) For more than three variables, in general no set of a's will be satisfactory. We have n a_i with which to fit $n(n - 1)/2$ σ_{ij}, and we are therefore short $n(n - 3)/2$ parameters. The question naturally arises of **fitting** a reasonable set of a's to the covariances observed.

Various criteria have been suggested in the psychometric literature, such as maximum-likelihood estimation assuming a multivariate normal population, or minimization of the sum of squares of the residual covariances. All were designed for the case of explanation by more than one general factor. For the application to size allometry, which usually requires only one general factor, I recommend the simplest algorithm, Sewall Wright's **consistency criterion**, which is explained in Bookstein et al. (1985:sect. 4.2.3). The algorithm is presented there for fitting residual factors as well. For the particularly simple model here, the algorithm reduces to a least-squares rank-1 fit to the off-diagonal entries of the covariance matrix, one of the family of broadly similar computations reviewed in Section 2.3. That first factor may be computed iteratively by the following algorithm:

(1) Set a starting guess $\{a_i\}^{(0)} = \{1\,1\, \cdots\, 1\}$ for the pattern of factor loadings (regression coefficients) suiting a set of K distances.

(2) For any estimate $\{a\}^{(k-1)}$ of this vector of coefficients, construct each element of the next estimate $\{a\}^{(k)}$ by ordinary regression over columns of the covariance matrix (not cases of the data):

$$a_j^{(k)} = \sum_{i \neq j} \sigma_{ij} a_i^{(k-1)} / \sum_{i \neq j} \left(a_i^{(k-1)} \right)^2.$$

(3) Normalize the vector $\{a\}^{(k)}$ by scaling the variance of the factor estimate $\Sigma a_i \hat{X}_i / \Sigma a_i^2$ to 1 $[\Sigma\Sigma a_i a_j \sigma_{ij} + \Sigma a_i^4 = (\Sigma a_i^2)^2]$, and return to step (2) until convergence.

The formula in step (2) supplies the coefficient for the usual regression through zero of the jth column of the covariance matrix, diagonal omitted, upon the corresponding entries of $\{a\}^{(k-1)}$. Note that there is no reference to variable values in this computation. The explained sum of squares *of the* σ_{ij}, totaled over the K regressions (one per row or column of the covariance matrix), increases at each step; hence the algorithm must converge. In practice it does so very quickly.

For more on least-squares fits to parts of covariance matrices, see Section 2.3.2. In my view, these are the only algorithms worthy of application to covariance structure analysis in morphometrics. Factor models should be fit to biological data only when details of the modeling are of no consequence. One needs to be considering only a very small number of factors, having names known in advance and collectively explaining a very high fraction of the observed covariance structure. In practice, this means least-squares fits of low rank: simple explanations by one or two factors. Concepts of "likelihood," factor rotation, and other statistical paraphernalia are best ignored.

4.2.2.1. Transformation to the logarithm. —

Size data usually should be transformed to the logarithm before they are submitted to statistical analysis. This maneuver not only guarantees the connection with our methods of shape analysis, Chapters 5–7, but also is convenient in the treatment of multiple distance measures outside the coordinate representation. Whatever size S is to be, the dependence of each of our observed distances (or their transformations) on it will be that of the factor model, having the form

$$d_i = \mu_i + a_i S + e_i, \tag{4.2.1}$$

where d_i is the ith distance measure or transform, μ_i is a correction (possibly including group effects) for the mean of d_i (as discussed later), a_i is a positive "loading" or hypothetical regression coefficient, and e_i is an error term independent of S and all the other e's. In an analysis of a single group, the first principal component of log-transformed data almost fits the requirements of S in this model. (The only difficulty, a minor one, is that if S is taken exactly equal to the first principal component, the error terms e_i cannot be quite uncorrelated.) For a set of distance measures, the first component normally is characterized by consistently positive loadings corresponding to joint increases (or decreases) of all variables. Whenever growth is expressed as a joint upward trend of all variables, this component usually is interpreted as the "underlying" growth trend; in the current terminology, it is a factor for General Size. **Allometry** (change of shape with change in size) is indicated by unequal loadings (regression coefficients) of variables on this first component; biological interpretation of allometric data proceeds using both slopes and intercepts of the regressions. For instance, when slopes a_i are equal in two groups, or nearly equal, then the intercepts μ_i of the regressions, referred to pooled mean size, serve as "adjusted means" describing group-specific differences in shape.

On this model the log transform corresponds to a certain special null hypothesis, namely, **isometry**. In the case of growth without change in shape – strict Euclidean similarity – we would prefer that the coefficients a_i indicate equivalence of the responses by some numerical equivalence of their own. For such perfectly isometric data, if the dependent variable of equation (4.2.1) is the raw distance measure, then each distance will have a regression coefficient (on S or any other predictor) proportional to its own typical or mean value. We would like isometry to appear instead as a collection of coefficients that are equal; so we must correct each loading for that variable's own scale, by dividing out its mean.

This division results in a derived variable d_i/μ_i whose regression coefficient on S closely approximates the regression coefficient of $\log d_i$ upon this same predictor. [For $x_1 \sim \mu$, $x_2 \sim \mu$, we have $\log x_1 - \log x_2 \sim (x_1 - x_2)\,d(\log x)/dx|_\mu = (x_1 - x_2)/\mu$. This is the same formal maneuver involved in the derivation of the differential form of Huxley's model, $dy/y = k\,dx/x$. The allometric constant k of Huxley's equation $y = bx^k$ is the ratio of the two loadings a_y, a_x in the factor model.] The further transformation to correlations destroys this equivalence of loadings and regression slopes; hence morphometric factors should be extracted from the covariance matrix, not the correlation matrix, of log distances.

Other justifications of the log transformation and the use of covariances rather than correlations may be found in Bookstein et al. (1985:sect. 2.2.1). Factor analysis of the covariance matrix of log-transformed interlandmark distances is the only variety of factor analysis consistent with the statistical analysis of the space of shape coordinates to be introduced in Chapter 5. Changes in shape coordinates are always measured as fractions or percentages of starting length. Our main model of shape change, indeed, is a formal analogue to simple allometry. Each shape or size variable is represented by its regression coefficient upon the change when the change is interpreted as a deformation; these coefficients may be computed geometrically, without any consideration of variance or covariance. Those variables are emphasized for which the corresponding loadings are highest and lowest, or else precisely zero, out of the universe of all possible size and shape measures. When data come in the form of discrete landmark locations, these preferred variables can be explicitly constructed in the form of a finite list once the data are examined. In advance of the analysis, one need not have guessed at particular size and shape variables at all.

4.2.3. Example: rat calvarial growth

Section 3.4.1 introduced a data set of eight landmark locations in 21 growing male laboratory rats observed eight times between the ages of 7 and 150 days. These data (Appendix A.4.5), originally gathered by Henning Vilmann (Copenhagen) with extraordinary care, will serve as a useful running example for comparison of several morphometric techniques. For this first exploitation, we compute 28 distance measures – all there are among the eight landmarks supplied – and then subsequently ignore the origin of the data in landmark locations. A single-factor model fitted to the

Table 4.2.1. *Regressions of 28 log interlandmark distances on log centroid size S (21 rats, 8 ages)*

Log distance[a]	Size loading	Total sum of squares (SSQ)	Explained SSQ			Cubic Regression	
			Linear[b]	Quadratic	Cubic	R^2	Error SSQ
Basion–Opisthion	.0644	1.100	0.691	.145	.006	.765	.259
Basion–IPS	.1261	2.705	2.591	.017	.003	.965	.094
Basion–Lambda	.0891	1.412	1.297	.001	.005	.992	.111
Basion–Bregma	.1270	2.706	2.626	.020	.001	.978	.059
Basion–SES	.2234	8.206	8.099	.029	.009	.992	.069
Basion–ISS	.2314	8.865	8.701	.051	.002	.987	.111
Basion–SOS	.2172	7.910	7.678	.010	.011	.973	.211
Opisthion–IPS	.1824	5.942	5.414	.017	.006	.915	.504
Opisthion–Lambda	.1011	1.892	1.670	.025	.025	.909	.173
Opisthion–Bregma	.1228	2.517	2.463	.007	.003	.982	.045
Opisthion–SES	.1900	5.890	5.863	.001	.003	.996	.024
Opisthion–ISS	.1828	5.485	5.442	.000	.000	.992	.042
Opisthion–SOS	.1436	3.504	3.376	.037	.004	.975	.087
IPS–Lambda	.0804	1.751	1.081	.075	.143	.742	.451
IPS–Bregma	.1157	2.291	2.202	.000	.014	.967	.075
IPS–SES	.1818	5.421	5.388	.005	.000	.995	.028
IPS–ISS	.1721	4.906	4.842	.013	.002	.990	.049
IPS–SOS	.1461	3.603	3.495	.053	.002	.985	.053
Lambda–Bregma	.1192	2.578	2.346	.042	.000	.926	.190
Lambda–SES	.1622	4.378	4.302	.047	.001	.994	.028
Lambda–ISS	.1269	2.807	2.647	.098	.001	.978	.061
Lambda–SOS	.0857	1.418	1.208	.106	.000	.927	.103
Bregma–SES	.1325	2.982	2.873	.023	.000	.971	.086
Bregma–ISS	.0712	1.102	0.840	.056	.002	.886	.115
Bregma–SOS	.1025	1.788	1.715	.002	.000	.960	.071
SES–ISS	.2060	7.304	6.921	.002	.045	.954	.336
SES–SOS	.2281	8.615	8.451	.045	.010	.987	.110
ISS–SOS	.2470	10.323	9.948	.123	.000	.976	.252

[a]IPS, Interparietal suture; SES, Spheno-ethmoid synchondrosis; ISS, Intersphenoidal suture; SOS, Spheno-occipital synchondrosis.
[b]Entries in this column are proportional to squares of the linear slopes in Figure 4.2.2.

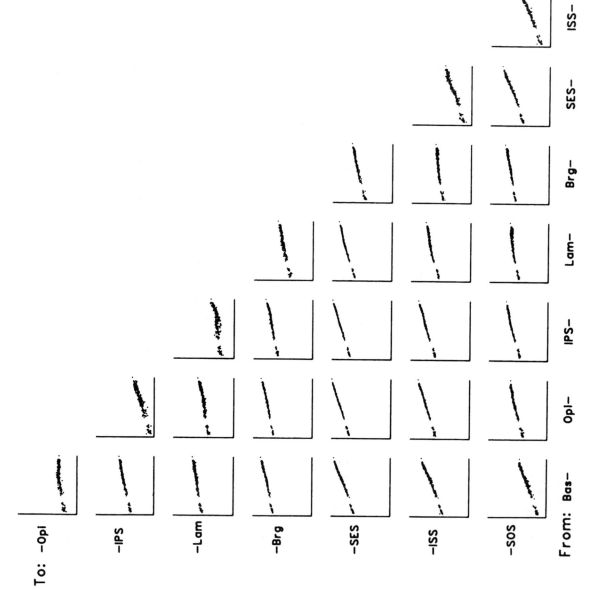

Figure 4.2.2. Scatters of 28 inter-landmark distances against Centroid Size. These are log distances. The slope of each regression is a relative growth rate. Rows, landmarks *to* which distances are measured; columns, landmarks *from* which distances are measured. Log S is the abscissa of all 28 scatters.

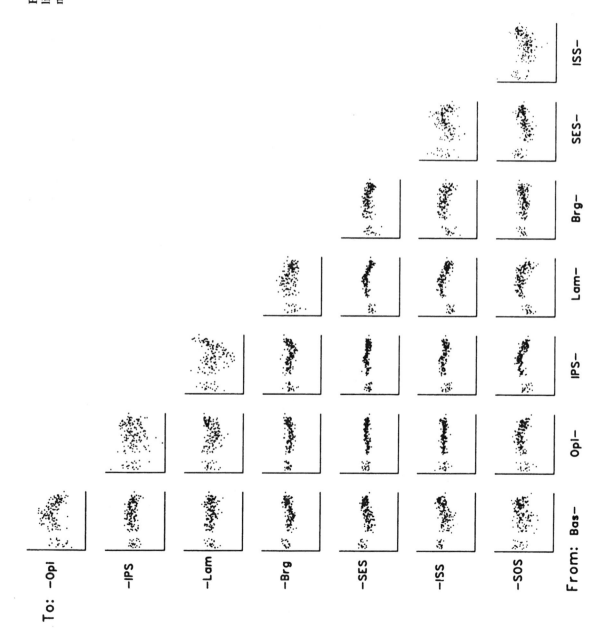

Figure 4.2.3. Residuals from log-linear allometry, 28 interlandmark distances.

105

covariance matrix of their logarithms has loadings as in Table 4.2.1; this factor accounts for 95.6% of the sum of variances (by comparison, the first principal component accounts for 95.8%). The correlation between the estimated first factor score and log S (Centroid Size) is 0.9997; clearly, Centroid Size is a satisfactory explanation of the covariances among the 28 log distances.

The model of size allometry corresponds to a particular structure of regressions of each variable against General Size. Figure 4.2.2 presents all 28 of these regressions in the form of scatters of log interlandmark distances (vertical) by log S (horizontal). The height of the scatter within its row on the page is the (log) mean length, the apparent slope of the scatter is the relative growth rate of that length, and the straightness of the scatter indicates constancy or inconstancy of that rate over growth from 7 days of age to 150 days. The 21 points at the left of each scatter represent the 7-day-old rats, which do not overlap in size with the 14-day-olds. Otherwise, the size ranges of successive waves of observation overlap. As the rats vary widely in calvarial size at the same age, the regressions are much tighter for prediction by size than by age (which would be the import of any analysis of variance of these same data using the wave of data collection as a discrete classifier). There is one unusually large animal at the last wave of observation, but his data lie close to all 28 regression lines.

The factor loadings a_i in Table 4.2.1 approximate the fitted linear slopes of each of these regressions. (If S were the first principal component of these distances, the coefficients would match the slopes exactly.) Note the considerable variety of slopes (from .0644, Basion–Opisthion, to .2470, ISS–SOS). These range over a factor of 3.83 in relative growth rate – a factor of $2^{3.83} \sim 14.3$ in doubling time. The regressions are, as a group, quite well behaved, but show a variety of deviations from linearity. For some distances, like Lambda–SES and Lambda–ISS, the deviation from linearity is mainly deterministic, absorbed in quadratic, cubic, and higher terms of a polynomial regression. For other distances, such as SES–ISS, the deviations seem mainly to be noise; for still others, such as ISS–SOS or Basion–Opisthion, there are quadratic or cubic effects *plus* noise. The largest error variances – that is, the fattest curves in Figure 4.2.2 – correspond to the shorter distances, mainly around the perimeter of this polygon of landmarks.

We can inspect these nonlinearities in greater detail by partialing out the dominant linear term from each allometric regression. In Figure 4.2.3 it is plain that different distance measures show patterns of residual variation that are variously curving or noisy. These residuals are no evidence for additional factors after the first. Instead, they indicate variations of developmental **timing** (Hopkins, 1966) in the growth of different regions of the calvarium in these rats. Some variables, such as Basion–Opisthion, grow fastest earlier; others, such as SOS–ISS, fastest later; still others, such as Lambda–IPS, grow quickly at both extremes of the age range but relatively slowly in the middle. These variations must average out, of course – any "net" nonlinearity would be absorbed in the estimate of S itself. I suppose one ought to standardize these variables for nonlinearity before computing any estimate of the underlying size factor; but for data so nearly linear as these, the additional delicacy makes no practical difference.

From the pattern of coefficients for length measures it is difficult to visualize the geometric origin of these nonlinearities; we shall return to a detailed consideration in Section 7.6.4.

The interpretation of these data as evidence for a single-factor model under conditions of slight nonlinearity is supported by the ordinary principal-component analysis. Figure 4.2.4 shows the scatters of the second and third components of the log distances against the first principal component, which is virtually identical with S and with the first factor score. These particular second and third components say nothing about rat skull growth. They are, rather, the second and third **Legendre polynomials**, the shapes that "automatically" represent two degrees of orthogonal polynomial deviations from the linear model. The group of seven-day-olds, whose disjunction ordinarily violates all the assumptions of component analysis, clearly fits the curving of models for the pool of older forms; otherwise, the data would require careful attention to atypical values (Reyment, 1990).

The extraction of multiple within-group factors takes a special form for landmark data. I have put off this discussion until the last section of my main text, Section 7.6, by which time we shall have tools for rendering the analysis quite independent of any a priori choice of distance or shape measures. The reader interested in further pursuing the factor analysis of distance measures unre-

4.2.3. Example

Figure 4.2.4. Scatters of the second and third principal components against the first (log S) for the same 28 log distances. These are merely the orthogonal polynomials of second and third degree.

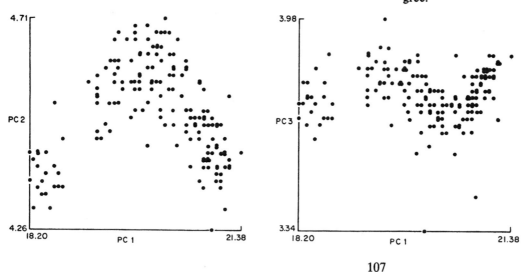

lated to landmark locations is directed to Section 4.2.3 of Bookstein et al. (1985), which explains the method I prefer, Sewall Wright's technique of primary and secondary size factors.

4.3. MODELS WITH TWO FACTORS: SIZE AND GROUP SHAPE

4.3.1. Path analysis versus discriminant analysis

We introduce the interpretation of group differences in size and shape by a simple simulation that highlights the contrast between discriminant-function coefficients and the quantities returned by path analysis in their stead. The simulation is as in Figure 4.3.1. We presume two variables, here called Length (L) and Width (W), and two groups, equal in number. The means of Length are 4 and 12 in these two groups; the mean Widths are 4 and 10. We presume a variance-covariance matrix of Length and Width *within* group as follows:

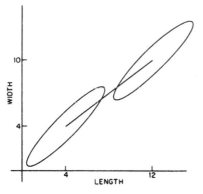

Figure 4.3.1. Simulation of two groups differing in both size and shape.

$$\Sigma_{within} = \begin{bmatrix} 13 & 12 \\ 12 & 13 \end{bmatrix}.$$

Then the correlation between L and W is $12/13 \sim 0.923$, the variance of $(L + W)$ is 50, and the variance of $(L - W)$ is 2. The within-group covariance ellipse has axes of lengths in the ratio $(50/2)^{1/2} = 5:1$, as drawn, at $\pm45°$ to the coordinate axes. For the pool of two groups we have

$$\Sigma_{total} = \Sigma_{within} + \begin{bmatrix} 4 \\ 3 \end{bmatrix}[4, 3] = \begin{bmatrix} 29 & 24 \\ 24 & 22 \end{bmatrix}.$$

(The vector [4, 3] is half the difference between the group means.) The pooled correlation between L and W is 0.950.

4.3.1.1. Path analysis of the group-difference problem. —

Often it is biologically sensible to interpret data like these as signifying the determination of form by two *factors*, Size and Group Shape, according to the path-decomposition principles of Sewall Wright (1954, 1968). Recall that in this class of models, all observed covariances represent the algebraic consequences of causal paths explicitly set down in a **path diagram**, here Figure 4.3.2, that represents the explanatory end to which the data analysis will be put. All the coefficients in the diagram – **path coefficients** – are regression coefficients relating one observed variable or postulated factor to another. In this example, as in that of the preceding section, the factor Size is declared to account for all the observable covariation between the two measures Length and Width *within* group. Additionally, another factor, identified as the

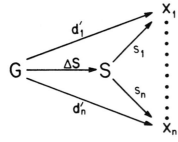

Figure 4.3.2. Path model for explanation of morphometric variables by differences in shape and size.

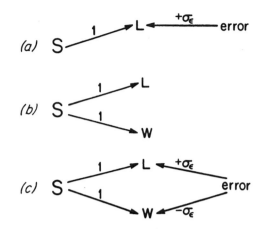

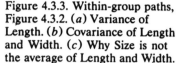

Figure 4.3.3. Within-group paths, Figure 4.3.2. (*a*) Variance of Length. (*b*) Covariance of Length and Width. (*c*) Why Size is not the average of Length and Width.

effect of Group alone, accounts for covariances *between* but not *within*. There are the same two classes of sites at which variance is injected into the model: true within-group variation of Size, and measurement errors in Length and Width separately. Write σ^2_{Size} for the variance of Size, and $\sigma^2_{\varepsilon L}$, $\sigma^2_{\varepsilon W}$ for the variances of the two measurement errors. Let Group be coded ± 1, so that its variance is 1.

According to the path diagram, there are no forms of influence of variables upon one another other than those mediated by these factors. One of these influences is of one factor upon another: The value of the Size factor is presumed to differ between groups, as indicated by the regression coefficient ΔS in the diagram. Group is presumed to have effects upon the mean values of the measured length variables independent of Size: This is what is meant by a factor for *group shape*. Finally, the measurement errors of Length and Width are assumed uncorrelated with each other and with Size.

The setup of the simulation, with mean differences and Σ both specified, provides enough information to identify almost all of the path coefficients in Figure 4.3.2. As in the preceding section, the variance of Length, which is declared to be 13, is accounted for by the sum of variances of its independent "causes," Size and error (Figure 4.3.3*a*): We have

$$13 = \text{var}_{\text{within}}(\text{Length}) = a^2\sigma^2_{\text{Size}} + \sigma^2_{\varepsilon L},$$

and also

$$13 = \text{var}_{\text{within}}(\text{Width}) = b^2\sigma^2_{\text{Size}} + \sigma^2_{\varepsilon W}.$$

The *covariance* of Length and Width is accounted for along the path joining them (Figure 4.3.3*b*) by products of path coefficients and variances:

$$12 = \text{cov}_{\text{within}}(\text{Length}, \text{Width}) = ab\sigma^2_{\text{Size}}.$$

109

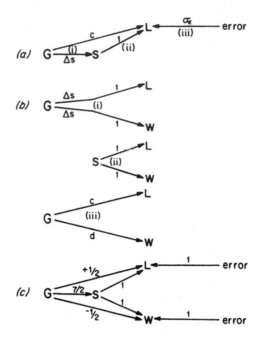

Figure 4.3.4. Between-group paths. (*a*) Variance of Length. (*b*) Covariance of Length and Width. (*c*) Completed path model.

In this simplistic setting, we cannot distinguish the values of a and b, or those of the two σ_ϵ^2, without further assumptions. For convenience, in the absence of any other information, such as correlations with other size measures, we take $a = b = 1$ and $\sigma_{\epsilon L}^2 = \sigma_{\epsilon W}^2$. It follows that $\sigma_{Size}^2 = 12$ and that $\sigma_\epsilon^2 = 1$. This latter quantity is the variance of Length and Width independently about values predicted by the joint size factor they share. If we had more than two observed size measures, their covariances would be sufficient to fix the ratio $a : b$ that we cannot identify here, as explained in Section 4.2.2.

The factor Size explaining cov(L, W) is not measured by the explicit formula (Length + Width)/2, although it is estimated by that average. The variable $(L + W)/2$ has a variance of 12.5 on our assumptions; that value is wrong. The prediction errors of Length and Width after regression upon $(L + W)/2$ are $(L - W)/2$ and $(W - L)/2$, which are perfectly negatively correlated. $(L + W)/2$ is instead the **first principal component** of this pair of variables. It plays the role of Size in the *different* path model shown in Figure 4.3.3*c*, a model that, for all its familiarity, is basically without biological meaning: It is freely rotatable, and there are no error terms. The formula $(L + W)/2$ differs from Size by the mean of two measurement errors. As each is of variance 1, the mean has a squared standard error of 0.5, and so the variance of the factor is 12 only.

We turn next to the effects of Group on Size and its indicators. The variance of Length *pooled over* groups, 29, is accounted for by the three terms corresponding to the three paths in Figure

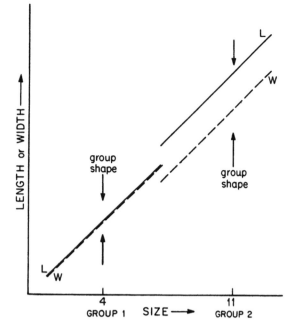

Figure 4.3.5. Summary of the relationships of the two postulated factors. The model in Figure 4.3.2 corresponds to the set of four regressions here ("size variable" on Size, separately by variable and by group). The groups differ by 7 units of Size and by 2 units of Shape ($L - W$) at constant Size.

4.3.4a. We have

$$29 = \text{var}_{\text{total}}(\text{Length}) = \underset{\text{(i)}}{(\Delta S + c)^2 \text{var}(\text{Group})} + \underset{\text{(ii)}}{\sigma_{\text{Size}}^2} + \underset{\text{(iii)}}{\sigma_\varepsilon^2}$$

$$= (\Delta S + c)^2 + 13.$$

Likewise,

$$22 = \text{var}_{\text{total}}(\text{Width}) = (\Delta S + d)^2 + 13.$$

The between-group covariance of Length and Width is accounted for by the three paths in Figure 4.3.4b: We have

$$24 = \text{cov}_{\text{total}}(\text{Length}, \text{Width})$$

$$= \underset{\text{(i)}}{\Delta S^2 \text{var}(\text{Group})} + \underset{\text{(ii)}}{\sigma_{\text{Size}}^2} + \underset{\text{(iii)}}{cd\,\text{var}(\text{Group})}$$

$$= \Delta S^2 + 12 + cd.$$

From these three equations in ΔS, c, and d there follow $\Delta S = 3.5$, $c = 0.5$, and $d = -0.5$. (To indicate the effect of a change in Group, each must be multiplied by 2, as Group was coded ± 1.) The fully identified path model is shown in Figure 4.3.4c. The groups are distinguished by a size difference of 7 units and a shape difference of 2 units at constant size, as shown in the form of the regressions underlying the model, Figure 4.3.5.

111

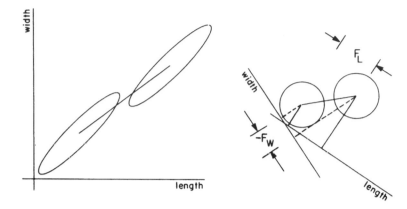

Figure 4.3.6. Origin of the discriminant-function coefficients.

4.3.1.2. Discriminant-function analysis. —

For this same simulation, the usual Fisherian discriminant function is proportional to $[8, 6]\Sigma_{\text{within}}^{-1}$, which is (up to a factor of the determinant of Σ) the vector of **discriminant-function coefficients** $[32, -18]$. This vector, as indicated in Figure 4.3.6, is derived by orthogonal projection of the vector of group mean differences onto the images of the Length and Width axes after the matrix Σ_{within} has been circularized.

By definition, this discriminant function satisfies the criterion of the largest ratio of between-group to within-group variance. The R^2 of the multiple regression of Group on Length and Width is 0.86, and the discriminant function is the predicted value from this multiple regression. The squared correlation of Group with pure Size, Length + Width, is only 0.80; with Width alone, 0.73; with Length alone, 0.83.

Yet however precise the discrimination between groups 1 and 2 by way of this discriminant function, its *coefficients* are without value for biological explanation. The underlying path model decomposed the vector $(\Delta L, \Delta W)$ of mean changes into the sum of two effects based on Group: the Size effect $(\Delta S, \Delta S)$ and the Group Shape effect $(0.5, -0.5)$. The discriminant analysis gives us only $(\Delta L, \Delta W)$, the difference of centroids with which we began (not much modeling there!), multiplied by the matrix Σ^{-1} rather than decomposed.

The source of this confounding is the optimization embedded in discriminant analysis (and also its generalization to many groups), which requires inversion of a correlation or covariance matrix. The path model for this step, Figure 4.3.7, is biological nonsense; L and W are not, after all, causally responsible for group assignment.

The difference between the path-analytic (Figure 4.3.2) and discriminant-analytic (Figure 4.3.7) approaches to the description of Figure 4.3.1 may be viewed as well in the geometry of that

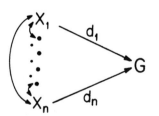

Figure 4.3.7. Path model for the discriminant function. These paths do not correspond to biologically meaningful processes.

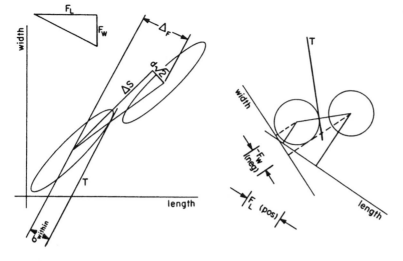

Figure 4.3.8. Comparison of two models upon the original diagram, Figure 4.3.1. The direction *T* represents a level line of the discriminant function. The path coefficients have been attached to the vectors they represent.

figure. The discriminant function (Figure 4.3.8, constant along lines parallel to *T*) is aligned with the normal to the within-group scatter ellipse at the point where it is pierced by the line connecting the group centroids. (Compare the construction in Figure 4.3.6.) The path coefficients are based on a model stating that the "width" of that ellipse is pure noise, as is some fraction of the length. The path analysis therefore relates the observed group differences to the long axis of the within-group ellipses only, together with a residual of Group Shape effect expressing the subsample means but making no reference to the within-group structure at all.

Paradoxically, even though discriminant analysis produces only a single linear combination, rather than the two factors of the path model, its difficulty is that it is assuming *too much* of the data, rather than too little. The discriminant analysis corresponds

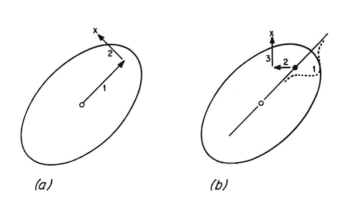

(a)   (b)

Figure 4.3.9. Comparison of within-group scores, discriminant-function and path models. (*a*) In the principal-component model underlying multiple regression, as in discriminant-function analysis, the location of any sample point is the sum of two effects, each a reliable score. (*b*) In the factor model, any data point is a sum of three perturbations about the mean, corresponding to the three ultimate variances in the path diagram. In this example, two of these are error variances, and only one is a meaningful case score.

113

to the two-dimensional interpretation of the *within-group* scatter shown in Figure 4.3.9*a*. Each point is interpreted as the resultant of two effects, both equally meaningful: a displacement from the mean by some number of units along component 1 (Size), and another displacement from the mean by a different number of units, along component 2 (Shape). The discriminant analysis normalizes *both* of these "dimensions," in the process irresponsibly inflating the representation of shape in the coefficients (as size is foreshortened 25-fold).

In the path model, on the other hand, we interpret only those aspects of covariance for which we have corresponding biological processes. Each point of the same scatter is now interpreted as the resultant of *three* components, Figure 4.3.9*b*: one value of true Size (incorporating a correlation with Group, i.e., a group difference), and two values of pure noise that do not support any interpretation. The approach through path analysis regresses out only factors identified in advance of the computations and supplies coefficients corresponding much more closely to the biological processes that determine form.

Discriminant-function analysis is not a morphometric technique, as morphometrics was defined in Chapter 1. Neither is the extension to multiple groups, **canonical-variates analysis**. They are based on no hypotheses about biological processes, whether or not expressible geometrically, and do not produce biometrically meaningful coefficients. This critique is reiterated and extended in Crespi and Bookstein (1989), in Rohlf and Bookstein (1987), and in Reyment et al. (1988). The technique is particularly unwise in the application to samples of forms associated with time series. The canonical variates extracted from analysis of temporal series of group forms tend to be dominated by "trends"; but these appear with unexpectedly high probability even under conditions of meaningless drift. See Appendix A.3.2.

The belief that discriminatory analysis is a form of explanation is a common illusion, one not restricted to the natural sciences. Discriminant-function coefficients pay no attention to the possible multiplicity of biological processes underlying an empirical group difference; the matrix manipulation optimizing "separation" is the wrong formula if one's purpose is understanding instead. Briefly, the solution to this conceptual difficulty by recourse to path analysis replaces the *multiple* regression underlying the discriminant function, a regression jointly linear on *all* of the predictors, by a series of *simple* regressions on only the factors known to underlie the group separation. In a typical example, these factors will include Size and one or more dimensions of Group Shape (e.g., taxon, sex, habitat, mortality). For a related technique that restricts one to regressions upon the space of the first few principal components, without necessarily identifying them as factors, see Campbell (1982).

114

4.3.2. Example: two strata of *Brizalina*

Section 3.4.3.1 explained the location of six landmarks for the creature *Brizalina*, a Miocene foraminiferan that Richard Reyment found in several strata along a core from Cameroun. I shall restrict the current discussion to two of the five strata listed in Appendix A.4.4 and to four of the landmarks from that set, those on the "axis" of the form and pertaining to the final chamber. This little data set quite clearly demonstrates the difference between discrimination and explanation. In subsequent chapters, once the shape coordinates are introduced, we shall reanalyze the same subset of these data more elegantly; the more sophisticated conclusions recapitulate those of the path analysis, not the discriminant-function analysis. See also Marcus (1990).

The various coefficients involved in these analyses have been assembled in Table 4.3.1. (The logarithm of the appropriate magnification case by case, as tabulated in Appendix A.4.4, has been subtracted from each log distance prior to all further computations.) It is plain that the specimens of the fourth stratum are larger than those of the second, on average, on all six of these distance measures. The differences for measures of the chamber, distances *A–C*, *A–D*, and *C–D*, are considerably larger than those for distances to *B*; it will be seen that the discriminant function says nothing other than this. Within groups, the correlations among these six variables are considerable. The first principal component "explains" 87% of the total within-group variance; the third through sixth components, a total of 3%.

The discriminant function for this pair of strata cannot be computed meaningfully using the full set of all six distances. The

Table 4.3.1. *Analysis of two strata of Brizalina by path analysis and discriminant analysis*

Log distance[a]	Mean		Discriminant function		Path analysis	
	Stratum 2	Stratum 4	Coefficient	Loading[b]	Size loading	Group Shape loading
A–B	3.444	3.826	−1.976	0.247	0.330	−0.240
A–C	2.539	3.262	2.857	0.657	0.372	0.371
A–D	2.063	2.689	—[c]	0.561	0.379	0.096
B–C	3.261	3.576	4.316	0.010	0.469	−0.245
B–D	3.548	3.927	−4.952	0.257	0.444	−0.226
C–D	2.288	3.009	0.541	0.708	0.437	0.199

[a]*A*, aperture; *B*, proloculus; *C*, proximal point of ultimate chamber; *D*, bulge point of ultimate chamber.

[b]Correlation of the discriminant function with each of the measured distances.

[c]The joint distribution of six distances among four points in a plane is nearly singular. The distance of short mean length was omitted from the list of predictors.

4.3. Size and group factors

distances on four points in a plane have only $2 \times 4 - 3 = 5$ geometric degrees of freedom; as we used all six, there results a nearly singular distribution the covariance matrix for which ought not to be inverted. I omitted the distance of smallest mean, that from aperture (A) to bulge point (D), and proceeded with the ordinary discriminant-function analysis. The coefficients seem quite meaningless. None of them are significant separately, owing to the considerable correlation among all these size measures, but the overall equivalent regression ($r = 0.768$) is significant at $p \sim$ .002. The canonical loadings (see the table), by contrast with the coefficients, are modestly interpretable: Those involving landmark B (proloculus) do not seem to count for much. The score that best separates the groups appears to be "expressing" only the log size measures that apply to the ultimate chamber itself: a measure of its (absolute) size. These loadings are nearly monotone with the mean differences on the strata variable by variable; of course, we needed no matrix manipulations to compute *those*. In fact, this particular discriminant function is more than half size: Its correlation with that covariate is about 0.78.

The path analysis I am suggesting as substitute for the more familiar discriminant-function analysis begins with computation of a factor for pooled within-group size. In view of the strength of the first principal component (PC), as mentioned earlier, we may adequately approximate it by the first PC score of the covariance (not the correlation) matrix. The loadings appear approximately equal, furthermore, in which case the PC score *is* the estimated factor score anyway. (This sample is too small to test for failure of isometry.) These factor loadings, although computed by a within-group analysis, are applied to reconstruct a measure of General Size that takes the group mean differences into account: the actual linear combination

$$\text{Size} = 0.330 \log|AB| + \ldots .$$

The correlation of this score with stratum (a binary indicator in this subsample) is 0.607.

Next, analyses of covariance, adjusting for size, are computed for each of the log distances. According to the usual tests, there are no differences in slope between the groups (not a surprising finding in samples this small), and so the adjusted mean differences can be taken as the vertical separations of parallel allometries, one per group, with coefficients depending on the dependent variable (the log distance). These adjusted mean differences, called Group Shape loadings in the table, are assembled in the last column. They could be tested collectively for the "significance" of any adjusted mean shape difference as a vector with five degrees of freedom (as the covariate is the weighted sum of all six); but this test is superseded by the T^2 for shape difference demonstrated in Section 5.4, and so will not be pursued here. The

116

adjusted mean differences have no more relation than the discriminant loadings to the coefficients for the linear discriminant function; for instance, the two largest discriminant-function coefficients correspond to the largest *and the smallest* path coefficients for the group shape factor.

If the log distances were combined into a *second* factor score using these adjusted mean differences as coefficients – $H = -0.240 \log|AB| + \ldots$ – then "prediction" might proceed by multiple regression upon the pair of factors, S and H, together. The separate correlations of H and S with stratum are 0.565 and 0.607, and the multiple correlation is 0.678, by comparison with the 0.768 achieved by the optimal discriminator. For this problem of the two strata of *Brizalina*, the cost of the path model is a decrease of some 13% ($.768^2 - .678^2$) in "variance explained." But it is covariance, not variance, that the morphometrician ought to be trying to explain; and the purpose of the analysis is to produce not the scores for H but its loadings, the numbers printed in the table. There has been a considerable increase (from zero, in fact) in the interpretability of the coefficients for the function that describes the group separation. Each number in the rightmost two columns of the table is a path coefficient having its own role to play in a scheme of linked regressions. The coefficients of one set – those of S – have biological meaning in terms of the allometric model; here they indicate nothing beyond isometry. The meaning of the other set, the loadings on Group Shape, is hinted at here in the fact that the two algebraically largest loadings, for the distances $A-C$ and $B-C$, refer to the same point with opposite signs. Interpretation of this coincidence within the context of the path analysis is the concern of the next subsection. In Chapter 6 we shall generate a most powerful way of expressing this same contrast by demonstrating a specific conventional shape variable with which it is correlated just about 1.0. In this way we shall show that the change refers quite explicitly and directly to one familiar parameter of these forms, the conical angle.

It may be helpful to review the steps in this example, the provenance of the quantities in Table 4.3.1 and their meaning or lack of meaning. The data comprise six strongly correlated log size measures for each of two groups of specimens. We suspect that the groups differ in some combination of size and group-specific shape, a combination the effects of which we wish to describe variable by variable. The coefficients of a conventional discriminant function could not possibly serve that role even if these particular variables did not have one eigenvalue vanishing almost exactly (owing to the restriction of the data to a plane) and another that is dangerously small. The discriminant-function loadings, whose total is distinctly positive, show salience for all distances except those to landmark B, proloculus. This pattern suggests the very misspecification that the path models are intended to correct: The group difference seems to have some

117

element of size to it, but also some residual shape aspects. It is better to estimate these separately from the outset. The first step in the path modeling is to estimate a within-group General Size factor. For these data, the familiar first-principal-component score appears quite adequate in that role. The path model expresses each log size measure as the sum of an allometric dependence on General Size (which is allowed a mean difference between groups) together with its own mean difference between groups adjusted for Size. These adjusted mean differences, as produced by the standard analyses of covariance, are equal and negative for all distances to B, while the value for the diameter $|AC|$ of the final chamber is especially large and positive. This exhausts the information available from covariances among the distances analyzed; to learn more, we shall have to inspect their means (i.e., the typical landmark configuration) as well.

Crespi and Bookstein (1989) present two more examples of this technique. Their applications involve a grouping variable that is an estimate (perhaps the noisiest possible) of relative fitness: survival of a stressful event. The data are from two great "natural experiments" on selection by storm kill, Lande and Arnold's pentatomid bugs and Bumpus's house sparrows. We argue that only the path model can lead to appropriate hints about the factor truly undergoing selection. For the bugs, this seems to be wing loading; for the female birds, general size; and for the male birds, relative wing size. In all these instances, the regression coefficients produced by a conventional discriminant-function analysis conflate selection on shape and selection on size in a single score. The discriminations are further sullied by near-collinearities among the predictors in both examples. But that "problem" expresses precisely the understanding of multiple dependences upon a single size factor that underlay the selection of variables to measure in the first place. I find it strange that so many applications of multivariate morphometrics would interpret the most frequent nontrivial finding, size allometry, as the "defect" of multicollinearity. Surely the problem lies in the modeling, rather than in the data.

4.3.3. Cross-ratios: from log size residuals to shape measures

Let us return to the details of the path modeling for *Brizalina* and now reinterpret these analyses of covariance in light of the fact that the underlying variables are all log distances. Each entry in the rightmost column of Table 4.3.1 may be thought of as a difference in expected values of one of the dependent variables $\log d_i$ at the pooled geometrical mean size. (Properly, "size" here is allometric, not geometric; but we can ignore this small difference in interpretation except for data of unusually striking allometry.) Then differences of these among the separate analyses of covariance tabulated here are expected values of *differences* of the

118

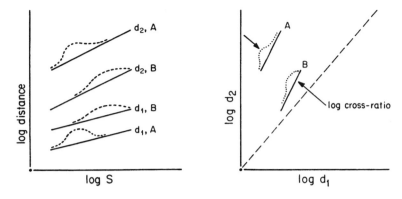

Figure 4.3.10. Interpretation of the contrast of two adjusted shape differences as the expected logarithm of a cross-ratio. Left: Two adjusted mean differences for log distances d_1, d_2 and groups A, B. The distances show allometries of different slope with respect to log size S. Right: The same in the $\log d_1$–$\log d_2$ plane, with log S suppressed. The log cross-ratio is the separation between these lines in the direction shown.

log d_i at that same geometric mean size. But the difference of log d_i and log d_j is $\log(d_i/d_j)$, the logarithm of a "shape variable." For instance, the difference between the adjusted mean differences 0.371 and -0.245 for the distances $|AC|$ and $|BC|$ in the table is the adjusted mean difference of $\log(|AC|/|BC|)$. The expected value of $|AC|/|BC|$ differs by a factor of $e^{0.371-(-0.245)}$ ~ 1.85 between the shapes typical of the groups at a pooled mean size. Every other difference of entries in that column of the table is likewise the adjusted mean difference of a log ratio of interlandmark distances, sides of a triangle or a quadrilateral, between the groups.

As Figure 4.3.10 shows, however, this expected value is now independent of the size used for "adjustment," as long as within-group allometric slopes are the same in the two groups. Because the value 1.85 is an expected ratio of ratios, $(d_{1P}/d_{1Q})/(d_{2P}/d_{2Q})$ being the same as $(d_{1P}/d_{2P})/(d_{1Q}/d_{2Q})$, I call it a **cross-ratio**. (The subscripts P and Q stand for the two strata involved, and 1 and 2 stand for the particular distances.) The log of the cross-ratio is the separation of the parallel lines (representing within-group allometry) in the 45° direction indicated in the figure. The choice of algebraically largest and smallest adjusted mean differences from the path model guarantees that this pair of lines manifests the greatest separation in the direction of their cross-ratio regardless of the slope of the lines separately (which is the ratio of their loadings on General Size). In the application to strata 2 and 4 of *Brizalina*, of the 15 possible ratios for six distances, $\log(|AC|/|BC|)$ has the largest mean difference between the strata – the largest log cross-ratio.

By scanning the rightmost column of Table 4.3.1 for its largest and smallest entries, then, we have in effect sampled 15 shape variables, the ratios of six distances in pairs, before selecting one as showing the largest mean log difference between the groups. This is much too arbitrary a procedure to be of reliable biometric use even in an exploratory fashion. (Compare the discussion of the same model with allometry suppressed, Section 6.4.3.) In entering into the path analysis, we gave no hint that the ratios of the original variables were of interest to us a priori as "aspects of shape." Furthermore, we have made no use of the fact that there are *landmarks* at the ends of the ruler responsible for the distance measurements. These distances are not the anonymous integrals explained in Section 3.1.1; for instance, the landmarks have typical locations as well as covariances. We need not have measured distances at all to get at shape: We could have approached the matter instead by considering angles, circumcircles, ratios of areas, or diverse other quantifications. For instance, noticing in Table 4.3.1 that all distances from landmark B have about the same adjusted mean difference between the strata, we might wish to aggregate them somehow before interpreting. Would measuring the distance from B to the centroid of A, C, and D make the contrast "more significant"? But the path analysis has no access to the algebra of combinations of distance measures, as reviewed in Section 4.1. What about all *those* variables? Surely some pair of *them* might have an expected cross-ratio even larger than 1.85? As it happens, in this example the answer is "No." Because the distances $|AC|$ and $|BC|$ are at nearly 90° in both forms, their ratio very nearly bears the actual extremum over the space of all shape measures (Section 6.3). But in general the extremum of the cross-ratio is not associated with a pair of simple interlandmark distances in so straightforward a fashion (see Section 6.4).

Then although the path analysis of Size and Group Shape leads to a tentative interpretation of adjusted group differences in terms of shape, we can go no further unless we consider more information than just the covariances. We are blocked unless we can make some further use of geometry. *The path analysis squeezes out as much explanation as can be had from a vector of size measures; if the size measures are interlandmark distances, then that analysis is not informed enough*. The path analysis "doesn't know" that the ratio $|AC|/|BC|$ having the extreme adjusted log mean difference involves the same landmark at the end of two different distances that are nearly perpendicular. If it is our aim to discover shape variables that best explain group differences – that not only show patterns of log cross-ratio between groups but also suggest biological processes explaining those patterns – it is inappropriate to restrict ourselves to the raw landmark distances, or their logarithms or their allometric residuals, as variables. In effect, this restricts the spectrum of our shape variables to the distance ratios alone, and we shall see, by theorem, that that restriction is most unfortunate in most practical cases.

The next chapter pursues this line of thinking to a considerable, and ultimately satisfactory, length. In effect, Figure 5.4.6 is one of the "correct" illustrations for the problem of discrimination posed in the preceding section. It will be shown that ratios of interlandmark distances are indeed a reasonable *basis* for a space of shape variables, and yet that the findings they support are not profitably pursued to understanding in their terms. To adumbrate the potential biological meaning of shape differences between groups, or any other explanatory factor covarying with form, it is necessary to reattach the covariances of the distances to the information about mean landmark locations. To test whether there is shape difference, we do not need this additional information; but to describe findings in any insightful way we must start over by another formalism. For this reason, Chapter 5 begins with a seemingly arbitrary quantification of shape as arising from standardization of a *geometric*, not an *allometric*, size variable (Bookstein, 1989*c*). Size in this sense is an operationalization of geometric scale rather than any sort of a priori explanation. This idea originated with Mosimann (1970), but the application to landmark data is so algebraically enriching as to justify the special notations required. The insights into allometry borne in the coefficients of the first principal component of a set of log distances – that is, in the coefficients of "allometric size" – will inhere in the covariances of geometric size with the space generated by the ratios of those same distances.

The distance ratios upon which we shall concentrate our attention involve not only the distances between landmarks in pairs; we must consider them in fairly free combinations. By doing so, it will be seen, we cover the statistics of all other possible homologous shape measures as well: angles, ratios of area, and the like. Only if we had surveyed the adjusted mean differences for all possible log size measures would it be appropriate to presume that the contrast of the largest with the smallest would represent an underlying cross-ratio that would be reasonably definitive of "the" effect under study. Even that extremum would be a fair description only in the application to triangles or to the "fuzzy triangle" representing the uniform component of a more complex transformation. Otherwise, to more complex configurations of landmarks correspond more complex descriptions. Chapter 5 is devoted to the geometrical equivalent of the rightmost column of Table 4.3.1 for this complete space of shape measures; Chapter 6, to the manner in which the geometry of the typical form combines with the information from covariances in interpreting findings for particularly simple cross-ratios. Chapter 7, finally, will combine information from the mean landmark configuration with information from their covariances into features of shape comparison in the general case.

4.4. A COMMENT ON "SHEARING"

In the preceding exposition, we constructed a General Size factor by within-group computations, and then regressed an estimate of it out of each observed variable in separate two-group univariate

4.4. "Shearing"

Figure 4.4.1. Path diagram of "size adjustment" for multiple groups in the absence of an a priori size measure (Rohlf and Bookstein, 1987:Fig. 3). *S*, within-group Size, having variance and also mean differences by group; *H*, Group Shape factors (of count one less than the number of groups) predicting Size and also shape at constant Size, without any within-group variance.

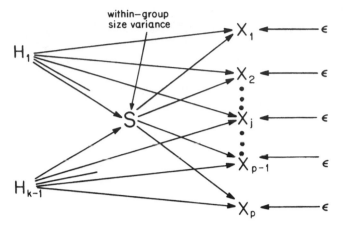

analyses of covariance. After this size adjustment, the remaining mean differences in morphometric variables were taken as elements in a vector of loadings for what was called a Group Shape factor. Contrasts among these loadings suggested biological hypotheses about mechanisms responsible for the group separation observed in nature.

When there are more than two groups, or when groups are not defined a priori, an alternative method is available (cf. Humphries et al., 1981; Bookstein et al., 1985:sect. 4.3; Rohlf and Bookstein, 1987) in which the ANCOVA step is omitted. The coefficients of Group Shape factors are not assembled by compilation of separate adjusted group mean differences; they are constructed, instead, by regressing within-group Size out of successive principal components of a pooled covariance matrix, and applying the same regression formula to the loadings (coefficients) of the components. The previously published explanations of this technique have been inconsistent (even though I am one of the authors of each); in this note it is my intention to set the technique to rest. Those who have not previously encountered this technique may skip the following remarks.

The multivariate maneuvers previously called "shearing," which differ in minor details, all attempt to construct interpretable patterns of coefficients; they are not intended, for instance, to generate any particularly interesting ordination of specimens. The nature of the explanation supplied is implied by the path model in Figure 4.4.1. Covariances among the observed morphometric characters are explained, within group, only by Size; between groups, by mean differences in Size and by other factors ostensibly constant within groups. Fitting such a model is problematic, and not merely owing to the usual choice between likelihood and least-squares methods. Rather, to make the explanation most useful, we wish Size to explain as much covariance as possible among the morphometric characters *within* group; but, also, we wish as much as possible of the observed group differences, exclusive of size, to be along variables relatively constant within groups. The computation needs to balance these two criteria.

There appears to be no straightforward way of fitting any such model in closed form. To "shear" (the metaphor arises from a certain transformation of scatter plots, as discussed later) is to partial within-group Size out of the between-group principal components. It is a compromise between the pair of competing optimizations just reviewed; it is most appropriate when within-group components of variability after the first are practically orthogonal to the first few dimensions of variability among the group means. Under such circumstances the kth pooled principal component may be considered to be a proxy for the $(k-1)$st Group Shape factor except for their joint confounding by within-group Size. The shear is based on identification of the span of pooled components 1 and k with the span of S and the $(k-1)$st Group Shape factor, whose loadings are thus reconstructed by regressing an estimate of S out of the kth principal-component score and its loadings. In the geometry of the scatter, the first versus the kth components, this change is a linear transformation; if the first principal component remains horizontal, the change is a shear with axis vertical. The net residual of the data from prediction by these pairs of components has certain optimal properties, deriving from those of the principal components with which they begin; but it does not follow that the associated allometric regressions have minimum residual – the effect of Group is not necessarily squeezed down to a constant. In other words, the factor score or scores associated with sheared principal components are of no particular utility, only the loadings.

The method of shearing may be considered one in a series of attempts (the first seems to have been that of Burnaby, 1966) to produce ordinations of forms "adjusted for size." It was typical in morphometrics of that period for a pair of vectors of variables to be aggregated into a measure of *multivariate* "distance," usually a sum of squared differences (possibly following upon univariate or multivariate normalization of covariances). The resulting matrix of "dissimilarities" would be passed to various manipulations of numerical taxonomy (Blackith, 1965; Sneath and Sokal, 1973). If size variation is "irrelevant" to those dissimilarites, one wants to measure "distance" in a space orthogonal to Size. The pursuit of such a "corrected" "distance," by shearing or any other method, is doomed for a different reason than that reviewed in the contrast of discriminant analysis and path analysis just concluded. In the application to numerical taxonomy, the intent of the dissimilarity scores is to serve as surrogate for evolutionary time. For realistic models of evolutionary change, the coefficient of variation of such aggregate measures is quite enormous *irrespective of sample size* – it is a matter of the sampling of *variables*, and the relevant standard error of the mean is approximately $.40/\sqrt{K}$, where K is the count of morphometric indicators.

4.4. "Shearing"

To restrict the "distance" measurement to a space of shape variation alone is to reduce this count K by *only one*. To the extent that the measure of Size thus suppressed was a factor for all the components of "distance," the effect of shearing is to replace a χ^2 on one degree of freedom by a χ^2 on $K - 1$ degrees of freedom. Selection effects owing to the perceptual psychology of the taxonomist can inflate these variances further. For data sets of any realistic richness, whether measuring size or shape, this irreducible error in the measurement of similarities intervenes to block any inferences beyond the trivial. Felsenstein (1985) argues similarly for the dominance of character-sampling noise under a quite different construction of "distance." As the argument supporting these assertions is slightly oblique to the main theme of this volume, it is relegated to Appendix A.3.

5
Shape coordinates

The preceding chapter reviewed the statistical space of size measures appropriate to a data set of landmark locations. For modest sample ranges, the variability of a rich collection of alternative measurements – the distances between any pair of weighted averages of landmark locations, and all of their linear combinations – could be expressed by variations in a much simpler set of size measures, the distance between landmarks in pairs. But shape differences could be represented only very clumsily in such a system, by linear combinations of size variables emerging from path models explicitly incorporating a factor of log General Size. For data that are landmark configurations, there is a better approach to shape variation, still beginning with the space of distance measures, but working with ratios of distance measures instead of linear combinations. For triangles, we shall introduce specific pairs of variables, the shape coordinates, that span all the distance ratios, in fact, all the measurements of triangular shape that maintain the distinctions among the three vertices. (These coordinates have already been demonstrated in Chapter 1.) We shall postulate a simple and realistic null model for variation of these shape coordinates, the consequence of an assumption of unstructured noise in the locations of the landmarks separately. On this model, there is one single size variable that ought to underlie studies of allometry; it replaces the data-based first principal component used in the preceding section. The formalism of shape coordinates permits the computation of mean shapes for configurations of any number of landmarks and permits the testing of these configurations for group differences, correlations with exogenous covariates, size allometry, and the like, all in an unambiguous fashion, using familiar multivariate statistical methods. Reporting findings of this sort will be the concern of the following two chapters.

By a **shape variable** we mean any measurement of the configuration of landmarks that does not change when your ruler stretches

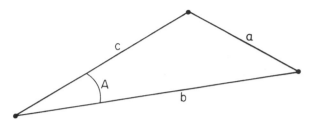

Figure 5.1.1. Angle as a nonlinear
transformation of length ratios.

or shrinks – that does not change its value when all lengths are multiplied by a scale factor *s*.

The best formal characterization of shape variables derived from size variables is one implied in Mosimann (1970, 1975). If $\mathbf{X}$ is any list of size variables $X_1, \ldots, X_k$, and $g(\mathbf{X})$ is any numerical (scalar) function of $\mathbf{X}$ such that $g(\alpha\mathbf{X}) = \alpha g(\mathbf{X})$, then a shape variable is any of the ratios $\mathbf{X}/g(\mathbf{X})$, or their linear combinations. Here $g(\mathbf{X})$, which has dimension one in physical scale, is called the size variable underlying the shape vector $\mathbf{X}/g(\mathbf{X})$: For instance, $g(\mathbf{X})$ might be ΣX_i, or $\sqrt{\Sigma X_i^2}$, or X_1, or something odder. Mosimann's papers deal with relationships of shape and size under changes of the choice of *g*. His interpretation is broad enough to apply to most studies of biological size and shape, whether based on landmarks or on outlines, and in fact extends quite a bit further; we shall not need the extensions here, but only the application in which $\mathbf{X}$ represents the vector of all distances between landmarks in pairs, as scrutinized in Section 4.1.

This definition is perfectly consistent with the less statistical characterization of geometrical shape as "the properties of a figure that are not changed by translation, rotation, or rescaling" (Bookstein, 1978:chap. 2). We shall take up this latter characterization in Section 5.6. Until then, it is natural to restrict one's attention to shape measures that derive from notions of size measurement – indeed, for landmark data this is just about all one can do – and it does not matter for statistical analysis whether we subject the ratios to additional transformations as long as the transforms are invertible in the vicinity of the mean form. (For instance, measuring an angle by its sine is useful unless the angle averages nearly 90°.)

Angles, in particular, may be considered nonlinear transforms of their own trigonometric functions (sine, cosine, etc.), which are, in turn, ratios of quadratic forms in measured lengths. For instance (Figure 5.1.1), according to the law of cosines, $a^2 = b^2 + c^2 - 2ab \cos A$. Then $\cos A = (b^2 + c^2 - a^2)/2bc$, a ratio of quadratic forms in the sides of the triangle. (The angle *A* is just the "arc-cosine" of this fraction – think of it as an arbitrary, and statistically rather inconvenient, nonlinear transformation.) Hence (recall Section 4.1) under conditions of modest variation its statistics will reduce to linear combinations of changes in the interlandmark distances. For this cosine, for instance, using the usual

$$\left[2bc\Delta(b^2 + c^2 - a^2) - (b^2 + c^2 - a^2)\Delta(2bc)\right]/4b^2c^2$$

$$= \left[2bc(2b\Delta b + 2c\Delta c - 2a\Delta a)\right.$$

$$\left. - 2(b^2 + c^2 - a^2)(b\Delta c + c\Delta b)\right]/4b^2c^2$$

$$= \left[2c\Delta b(b^2 - c^2 + a^2)\right.$$

$$\left. + 2b\Delta c(c^2 - b^2 + a^2) - 4abc\Delta a\right]/4b^2c^2.$$

There is nothing especially interesting about this expression except that if we plug in a change of size by a factor $(1 + \lambda)$, without change of shape – $\Delta a = \lambda a$, $\Delta b = \lambda b$, $\Delta c = \lambda c$ – we find that $\Delta \cos A$ is identically zero: The monomials b^3c, c^3b, a^2bc all cancel. (The "effect" of a size change must be zero by definition of shape variables. The algebra is a special case of Euler's theorem for homogeneous functions: Widder, 1961:20.) We would thus seem to be back nearly where we were at the end of the last chapter, examining columns of coefficients relating size and shape measures (there, one size variable and multiple shape residuals; here, one shape variable and multiple size measures) and an algebraic constraint expressing a crucial definition, either of size or of shape. We could talk about the algebra of any combination of changes in measured lengths whose coefficients total zero, and about the statistics of those combinations; but it is far from obvious how to explore those combinations systematically (because there is already one set of arbitrary coefficients in the definition of the size variables $|\Sigma c_i Z_i|$). Set forth in this abstract way, the collection of ratios of size variables cannot easily be assigned any particular statistical organization. Such a structure is assigned in three steps beginning from a different starting point.

We begin not with the ratio representation $\mathbf{X}/g(\mathbf{X})$ of shape but with the shape of a single triangle expressed in a way that does not look much like a set of distance ratios at all. By definition, our space of shape measurements is independent of the scale of the landmark configuration under study. You probably imagined this freedom as corresponding to an *object* changing its scale, but as Mosimann's approach implies, it is more useful to hold the object fixed and think of measuring it with a *ruler* changing its scale. We are free to presume that each case of the data set is measured with a different ruler. Each ruler is calibrated so that one particular size measure, which is ours freely to choose arbitrarily, has been set constant. As long as our biometric reportage is protected from consequences of the arbitrariness of that choice, the study of shape variation is equivalent to the study of the variation of the observed landmark data after that constraint has been imposed. In the first step, we impose a constraint of just this sort to represent each triangular shape by a pair of standardized Cartesian coordinates, the **shape coordinates** of the triangle. In the second step, we prove that the statistical properties of this representation are essentially independent of the arbitrary choice of size measures underlying the construction. In the third step, we prove that recourse to these shape-coordinate pairs makes it unnecessary to consider any other shape variables. To any baseline, the shape-coordinate pair encodes sufficient information to span the statistical space of all ratios of distances among constructed landmarks (Section 4.1). In accordance with the preceding discussion, that space will then automatically also incorporate the statistics of angles, altitude ratios, ratios of circumcircle to incircle radius, and the like. In Section 5.2 the sufficiency will be shown true of more extensive landmark sets than triangles. We can get at the statistics of all homologous shape measurements, whatever the count of landmarks, via shape coordinates of triangles.

Much of the material in Sections 1 through 5 of this chapter was published previously (Bookstein, 1986a).

5.1. FOR A SINGLE TRIANGLE OF LANDMARKS

Consider the simplest morphometric data structure, a **triangle** of landmarks *A*, *B*, and *C*. This section shows how to construct a picture of all possible measurements of that triangle that are distinguishable, no matter how small the variability of its shape. That picture will look just like a circle of directions through any vertex of the triangle, a vertex that the biologist is free to imagine as "moving" while the other two are treated as "fixed" up to change of scale. If we can carry out statistical analyses in a way that is sensitive to changes in any direction out of this circle of directions, and that detects changes in any of those directions with equal efficiency, then there is no need to specify any particular set of shape variables (set of directions) at all. We shall be particularly interested in pairs of shape variables that correspond to perpendicular diameters of this circle. They will prove to be uncorrelated under a certain model of independent variation in landmark locations separately. We shall see that changes of shape that hold one of such a perpendicular pair constant, on the average, can be best described by the other of that perpendicular set of variables. The shape-coordinate pairs themselves are perpendicular in this sense. Many other pairs of familiar variables are likewise paired in this way; they can all be thought of as shape-coordinate pairs to some other, usually less familiar, baseline.

5.1.1. The two-point registration

As was just explained, for purposes of shape measurement, we are free to standardize the scale of a landmark configuration in any

128

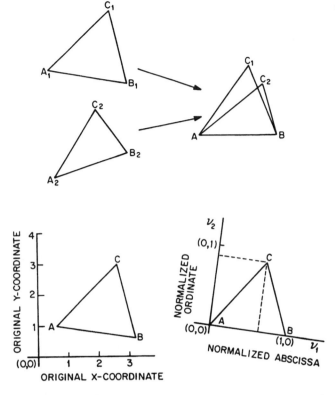

Figure 5.1.2. Shape coordinates as the output of a custom digitizer for triangles. When triangles are scaled so that the separation between one pair of landmarks is constant, then the triangle may be considered to have been set down with both of those landmarks fixed in position. Information about the shape of the original triangle devolves wholly upon the position of the third landmark. Its Cartesian coordinates are called the **shape coordinates** of the triangle to the **baseline** of the two landmarks whose locations were arbitrarily fixed in this way.

way. Let us slyly choose as our size measure for this (arbitrary) standardization the distance between one particular pair of landmarks A and B in every form of a data set of triangles. After this standardization, A and B are at a constant separation – call it 1 unit. We can then imagine that our forms were set down for digitizing so that A and B were always at the same exact locations: point A at the location $(0, 0)$ of a Cartesian digitizing tablet, and point B at the point $(1, 0)$, 1 unit to the right along the x-axis.

When two landmarks of the original triangle are restricted in this way, the information about the shape of the original triangle must be encoded in the only aspect of the data that remains free to vary: the location of the third landmark. The Cartesian coordinates of that landmark, when the other pair are both fixed, are called **shape coordinates** of the original triangle. More precisely, the coordinates shown in Figure 5.1.2 are called "the shape coordinates of landmark C to the $A - B$ baseline." Other choices of baseline lead to other values of the shape coordinates; we shall see that they lie in very simple relationship to each other.

Those of you who know complex analysis will recognize the shape-coordinate construction as the representation of the triangular shape by the the quantity $(C - A)/(B - A)$. In this formula the landmarks A, B, and C are treated as numbers in the complex plane, quantities $(x + yi)$, where i is the square root of -1. The formula is complex-linear in C and sends the complex number A to $(A - A)/(B - A) = 0$ and the complex number B to $(B - A)/(B - A) = 1$. For the rest of you, if A was digitized at coordinates (x_A, y_A), B at (x_B, y_B), and C at (x_C, y_C), then after a standardization moving A to $(0, 0)$ and B to $(1, 0)$, point C is necessarily assigned the coordinates

$$\nu_1 = \frac{(x_B - x_A)(x_C - x_A) + (y_B - y_A)(y_C - y_A)}{(x_B - x_A)^2 + (y_B - y_A)^2},$$

$$\nu_2 = \frac{(x_B - x_A)(y_C - y_A) - (y_B - y_A)(x_C - x_A)}{(x_B - x_A)^2 + (y_B - y_A)^2}. \tag{5.1.1}$$

In this manner the shape coordinates (ν_1, ν_2) may be computed by any conventional statistical package, whether or not it comprehends Cartesian coordinates or complex numbers. (Note to typists: Take care that the second product is indeed *added* in the numerator of ν_1, but *subtracted* in the numerator of ν_2.)

5.1.2. A change of baseline rotates and rescales shape scatters

The construction thus far explicitly selects two landmarks to use for the baseline. What is the effect on the observed shape-coordinate pair (ν_1, ν_2) of changing the pair selected to be fixed in this way? In one aspect, absolute location, the change may be quite large. Figure 5.1.3 shows three sets of shape coordinates for the same scalene triangle: The coordinate of A to baseline BC, the coordinates of B to baseline AC, and the coordinates of C to baseline AB are all different. There are likewise three other sets of shape coordinates corresponding to the same baselines taken with reversed sense. These shape coordinates – A to baseline CB, B to baseline CA, and C to baseline BA – correspond to a rotation of the first group by 180° around the point $(0.5, 0)$, the center of the baseline. This midpoint will be encountered again in connection with size-shape covariances, the subject of Section 5.5.

For purposes of statistical analysis, however, we do not deal with the absolute positions of triangles in shape-coordinate space; our concern is rather with modest variations of shape about a typical, expected, or mean position in that space. Under those conditions, alternate sets of shape coordinates lie in a most convenient relationship to one another:

Scatters of different sets of shape coordinates for the same triangle of landmarks differ from each other mainly by translation, rotation, and rescaling.

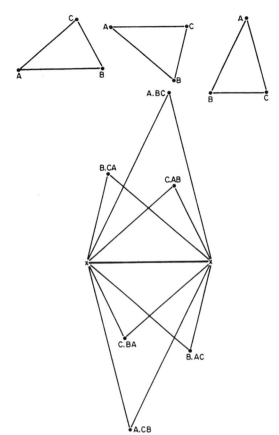

Figure 5.1.3. Six sets of shape coordinates: the same triangle *ABC* to six different baselines. Notation: *A.BC*, shape coordinates of point *A* to a baseline from *B* to *C*, and similarly the others.

I cannot find a simple proof of this assertion that does not involve **complex analysis**, the calculus of complex numbers. In that notation the proof is nearly trivial. If the two sets of shape coordinates are $(C - A)/(B - A)$ and $(A - C)/(B - C)$, for instance, the second is an analytic function of the first: We have

$$\frac{A - C}{B - C} = f\left(\frac{C - A}{B - A}\right),$$

with $f(z) = z/(z - 1)$. Other analytic functions, all derived from the permutation group of the projective cross-ratio (Schwerdtfeger, 1962), correspond to other permutations of the landmarks in the formula. But analytic functions are *conformal* mappings – their derivatives are similarity maps in the small. The effect of an analytic function is mainly to translate, rotate, and rescale small regions of the complex plane. Hence the effect of changing one's choice of baseline in the formulation of shape coordinates is principally to translate, rotate, and rescale their ordinary statistical scatter. This leaves unaffected any multivariate statistical analysis of the pair of coordinates as it relates to other aspects of a biometric design. Here the word "multivariate" refers

131

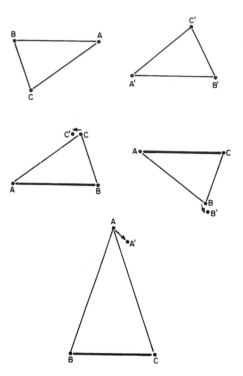

Figure 5.1.4. Three pictures of the same shape difference: two triangles superimposed to each of three baselines. Sections 5.3.1 and 6.3.4 deal with the geometrical invariants linking these three separate pictures.

to two variables, the two dimensions of the shape-coordinate scatter.

This demonstration may be extended to show that the replacement of the *AB* baseline by a baseline through any pair of computed landmarks – say from *A* to the point one-third of the way from *B* to *C* – is likewise a mere similarity transform of the resulting scatter of shape coordinates.

5.1.2.1. How much rotation and rescaling? —

We have $d[z/(z-1)]/dz = -1/(z-1)^2$. To the baseline *AB*, the quantity $(z-1)$ is the side *CB* of the triangle after the two-point registration. Hence (according to the interpretation of complex multiplication as a rotation and rescaling) change of baseline rescales the shape-coordinate scatter, to first order, by the inverse square of the ratio of change in baseline length, and rotates it by twice the reflection of the angle between the old and the new baselines. This latter aspect of the change, the angle doubling, will be encountered again in Section 6.2.

Figure 5.1.4 shows this description for one particular pair of triangles, and Figures 5.1.5 and 5.1.6 show example of this very convenient invariance for real data manifesting two different extents of shape variability. The error of the approximation here – the extent to which the effect of change of baseline is nonlinear – is determined by the largest "diameter" of the scatter

132

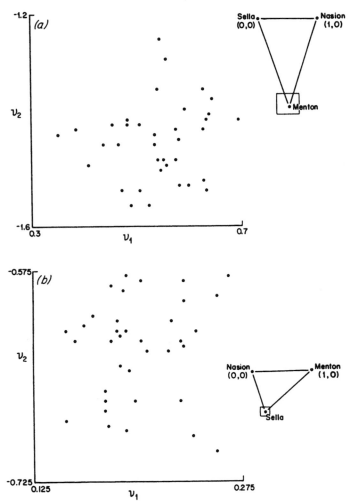

Figure 5.1.5. Scatter of pairs of shape coordinates for the triangle Sella–Nasion–Menton to two different baselines. (*a*) Menton to baseline Sella–Nasion: boy standing normally. (*b*) Sella to baseline Nasion–Menton: boy face-up. The data are the 36 age-8 forms (pinheads) of the boys in the cranial-growth example (Section 6.5.1).

as measured quite peculiarly, using a protractor scaled to the log tangent of the half-angle, instead of a ruler. This and other aspects of the classic non-Euclidean geometry of the shape coordinates are discussed in Appendix A.2.

5.1.3. Shape variables as directions in the shape-coordinate plane

So far we have used points in the shape-coordinate plane to represent triangular shapes; this section shows how directions through points in this plane represent shape variables measured on triangles. These directions will actually be coded "at 90°" – for any shape variable we shall compute the direction in which it does *not* change, and then assign to this variable the perpendicular direction, corresponding to its gradient. By reversing this procedure we can look at variability or change of shape first, by

5.1. One triangle

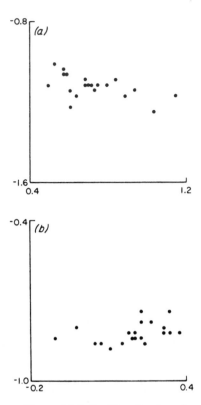

Figure 5.1.6. Scatter of pairs of shape coordinates for 20 sample mean forms of *Globorotalia truncatulinoides*. (*a*) Landmark #3 (tip of the axis) to a #1 – #2 baseline. (*b*) Landmark #1 to a #2 – #3 baseline. These data will be analyzed for size allometry and ecophenotypy in Section 6.5.2.

statistical analyses that generate reports implicating directions like these, and worry later about the variables that "name" them.

Because all information about the shape of a triangle is encoded in its position in the shape-coordinate plane, we must be able to reconstruct the value of any preassigned shape variable from this pair of coordinates. We may therefore write any shape variable as a scalar (real-valued) function of the shape coordinates, say $H(\nu_1, \nu_2)$.

Now, in general, smooth real-valued functions of a point in a plane are constant along whole extended *curves* of that plane (Figure 5.1.7*a*). For "sufficiently small" shape variation, we can model these curves as straight lines at nearly equal spacings (Figure 5.1.7*b*). H is (approximately) constant along the lines of this family, and it varies most rapidly in the direction perpendicular to them, along the vector that is the **gradient** of the shape variable H. For statistical purposes, any shape variable may be treated as equivalent to projection along the line of shape-coordinate space in the direction of its gradient. That is, change in any shape variable can be considered to be an expression $a_1\nu_1 + a_2\nu_2$, a suitable linear combination of any pair of shape coordinates in the vicinity of a mean form. This is true whatever the baseline of the coordinates. Of course, the a's may be expected to vary from point to point as well as from shape variable to shape variable.

By reversing the thrust of this equivalence (Figure 5.1.7*d*), we may refer to directions first, shape variables second. Any direction – defined, perhaps, by the little vector connecting two pairs of shape coordinates for two different group means – determines two classes of variables. One class, the **covariants** of the direction, includes the variables for which the assigned direction serves as gradient; the other class, the **invariants**, are the variables for which the assigned direction is tangent to their level curves, perpendicular to the gradient. In the context of biological explanation, which is the ultimate goal of all this maneuvering, it is as if we automatically ask two questions whenever we examine change in shape of a single triangle: not only "What most changed?" but also "What exactly didn't change?" The 90° rotation between gradient and level curves may be reinterpreted as an **involution** (association that is its own inverse function) pairing classes of variables at a given point of shape space by perpendicularity of their gradients. For two directions of shape space having gradients at 90° in the vicinity of a mean form, covariants of one of the directions are invariants of the other. (This is the same 90° as that separating the principal axes of the tensor representing a single shape change, as will be discussed in Chapter 6. But these are not the same directions as those principal axes. The relevant construction is in Figure 6.2.8.) We shall encounter another involution, this one pairing points rather than directions, in Section 5.3.2.

There is one major exception to this generalization. At the center of an equilateral triangle, ratios of symmetric size variables,

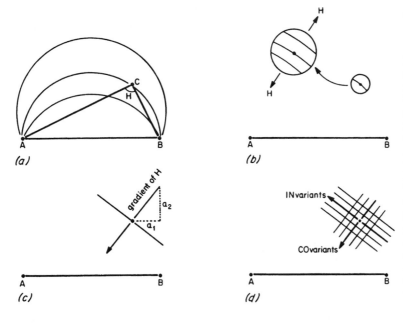

Figure 5.1.7. Interpretation of a shape variable H as a direction in the shape-coordinate plane. (*a*) The value of H (in this instance, the angle at landmark C) is constant along certain curves (in this instance, circles through A and B). (*b*) Enlargement of this scheme in a small neighborhood of the sample mean shape. The curves of constant shape variable H are indistinguishable from a family of equally spaced parallel lines. (*c*) The shape variable specifies an orientation of coordinates in this plane. One axis is along the direction of no change in the shape variable, and the other is along the direction of its gradient. The ratio $a_1:a_2$ specifies the linear combination of shape coordinates ν_1, ν_2 equivalent to the indicated shape variable in this vicinity. (*d*) Conversely, any direction of observed change in shape space specifies a coordinate system for shape variables. The shape variables with gradient along the assigned direction are the **covariants** of the shape change; the variables with level lines along the assigned direction (gradient perpendicular to that direction) are the **invariants** of the observed change. Compare Figure 6.3.3 and the associated table.

such as perimeter, area, or radii of inscribed or circumscribed circles, correspond to *three* directions of invariance and three of covariance. Such measures have a gradient of zero there, and the "curve" under discussion reduces to a point.

Certain symmetric shape variables that are *not* ratios of homologous size variables are the subject of study in other branches of spatial statistics. For instance, the variable that is the largest angle of a triangle is important in characterizing collinearities among points (e.g., stars on an astronomical plate) in the absence of any notion of "homology." The most general statistical context for work with unlabeled points is the brilliant recent development of shape manifolds by David Kendall and his colleagues. This tie will be discussed at length in Section 5.6.

5.1.3.1. Some useful pairs of shape variables in involution. —

We have defined pairs of shape variables in involution as those having gradients at 90°, so that one variable is a covariant of changes to which the other is invariant. Figure 5.1.8 shows three pairs of such variables that will be exploited later for the reporting of arbitrary shape changes in biologically suggestive terms.

The second coordinate ν_2 of shape space is the height of the triangle when scaled to constant baseline length; it therefore represents, all by itself, the **aspect ratio** of the triangle, the ratio of height to baseline length. The gradient of this shape variable is vertical. A variable having that direction for its level lines has gradient parallel to the axis of the other shape coordinate, ν_1; this

135

5.1. One triangle

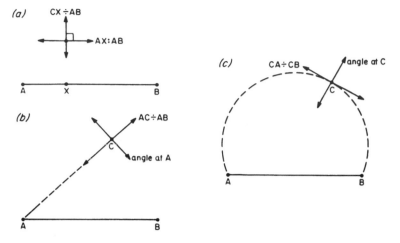

Figure 5.1.8. Three familiar pairs of shape variables that are in involution. (*a*) Ratio of height to baseline length; relative position of movable landmark along baseline. Compare Figure 6.3.3, left column. (*b*) Angle at a baseline landmark; ratio of one side to baseline. (*c*) Angle between sides; ratio of lengths of sides. Compare Figure 6.3.3, right column.

measures the **relative position of the moving landmark along the baseline**. This pair of variables is thus in involution (Figure 5.1.8*a*).

Reasoning similarly, we may see that the direction *AC* through point *C* in the two-point registration is the gradient of the length of that edge of the triangle when *AB* is held constant – that is, the **ratio of sides** *AC*:*AB* (Figure 5.1.8*b*). The **angle** *CAB* is constant along that direction and therefore has gradient at 90°, suggesting the "torque" of the tangent to a circle around *A*.

Changes in baseline, we have seen, mainly rotate and rescale shape scatters, and so leave unchanged the relation of involution between shape variables. The previous finding is therefore general (Figure 5.1.8*c*). The ratio between two lengths sharing an endpoint (*AC*:*BC* in the figure) has gradient at 90° to that of the angle between those two segments considered as vectors. Because angles are constant along circles through three points (Figure 5.1.7*a*), the gradient of the ratio of sides must be along tangents to circles through the two baseline points, as shown in Figure 5.1.8*c*. This particular involutory pair, most important (because most efficient) when the angle at *C* is 90°, will be encountered again in Section 6.3.

Because for statistical analysis it does not matter which baseline we choose, a proposition to be proved in the next section, we ought to be able to see all three of these pairs as perpendicular no matter which landmark is "movable." The different variables – ratios, angles – make specific angles *with each other*. These angles are functions of the mean shape of the triangle. But the resulting set of labels of the directions out of any vertex merely rotates when we change to another baseline (Figure 5.1.9).

Different shape variables are correlated to different extents. Under the "null model" to be introduced in Section 5.3, the expected correlation between two shape variables upon a single triangle is nearly equal to the cosine of the angle between their

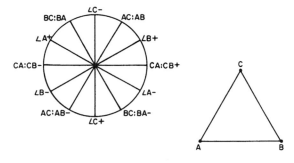

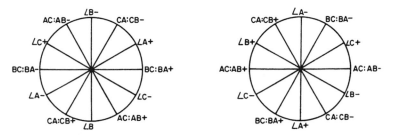

Figure 5.1.9. Six useful variables superimposed for an equilateral triangle. Each circle represents the set of directions of shape variability when the other two vertices serve as baseline. Changing the baseline direction by 60° clockwise rotates these wheels of variables by 120° counterclockwise.

gradients near the mean form. Pairs of variables in involution are thus the most efficient ways to represent the space of measures of a triangle for most applied purposes. The shape coordinates v_1 and v_2 are one such most efficient basis. We shall see later that any pair of shape variables in involution may be thought of as the shape coordinates to one of two baselines between constructed landmarks along the sides of the triangle.

5.2. RATIOS OF SIZE VARIABLES FOR ANY NUMBER OF LANDMARKS

We have just demonstrated, in connection with Figure 5.1.7, that "in the small," any shape measure of a single triangle may be expressed as a linear combination of the shape coordinates (v_1, v_2) of that triangle, so that the complete multivariate statistical analysis of the form of that triangle may proceed by way of that single pair of variables. We shall return to the mechanics of this multivariate analysis in Section 5.3. First, however, it is convenient to establish a generalization of this result.

> **For small variation in a configuration of any number of landmarks, any ratio of size variables has the same statistical behavior as some linear combination of the shape coordinates of any set of triangles that rigidly triangulates the landmarks.**

5.2. Triangles are enough

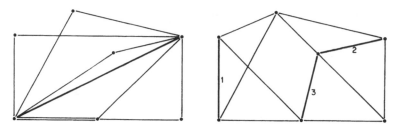

Figure 5.2.1. Two of the many possible sets of shape coordinates that span the ratios of size variables on seven landmarks, a space having 10 degrees of freedom. Left: Five landmarks to one baseline. Right: Two landmarks to baseline 1, two to baseline 2, and one (a duplicate) to baseline 3.

This means that it is not necessary to measure any particular shape variables *at all* for a configuration of however many landmarks; a complete multivariate analysis of those data may proceed in terms of shape coordinates alone. The shape coordinates, furthermore, may involve any set of triangles that permits the rigid reconstruction of the original landmark configuration. Two possibilities for seven landmarks are shown in Figure 5.2.1; there are many others.

5.2.1. Example: ratio of two interlandmark distances

The geometry by which shape coordinates combine to span the differentials of arbitrary ratios of size variables involving more than three landmarks is sketched in Figure 5.2.2 for the ratio between a pair of interlandmark distances. Using for baseline the pair of landmarks whose distance serves as denominator for the

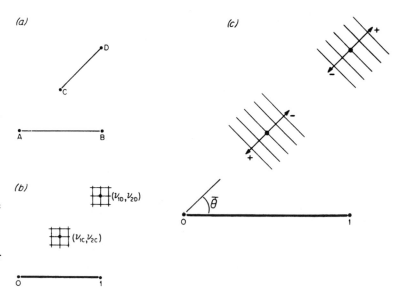

Figure 5.2.2. A ratio of two interlandmark distances is expressible using shape coordinates of triangles. (*a*) Two interlandmark distances AB, CD. (*b*) The shape coordinates of the endpoints of the second when the first is used as baseline. (*c*) The change in the relative length CD/AB of the distance between the two movable landmarks is the sum of linear projections of changes in their shape coordinates separately, as shown.

138

ratio, we interpret the ratio in question as the scaled distance between the shape coordinates for the two landmarks whose distance serves as numerator. A change in that distance clearly is the sum of changes in the two shape coordinates separately along a pair of directions lying at 180°. In terms of the mean angle $\bar{\theta}$ between the segments, change in this shape variable is very nearly identical with $(\nu_{1C} - \nu_{1D})\cos\bar{\theta} + (\nu_{2C} - \nu_{2D})\sin\bar{\theta}$, clearly an element of the space spanned by the shape coordinates of those two triangles. This value is the difference of the two projections $(\nu_{1C}\cos\bar{\theta} + \nu_{2C}\sin\bar{\theta})$ and $(\nu_{1D}\cos\bar{\theta} + \nu_{2D}\sin\bar{\theta})$, the readings of a ruler for the two "movable" landmarks separately in the direction $\bar{\theta}$ with respect to the baseline, as shown.

The idea that will generalize here is as follows: By a "shape variable" we mean the ratio of two size variables, and size variables are combinations of distances between constructed landmarks (Section 4.1). We shall take these ratios one distance at a time in numerator and denominator; but we can make the denominator appear to go away by using shape coordinates along a baseline from one of its two constructed landmarks to the other. The numerator is then the distance between a pair of constructed landmarks. Place a ruler down between those landmarks; distance measured along the ruler is the difference of the projections upon its direction of the two movable pairs of shape coordinates. But each projection is (nearly) linear in the shape coordinates; hence so is the ratio; hence so is any weighted sum of these ratios – but that covers all the shape variables.

5.2.2. Proof

Turning this sketch into a proof in the general case goes most quickly using the formalism of complex numbers and absorbing the construction of those constructed landmarks directly into the algebra. The following version is taken from Bookstein (1986a). Recall from Section 4.1 that the size variables we are considering can be written as linear combinations $|\Sigma a_i Z_i|$, where the Z_i represent the landmarks of the configuration as complex numbers, and where the coefficients a_i are real numbers that sum to zero.

A nineteenth-century notation, now obsolete, will nevertheless be useful here. Let us write the function of three complex numbers that is the shape-coordinate pair in the form

$$Q(A, B, C) = \frac{C - A}{B - A}.$$

Then the **differential** of the function Q, the change in its value corresponding to arbitrary small changes dA, dB, and dC in the values of A, B, and C, is

$$d\left(\frac{C-A}{B-A}\right) = \frac{(B-A)\,d(C-A) - (C-A)\,d(B-A)}{(B-A)^2}.$$

$$(5.2.1)$$

Our task is to prove that the linearized space of all ratios of admissible size variables $d(|\Sigma a_i Z_i| / |\Sigma b_i Z_i|)$, $\Sigma a_i = \Sigma b_i = 0$, is spanned by the sets of shape coordinates $dQ(Z_i, Z_j, Z_k)$. Because for scatters bounded away from the origin the absolute-value operator is linearly equivalent to projection along a line from the origin, it is sufficient to show that the shape coordinates span the space of complex shape ratios $d(\Sigma a_i Z_i / \Sigma b_i Z_i)$ with $\Sigma a_i = \Sigma b_i = 0$.

Rewrite this latter expression as $d[\Sigma a_i(Z_i - Z_1)/\Sigma b_i(Z_i - Z_1)]$ for any landmark Z_1. Ignoring a factor (a complex number: rotation together with rescaling) $[\Sigma b_i(Z_i - Z_1)]^2$, the value of the denominator in the usual formula, the differential then becomes

$$[\Sigma b_i(Z_i - Z_1)]\,d[\Sigma a_i(Z_i - Z_1)]$$
$$\qquad - [\Sigma a_i(Z_i - Z_1)]\,d[\Sigma b_i(Z_i - Z_1)]$$
$$= \sum_{i=1}^{K}\sum_{j=1}^{K}(a_i b_j - a_j b_i)\big[(Z_i - Z_1)\,d(Z_j - Z_1)$$
$$\qquad\qquad\qquad\qquad - (Z_j - Z_1)\,d(Z_i - Z_1)\big]$$
$$= \sum_{i=1}^{K}\sum_{j=1}^{K}(a_i b_j - a_j b_i)(Z_i - Z_1)^2 d\left(\frac{Z_j - Z_1}{Z_i - Z_1}\right)$$
$$\simeq \sum_{i=1}^{K}\sum_{j=1}^{K}(a_i b_j - a_j b_i)(W_i - W_1)^2 d\left(\frac{Z_j - Z_1}{Z_i - Z_1}\right),$$

where the W's are the expected locations of the Z's in some convenient coordinate system, the locations that supply expected values for the coefficients of the differentials in the formula. In any change of global coordinate system, rotation or rescaling of the terms $(W_i - W_1)^2$ is exactly canceled by the same changes in the denominator $[\Sigma b_i(Z_i - Z_1)]^2$ of the differential, the term omitted from all the formulas.

Thus, just as the distance differentials $d|Z_i - Z_j|$ span the space of all size variables, so the shape coordinates $d[(Z_k - Z_i)/(Z_j - Z_i)]$ span the space of differentials of all ratios of size variables. The space of shape variation on K landmarks has $2K - 4$ geometric degrees of freedom ($2K$ landmark coordinates, less four for the equivalence of forms by similarity: two dimensions of free translation, one of rotation, and one of rescaling). Hence any set of $K - 2$ triangles will do, as long as they exhaust the information of the landmark configuration, that is to say, as long as they form a rigid triangulation.

5.2.3. Implications

This theorem authorizes a far-reaching liberation of morphometric statistical analysis from reference coordinate systems. Many multivariate strategies are not changed much by linear change of basis; in particular, tests for group difference and for independence of vectors of measurements from other vectors have this property. The theorem implies that conclusions about differences of groups of landmark shapes are, in the limit of large samples or small variations, independent of the system of shape coordinates by which the landmark locations are represented. (The practical application of this approach to statistical-significance testing will be demonstrated in Sections 5.4 and 5.5.) The shape coordinates need not be chosen in any particular way, as long as the triangles to which they pertain form a rigid triangulation of the configuration. The coordinates need not, for example, have the same baseline. One can choose these representations rather freely to sustain graphical insights (e.g., our choice of the midline of the frontal facial photograph for the analysis in Section 1.2) or to suggest explanations from function (e.g., the registration upon the cranial base in Figure 7.6.6). In still other cases, the morphometrician might, while using the shape coordinates to carry out statistical computations, never present the findings by superposition at all: The thin-plate figures throughout Chapter 3 are of that sort, even though they could depend on shape coordinates for the computation of the average forms displayed. The choice of baseline is like the choice of a ruler from a drawerful – one picks for the convenience of the markings, confident of the invariance of one's findings. The theorem states, in the metaphor of the ruler, that everything you would find in the drawer would be equally straight, whether marked in millimeters or in inches.

5.3. A CIRCULAR NORMAL MODEL

Much of the analysis of shape coordinates in the examples to follow deals with the shapes of their distributions around a mean or a predicted form. In many applications, these distributions are rather nearly **circular:** The pair of shape coordinates has no direction of variation much greater than any other. In many of these examples, circular distributions correspond to no particular explanations, whereas other shapes in shape space (especially elliptical scatters) often express explanations of form by underlying factors. We may begin attaching statistics to these spaces, then, by constructing a plausible model in which biologically meaningless noise *is* circular in its effects on shape. As one extension, the separation between two groups, each circularly distributed in the shape-coordinate plane, may then be interpreted as indicating the presence of a mean group difference "plus" noise; as another extension, correlations of shape with size will be called the prediction of shape from size, "plus" noise; and so on. The persuasiveness of these reports will be enhanced if we can show that this "noise" of shape can arise from similarly uninformative "noise" at the landmarks severally, perhaps corresponding to mere jitter of the digitizing technician's hand.

At first this seems unreasonable. Put down three landmarks at their "mean" locations, vary each by a little circular bell of probability, then study the shape of the resulting triangle by replacing two of the landmarks right back where they started, so as to refer all the noise to the "relative position" of the third. How can there be no geometrically preferred direction of shape variability in the output of a computational process whereby one particular direction has been explicitly fixed (the orientation of the baseline)? The formulas for the shape coordinates, equations (5.1.1), involve two ratios to the same denominator – how can it be that they are not automatically correlated?

It is not difficult to convince oneself that something is suspect about these expectations. Recall from Section 5.1 that when we change the baseline in the shape-coordinate construction, the effect upon the sample scatter is merely a rotation and rescaling, not a change of shape; so the direction of the baseline apparently cannot be coded in the shape of that scatter. The only "shape" that maintains its form under arbitrary rotation is the ordinary circle, and so it is reasonable that the probability distribution we find has circular symmetry and, hence, expected correlation zero. But what probability process generates the circle we are seeing, and what determines its radius, the "size" of the shape scatter?

5.3.1. Origin of circular normals

The simplest explanation of the origin of these circular normal shape scatters appears to lie in a null model of **identical circular noise at each landmark location separately**. This section will show that regardless of the shape of the mean triangle, landmarks arising from data varying about these locations by small independent normal perturbations in each coordinate of each landmark, all of the same variance σ^2, generate a very nearly circular normal distribution of shape coordinates to any baseline, and the variance of that circular distribution of shapes is $\sigma^2 p^2/b^4$, where p and b will be defined presently. To say the shape coordinates are circularly normally distributed is to say that the two shape coordinates

142

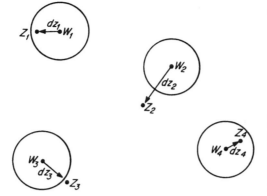

Figure 5.3.1. Null model for the generation of circular distributions in shape space: independent, identically distributed circularity of noise at each mean landmark location separately.

have the same variance and no covariance, whatever the mean shape of the triangle (even if the landmarks lie on a line), and whatever the choice of baseline.

This deduction may be demonstrated using any of the three principal forms of mathematical reasoning that run through this monograph: algebraic computations using the Cartesian coordinates, geometric constructions involving triangles, and manipulations of landmark locations as complex numbers with an arithmetic all their own. It is instructive to demonstrate the point using each of these methods and to show exactly how their implications all agree regarding the size of the circle one might expect to observe.

This triune derivation cannot be run backward. Many combinations of separately circular error variances at the three landmarks lead to the same distribution in shape space; from one circular distribution of shape one cannot reconstruct three separate radii in the original Cartesian plane. The model of identical variances landmark by landmark is the simplest; in the presence of four or more landmarks, one can estimate the radii separately, as discussed later. Of course, even for triangles, shape scatters may not be circular at all (Section 5.3.3).

To proceed with any of the approaches, we need to begin with a probability model for the generation of the original landmark location data. This will presume a set of three fixed points, the (true, population) **mean landmark locations**, about which the observed data vary by **independent, identically distributed (i.i.d.) measurement "errors" in each Cartesian coordinate separately**. These underlying measurement-error distributions are not observable in practice. In the absence of any evidence to the contrary, it is convenient to presume that they are distributed normally. Write the true mean locations as W_1, W_2, W_3, and let the observed landmark locations be $Z_i = W_i + dZ_i$, $i = 1, 2, 3$, where dZ_i is a small vector in the plane of the data. The components of dZ_i, should we need them, will be written as $(\varepsilon_{ix}, \varepsilon_{iy})$, $i = 1, 2, 3$. The

143

distribution of each pair of ε's is, under the normal assumption, itself a circular normal distribution, normal in every direction, with the same small variance σ^2, as implied in Figure 5.3.1. Let b be the baseline $|W_1 - W_2|$ of the true mean triangle, and set p^2 to the sum of the squared lengths of the sides of that triangle, $p^2 = |W_1 - W_2|^2 + |W_1 - W_3|^2 + |W_2 - W_3|^2$. We assume throughout that $\sigma^2 \ll b^2$ – that the landmark error variances are small in comparison with the baseline chosen.

5.3.1.1. Demonstration using algebra of the coordinates. —

Consider (Bookstein, 1984a) the deformation of $\Delta W_1 W_2 W_3$ into a triangle

$$W_1 + (\varepsilon_{1x}, \varepsilon_{1y}), \qquad W_2 + (\varepsilon_{2x}, \varepsilon_{2y}), \qquad W_3 + (\varepsilon_{3x}, \varepsilon_{3y}),$$

where $\varepsilon_{1x}, \ldots, \varepsilon_{3y}$ are i.i.d. $N(0, \sigma^2)$, σ^2 small. We show that the shape aspects of this deformation are those of the deformation of $\Delta W_1 W_2 W_3$ into the triangle

$$W_1, \qquad W_2, \qquad W_3 + (\nu_1, \nu_2),$$

where (ν_1, ν_2) is $N(0, p^2 \sigma^2 / b^2)$.

Without loss of generality, place W_1 at $(0, 0)$, W_2 at $(b, 0)$ on the x-axis, and W_3 at the general point (r, s) of the plane. The point here is to watch what is added to W_3 at every step in the course of undoing the noise at W_1 and W_2 coordinate by coordinate. Passages from step 2 to step 3 and from step 3 to step 4 are approximations accurate to first order in all ε's.

(1) The transformation (Figure 5.3.2a) of $\Delta W_1 W_2 W_3$ to

$$W_1 + (\varepsilon_{1x}, \varepsilon_{1y}), \qquad W_2 + (\varepsilon_{2x}, \varepsilon_{2y}), \qquad W_3 + (\varepsilon_{3x}, \varepsilon_{3y})$$

is the same (by translation of the second triangle) as

(2) the transformation (Figure 5.3.2b) of $\Delta W_1 W_2 W_3$ to

$$W_1, \qquad W_2 + (\varepsilon_{2x} - \varepsilon_{1x}, \varepsilon_{2y} - \varepsilon_{1y}),$$

$$W_3 + (\varepsilon_{3x} - \varepsilon_{1x}, \varepsilon_{3y} - \varepsilon_{1y}),$$

which is the same [by rotation of the second triangle clockwise by $(\varepsilon_{2y} - \varepsilon_{1y})/b$ radians] as

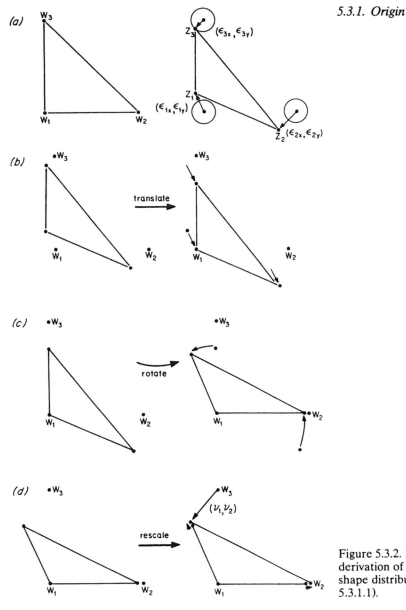

Figure 5.3.2. Diagram for the first derivation of circular normal shape distributions (Section 5.3.1.1).

(3) the transformation (Figure 5.3.2c) of $\Delta W_1 W_2 W_3$ to

$$W_1, \qquad W_2 + (\varepsilon_{2x} - \varepsilon_{1x}, 0),$$

$$W_3 + (\varepsilon_{3x} - \varepsilon_{1x}, \varepsilon_{3y} - \varepsilon_{1y}) + \frac{\varepsilon_{2y} - \varepsilon_{1y}}{b}(s, -r).$$

[The rotation moves all vectors by a fraction $(\varepsilon_{2y} - \varepsilon_{1y})/b$ of their distance from the origin in a direction 90° clockwise of that

145

distance. Then points near $W_3 \sim (r, s)$ are moved by appropriate multiples of $(s, -r)$.]

This differs only by a scale change $b/(b + \varepsilon_{2x} - \varepsilon_{1x})$, or $1 - (\varepsilon_{2x} - \varepsilon_{1x})/b$, from

(4) the transformation (Figure 5.3.2d) of $\Delta W_1 W_2 W_3$ to

$$W_1, \quad W_2, \quad W_3 + (\varepsilon_{3x} - \varepsilon_{1x}, \varepsilon_{3y} - \varepsilon_{1y})$$
$$+ \frac{\varepsilon_{2y} - \varepsilon_{1y}}{b}(s, -r) + \frac{\varepsilon_{2x} - \varepsilon_{1x}}{b}(-r, -s).$$

Collecting terms, this is the deformation of $\Delta W_1 W_2 W_3$ to the triangle $\Delta W_1 W_2[W_3 + (\nu_1, \nu_2)]$, where

$$\nu_1 = \varepsilon_{1x}\left(\frac{r}{b} - 1\right) + \varepsilon_{1y}\left(\frac{-s}{b}\right) + \varepsilon_{2x}\left(\frac{-r}{b}\right) + \varepsilon_{2y}\left(\frac{s}{b}\right) + \varepsilon_{3x},$$

$$\nu_2 = \varepsilon_{1x}\left(\frac{s}{b}\right) + \varepsilon_{1y}\left(\frac{r}{b} - 1\right) + \varepsilon_{2x}\left(\frac{-s}{b}\right) + \varepsilon_{2y}\left(\frac{-r}{b}\right) + \varepsilon_{3y}.$$

$$(5.3.1)$$

We shall refer back to this pair of approximations many times over the rest of this book.

Because the ε's are i.i.d. $N(0, \sigma^2)$, by assumption, we have

$$\text{var}(\nu_1) = \text{var}(\nu_2) = \frac{\sigma^2}{b^2}\left[(r - b)^2 + s^2 + r^2 + s^2 + b^2\right],$$

which equals σ^2/b^2 times the sum $p^2 = b^2 + (r^2 + s^2) + [s^2 + (r - b)^2]$ of the squared edge lengths of $\Delta W_1 W_2 W_3$. Rescaling one last time to set $|W_1 - W_2| = b$ to 1, we divide these variances by another factor b^2. By cancellation of cross-products of coefficients, we verify that $\text{cov}(\nu_1, \nu_2)$ is identically zero.

This demonstration is true for any pair of shape variables in involution (at 90° in the shape coordinates). Under the null model, any invariant/covariant pair have the same variance and correlate zero. The easiest way to see this is to rotate the baseline by the opposite of half the angle between either variable and the horizontal in the original shape-coordinate plane. There will result a new baseline that probably will link linear combinations of the original landmarks (like $.6Z_1 + .4Z_2$ and $.7Z_3 + .3Z_2$). To this new baseline, the invariant/covariant pair become vertical and horizontal. (Recall from Section 5.1.2 that changes of shape coordinates rotate twice as fast as the baseline, in the opposite direction.) Rotate the baseline 45° more and they will become horizontal and vertical instead. In either orientation, they play the role of ν_1 and ν_2 of the demonstration just completed. We shall see this same maneuver again in Section 6.2.2.

The zero correlation of pairs of shape variables in involution is a special case of a general relationship applying to circular models. Under the null model, in the vicinity of the mean form of a triangle of landmarks, the correlation expected between any two shape variables is equal to the cosine of the angle between their gradients in the shape-coordinate plane.

5.3.1.2. Demonstration using sums of rotations. —

The coefficients of equations (5.3.1) may be rearranged into three 2×2 matrices:

$$\begin{bmatrix} \dfrac{r}{b} - 1 & \dfrac{-s}{b} \\[2mm] \dfrac{s}{b} & \dfrac{r}{b} - 1 \end{bmatrix}, \quad \begin{bmatrix} \dfrac{-r}{b} & \dfrac{s}{b} \\[2mm] \dfrac{-s}{b} & \dfrac{-r}{b} \end{bmatrix}, \quad \begin{bmatrix} 1 & 0 \\ 0 & 1 \end{bmatrix}.$$

Each of these matrices is of the form corresponding to a Cartesian similarity operation (rotation and rescaling): diagonals equal, off-diagonals equal and opposite. We can express those similarity operations separately by simple vector constructions, as in Figure 5.3.3. The final set of shape coordinates is expressible as a deviation from the mean by a sum of three terms, each one corresponding to the deviation of one of the landmarks from its mean location, as follows.

The effect of perturbation in the location of landmark A is corrected as shown in Figure 5.3.3b. This landmark must be restored to the position at $(0, 0)$ assigned it in the shape-coordinate construction. We may consider the restoration to be the replacement of observed landmark C by the third vertex of the triangle on CB erected to be similar to triangle $A0B$. In effect, we stick a pin in point B, and rotate and rescale to restore A. The effect is to displace landmark C by a vector C_A that is the negative of the perturbation of landmark A rotated by the angle of the mean triangle at B and rescaled by the ratio of sides at B. The rotation of (r, s) about $(b, 0)$ adds in a vector perpendicular to $(r - b, s)$. Scaled by the length of the baseline, this results in the rotation matrix on $(r/b - 1, s/b)$ given in equations (5.3.1).

Similarly, the effect of undoing the perturbation at landmark B (Figure 5.3.3c) adds a perturbation C_B corresponding to the ratio of lengths at A and the angle of sides there. Finally, the perturbation at landmark C is simply added in.

But each of these perturbations is circular normal separately, a condition unchanged by rotation and rescaling; and the sum of independent circular normal variables is again a circular normal. If the standard deviation of each original ε is σ, then the standard deviation of the vector C_A is $\sigma |AC| / |AB|$, and that of the vector C_B is $\sigma |BC| / |AB|$. That of the contribution of the perturbation

147

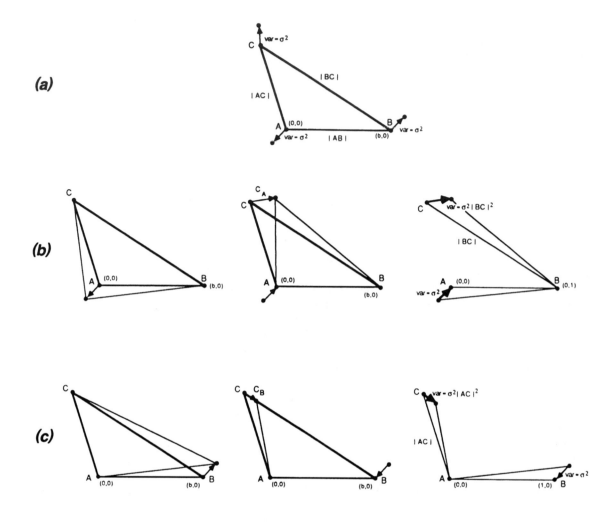

Figure 5.3.3. Shape coordinates as the sum of three different rotations/rescalings at the three landmarks of a triangle. (a) Three perturbations of landmark location. (b) Effect of correcting landmark A. (c) Effect of correcting landmark B. (d) The perturbation at landmark C is added unchanged to the vector sum of the other two corrections. (This figure was designed by Elena Tabachnick.)

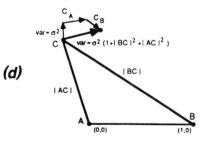

148

at landmark C remains, of course, $\sigma = \sigma|AB| / |AB|$. The varia-
tion of a sum of normals scales as the sum of their variances
separately; hence the net perturbation of shape coordinates is
distributed as a circular normal with variance

$$\sigma^2 \frac{|AC|^2 + |BC|^2 + |AB|^2}{|AB|^2} \bigg/ |AB|^2,$$

where the last division $|AB|^2$ restores the length of the baseline to
1. This expression is identical with the form $\sigma^2 p^2 / b^4$ arrived at in
the preceding section.

5.3.1.3. Demonstration by complex variables. —

Using the notation for differentials of the shape coordinates from
Section 5.2.2, we have

$$
\begin{aligned}
dQ &= d\left(\frac{Z_k - Z_i}{Z_j - Z_i} \right) \\
&= \frac{(Z_j - Z_i)(dz_k - dz_i) - (Z_k - Z_i)(dz_j - dz_i)}{(Z_j - Z_i)^2} \\
&= -\frac{(Z_j - Z_k) dz_i + (Z_k - Z_i) dz_j + (Z_i - Z_j) dz_k}{(Z_j - Z_i)^2} \\
&\simeq -\frac{(W_j - W_k) dz_i + (W_k - W_i) dz_j + (W_i - W_j) dz_k}{(W_j - W_i)^2}
\end{aligned}
$$

to first-order terms. The rotations and rescalings are all explicit in
the coefficients of the dZ's separately, and the variance of the
sum of independent normals is the sum $\sigma^2 p^2 / |W_j - W_i|^4$, as
before.

All these results are approximations. Although they are adequate for reasonably homogeneous biological data, it is possible to
pursue all these questions in full geometrical detail without any
approximation (see Section 5.6).

It is possible to suspend the assumption of equal variances for
the circular perturbations at the different landmarks of a data
base. The resulting distribution of shape coordinates will still be
circular normal. From four landmarks one can assemble four
different subsets of three; the shape coordinates of each triangle
are (presumably) circular with some variance. From these four

observed variances of the shape coordinates, a set of imputed original perturbation variances can be estimated by expressing the variance of each triangular shape as the sum of the three unknown variances, one for each landmark, scaled appropriately by the edge lengths. For more than four landmarks, the set of possible shape coordinates provides an overdetermined set of equations for the original measurement variances, and so should allow for statistical tests of the equality of their variances on the assumption of circularity. (Using interlandmark distances it is possible to pursue this issue even in the case of three landmarks; see Stoyan, 1990.) For an approach to failures of circularity, see the discussion of factors in Section 5.3.3; the failure of these deviations to be independent, in practice the more common finding, is treated in Section 7.6.

5.3.2. Covariances of different shape coordinates to the same baseline

That the shape coordinates of a single triangle do not manifest any effects of ratio correlation – that the variables ν_1 and ν_2 in equations (5.3.1) are uncorrelated in spite of sharing a denominator in equations (5.1.1) – is, like any other unexpected mathematical symmetry, a most pleasing phenomenon. It would be too much to expect, however, that this circularity would extend to comparisons of multiple shape coordinates to the same baseline. All shape coordinates of "third points" are subjected to the same explicit undoing of perturbations at the baseline landmarks. Although each pair of them may be distributed circularly, multiple sets of shape-coordinate pairs – shapes of separate triangles to the same baseline – are almost always correlated. As the baseline landmarks move apart or together, all the landmarks that are being scaled to their separation move closer or farther from the x-axis of the shape-coordinate construction; as the baseline rotates one way or another, all the landmarks rotate in the countervailing direction; and as the baseline is translated in one direction or another, all shape coordinates are translated in the direction opposite. All these processes induce correlations among shape coordinates corresponding to distinct landmarks even under the null model. These are all covariances about what is presumed to be a single group mean; yet other covariances are induced by group mean shape differences. The techniques that study group differences by conventional multivariate methods like Hotelling's T^2 (Section 5.4) automatically correct for these correlations.

Algebraically, the covariances of the shape coordinates are most easily derived from the equations (5.3.1) written twice, for shape coordinates (ν_{1k}, ν_{2k}) (landmark Z_k to a Z_1–Z_2 baseline) and (ν_{1m}, ν_{2m}) (landmark Z_m to the same baseline). From cross-prod-

$$\text{cov}(\nu_{1k}, \nu_{1m}) = \text{cov}(\nu_{2k}, \nu_{2m})$$

$$= \sigma^2[(r_k - 1)(r_m - 1) + r_k r_m + 2s_k s_m],$$

$$(5.3.2)$$

$$\text{cov}(\nu_{1k}, \nu_{2m}) = -\text{cov}(\nu_{2k}, \nu_{1m})$$

$$= \sigma^2[(r_k - 1)s_m - s_k(r_m - 1) + r_k s_m - s_k r_m].$$

Here σ is already scaled to baseline length $b = 1$, and (r_k, s_k) and (r_m, s_m) are the means of the shape-coordinate pairs (ν_{1k}, ν_{2k}) and (ν_{1m}, ν_{2m}). Notice that the matrix of these covariances is still of the form

$$\begin{bmatrix} a & b \\ -b & a \end{bmatrix},$$

a Cartesian rotation with rescaling. This is characteristic of the so-called *complex normal distributions* (Kent, 1990). We shall pursue these covariances further in Section 7.2.3, where they will be assembled into a matrix $\tilde{S}$ that can substitute for the covariances of shape coordinates under certain circumstances.

5.3.2.1. Uncorrelated shape-coordinate pairs: an involution. —

The equations (5.3.2) for the covariances relating two sets of shape coordinates have one interesting special case. For particular combinations (r_k, s_k) and (r_m, s_m), both of the covariance formulas yield zero. One formula is symmetric in k and m, the other, antisymmetric; then the fact of independence of the shape coordinates may be expressed as an **involution**, a mapping that interchanges the two points that are paired in this way.

One instance of this special case corresponds to the most symmetric four-landmark form, namely, a square of landmarks (Figure 5.3.4). The square must be assigned a baseline along one of its diagonals, as shown. The application of formulas (5.3.2) to mean shape coordinates $(0.5, 0.5)$ and $(0.5, -0.5)$ results in zeros. That is, the shapes of the two isosceles right triangles on the diagonal of a landmark configuration derived from a square by circular normal perturbations are independent, even though they share both baseline landmarks. As Figure 5.3.4b shows, the negative associations induced by changes in baseline length and orientation are precisely canceled, shape coordinate by shape coordinate, by the positive associations induced by baseline translation.

5.3. Circular normals

To express this absence of covariance in general, it is convenient to rephrase the covariance equations (5.3.2) in the form of a pair of multilinear equations that, given the values of r_k and s_k, may be solved for r_m and s_m:

$$r_m(2r_k - 1) + s_m(2s_k) = r_k - 1,$$

$$r_m(-2s_k) + s_m(2r_k - 1) = -s_k.$$

The solution for (r_m, s_m) in terms of r_k and s_k is the pair

$$(r_m, s_m) = \left[\frac{1}{2} - \frac{1}{2}\left(\frac{r_k - \frac{1}{2}}{4\,\text{dist}^2} \right), \ -\frac{s_k}{4\,\text{dist}^2} \right] \tag{5.3.3}$$

where "dist^2" is the distance $(r_k - \frac{1}{2})^2 + s_k^2$ from the point (r_k, s_k) to the point $(\frac{1}{2}, 0)$ at the middle of the baseline. It can be verified that this function is in fact an involution – that when it is applied to its own output, equation (5.3.3), the expression that is returned is just the pair (r_k, s_k) with which it began. Furthermore, the quantity "$4\,\text{dist}^2$" for the vector (5.3.3) is just the reciprocal of the expression "$4\,\text{dist}^2$" in the original (r, s) pair, and the numerators of the expressions (5.3.3) are proportional to the vector separating (r, s) from $(\frac{1}{2}, 0)$. It follows that the

Figure 5.3.4. Covariances between two landmarks induced by sharing a baseline upon two others. (a) Covariances induced by baseline (i) translation, (ii) rotation, (iii) scaling. (b) These sum to zero for opposite corners of the diamond (and other pairs of shape-coordinate pairs satisfying the involution condition derived in the text).

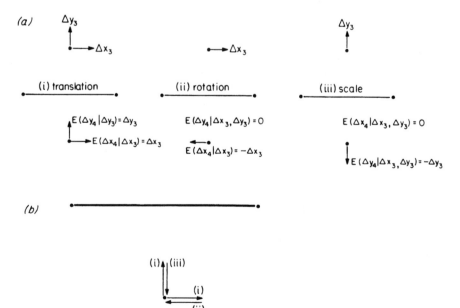

152

involution of zero shape covariance is equivalent to an ordinary **inversion** (Schwerdtfeger, 1962) in the circle of radius $(-\frac{1}{4})^{1/2}$ about the midpoint of the baseline. [The imaginary radius corresponds to the reflection of the ordinary inverse in that point: Shape coordinates above the baseline are in involution with shapes below the baseline, and conversely. I believe the role of the scale $\frac{1}{2}$ in this radius is the same as the $\frac{1}{2}$ that is the radius of the sphere of Kendall's "spherical blackboard" (1984); see Section 5.6.]

Involution exchanges the interior and the exterior of the circle of radius $\frac{1}{2}$ about the midpoint of the baseline. Hence, on the null model, the shape coordinates of a form whose mean lies outside the circle [cf. the isosceles right triangles using (1, 1); Figure 5.3.5] are in involution with a triangle having mean coordinates inside the circle, in this case the point $(0.4, -0.2)$, as can be verified from the formulas (5.3.3) or (5.3.2).

5.3.3. Factors for departure from circularity

We have just seen that circular shape distributions play a role in landmark-based morphometrics similar to that of normally distributed residuals in the classic analysis of scalars. Circular normal residuals often can be thought to have arisen "naturally" by processes characterized only by an error variance, not a signal. That circular shape scatters neither require nor provide much explanation is a useful observation: It implies that interpretable phenomena are likelier to be associated with the deviation of these scatters from circularity, a maneuver already familiar from ordinary multivariate statistics under the heading of **factor analysis**. The extension of factor analysis to configurations of several landmarks will occupy us in Section 7.6; here we make do with a few preliminaries that apply to the case of a single triangle of landmarks, a single pair of shape coordinates.

In a single-factor model (Figure 4.3.9), elliptical distributions are generated as the superposition of two processes: one, not necessarily causal, taking values normally distributed along a **line** in one's variable space (here, in the plane of the shape coordinates), and the other, independent of the first and necessary acausal, giving rise to circularly distributed noise. We can draw these distributions together (Figure 5.3.6c). Though it does not appear so in the figure, the sum of two normally distributed variables is another such, and so the distribution of the superposition really follows the contour of an ellipse rather than the schematic cigars that I have drawn.

In the applications to follow, the circular noise will arise from irreducible aspects of landmark digitizing error, developmental biological variability, and the like. The line distribution will be interpreted as a process in its own right: sometimes the irreducible indeterminacy of localization of a landmark along a

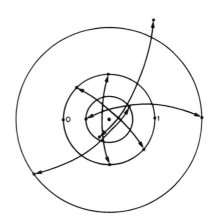

Figure 5.3.5. The general involution of uncorrelated shape-coordinate pairs is inversion in the circle of radius $0.5i$.

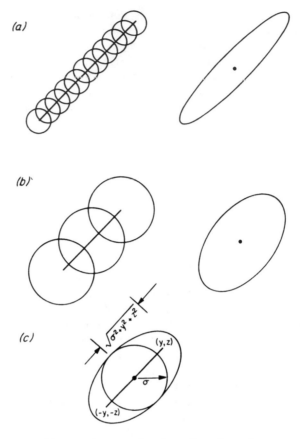

Figure 5.3.6. The single-factor model for the generation of non-circular shape scatters. (*a*) Large factor variance, small circular noise. (*b*) Small factor variance, large circular noise. (*c*) Geometry of the single-factor model fitted to an observed ellipse.

smoothly curving patch of outline (see the example to follow), which converts circular noise into "elliptical noise"; sometimes the effect of size variation (allometry) on expected shape; sometimes the effect of an exogenous, nonmorphometric covariate. All this is quite different from the more familiar language of linear regression plus "prediction error" often used to account for exactly the same elliptical distributions. If there is an "independent" variable at all, it is the factor score or its causal antecedents. And the "prediction error" is always larger than this particular circular part; it is inflated by the error of predicting that factor score itself.

Our algebra deals primarily with the observed covariance structure of the shape coordinates. We are modeling the covariance matrix

$$\begin{bmatrix} \sigma_{11} & \sigma_{12} \\ \sigma_{12} & \sigma_{22} \end{bmatrix}$$

of ν_1 and ν_2 around the mean shape as the sum of two terms, to

154

be given two separate interpretations: a contribution

$$\begin{bmatrix} \sigma^2 & 0 \\ 0 & \sigma^2 \end{bmatrix}$$

from circular perturbations at the landmarks separately, and a contribution

$$\begin{bmatrix} y^2 & yz \\ yz & z^2 \end{bmatrix} = \begin{bmatrix} y \\ z \end{bmatrix}[y \quad z]$$

from the factor along the long axis of the ellipse. This piece expresses two perfectly correlated direct effects of the factor just as if it took on only the values one standard deviation below the mean and one standard deviation above, with predicted (ν_1, ν_2) deviating from their means by $\pm(y, z)$. In symbols,

$$\begin{bmatrix} \sigma_{11} & \sigma_{12} \\ \sigma_{12} & \sigma_{22} \end{bmatrix} = \begin{bmatrix} \sigma^2 & 0 \\ 0 & \sigma^2 \end{bmatrix} + \begin{bmatrix} y^2 & yz \\ yz & z^2 \end{bmatrix}.$$

Then

$$\sigma_{12}^2 = (yz)^2 = (\sigma_{11} - \sigma^2)(\sigma_{22} - \sigma^2),$$

so that σ^2 satisfies the equation

$$\begin{vmatrix} \sigma_{11} - \sigma^2 & \sigma_{12} \\ \sigma_{12} & \sigma_{22} - \sigma^2 \end{vmatrix} = 0.$$

The error variance σ^2 must be an **eigenvalue** of the covariance matrix of the two shape coordinates. Clearly it is the smaller of these eigenvalues, the radius of the circle inscribed in the ellipse at its waist. The term

$$\begin{bmatrix} \sigma^2 & 0 \\ 0 & \sigma^2 \end{bmatrix}$$

represents the circle we have been drawing, located right at the center of the ellipse (Figure 5.3.6c), and the remainder $y^2 + z^2$ represents the excess squared length of the other principal axis of the ellipse, the long extension in the direction (y, z).

This decomposition bears interesting implications for a causal interpretation should the score on the factor aligned with (y, z) be associated with an exogenous variable. If the circular term corresponds to a process of noise, then the factor must represent the import for shape measurement of any other processes to which the factor score is attributed. Suppose, for instance, we claim that variation in the factor score underlying an elliptical shape-coordinate scatter is due to dependence on size, say by a coefficient η. Then (as shape coordinates depend on the score by regression coefficients y and z) the dependence of ν_1 and ν_2 on the score has coefficients ηy and ηz, in the same ratio. Thus the slope of the line representing the first factor is also the ratio of the coefficients by which the shape coordinates depend on size. That is, the vector (y, z) expresses the ratio of *simple* regression coefficients of the shape coordinates separately on size. Just as in Section 4.3.2, **there is no multiple regression involved in descriptions of the process for which a single factor accounts.** We shall see in Section 5.5 that multiple regression provides a statistical test for exogenous causation of the factor; nevertheless, it does not provide meaningful coefficients. This is exactly the same conclusion at which we arrive for the "prediction" of group by two size variables L and W in Section 4.3.1. When the ratio of simple regression coefficients does not approximate the direction of the principal axis of a scatter, then that predictor is not sufficient to account for the data even in the presence of a superimposed model of circular perturbation. There will be an example of this computation in Section 6.5.2.

5.3.4. Example: *Brizalina*

Section 3.4.3.1 introduced six landmarks for the foraminiferan *Brizalina*. Two of these landmarks, D and E, are "deficient" (Figure 3.4.5). They are defined as point on curves farthest from chords through the landmarks from which the curves spring, and so ought to have more measurement error parallel to that direction than perpendicular to it. Figure 5.3.7 shows this for the same specimens that were used to demonstrate the path-analytic approach to group discrimination by size variables (Section 4.3.2). The factor score for the long axis here is some combination of this measurement error with real differences in the shape of that chamber outline. Shape coordinates for the serially homologous landmark D to the AB baseline, long axis of the form, were published in Bookstein and Reyment (1989). Another example of error as factor will be shown in Section 6.5.1.6; a model with two factors (Size and directional error) is discussed in detail in Section 6.5.2.

5.4. AVERAGE FORMS AND COMPARISONS OF AVERAGES

We are now in a position to describe and demonstrate a first class of multivariate statistical procedures in shape space: the averaging of groups of shapes and the testing of differences between the

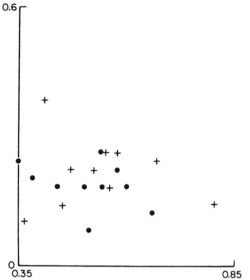

Figure 5.3.7. Shape coordinates for the penultimate-chamber landmark *E* of *Brizalina* to the *AF* baseline (cf. Figure 3.4.5); +, stratum 2; •, stratum 4.

groups for statistical significance. The problem of reporting those differences is the business of the two chapters following upon this one.

5.4.1. Machinery for averaging forms

Should one's data have arisen from deviations of landmark locations about a mean form – for instance, if the null model of the preceding section is true – then the most efficient way of averaging samples of homologous landmark configurations involves three steps (Figure 5.4.1):

1 Select a baseline for the construction of shape coordinates.
2 Compute the vector of mean shape coordinates to that baseline.
3 Draw out that configuration of landmarks with the baseline scaled to its sample average or log average size.

If the null model is assumed or observed to hold, the baseline selected ought to be the longest diameter of the form through the centroid, the diameter best approximating the first principal axis of the configurations case by case (Section 7.2.3). But whatever the baseline, different versions of this construction, corresponding to different baselines and triangulations, are statistically equivalent through terms of first order (Section 5.2), and differ only in the amount of nonlinearity induced by the absolute range of ratios

157

5.4. Average forms

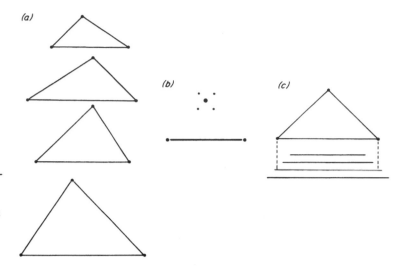

Figure 5.4.1. Steps in the averaging of landmark configurations. (*a*) Reduce to a basis of shape coordinates. (*b*) Compute mean shape coordinates. (*c*) Display that shape at the arithmetic or geometric mean baseline size.

of various lengths to the baseline length (reexamine Figures 5.1.3 through 5.1.6, or see Appendix A.2).

In the presence of knowledge about factors that contribute to the variation of form about its mean – size allometry, for instance, or covariance with some exogenous variable – the quantities being averaged might be the residuals of the shape coordinates after those predictors have been regressed out, and the resulting mean form, now having a smaller probable error in shape space, may be considered the expected average form "at mean size," "at mean temperature," or the like. We shall see examples of this in Section 6.5.

An alternative system of averaging was introduced by my group in an earlier publication (Bookstein et al., 1985). Our suggestion, intended to apply to the case of dependence of shape principally upon a size factor, involved regressing observed interlandmark distances (in the pattern of a truss) explicitly upon that factor, then computing a form corresponding to a least-squares relaxation of the predicted interlandmark distances (according to log-linear regression) at mean size. When data come in the form of landmark locations, there is no need for the additional complexity of working with distances and their regressions.

5.4.2. Testing for mean differences in shape

The formalism of the shape coordinates places the question of differences of mean landmark configuration in a multivariate statistical context that is, to first order, independent of all the arbitrary decisions (choice of triangulation, choice of baselines for each triangle) involved in actual computations. The situation is the same as in the statistical analysis of a single length variable.

We must choose a unit of measurement for the exercise, but once it is chosen, the biometrics of the study will be independent of that choice. The theorem of Section 5.2 states that all bases for shape space span the same set of shape variables, the ratios of the interlandmark distances. Then any multivariate procedure that is independent of change of basis will arrive at nearly the same findings for a particular group comparison, or other valid multivariate question, regardless of the manner in which the data have been reduced to shape space.

The usual test for such differences between two groups is Hotelling's T^2 (Morrison, 1990); for more than two groups, the statistic is Wilks' Λ (Rao, 1973) or one of its cousins (Anderson, 1958; Mardia, Kent, and Bibby, 1979). If shape scatters look roughly circular, with no striking outliers, and if one has no clear idea of what processes actually account for shape differences between groups, then one should *apply a packaged T^2 to a basis for the shape coordinates, and believe the printout*. Such advice assumes, perhaps harshly, that one has no real expectations of the nature of the form difference to be unearthed, its expected scale, its regional emphases, and so forth. In reality, one very likely assembled one's landmarks with such expectations clearly in mind (cf. the justification of the eyebrow points, Section 3.4.4.1). The alternative, innocent nescience, uses up $2K - 4$ degrees of freedom in the covariance matrix underlying the T^2, and thus for a rich landmark set demands a considerable sample size. Still, it is the most honest approach; most alternatives are at risk of turning into ad hoc ransacking. For instance, one might be tempted to get around this diminution of effective degrees of freedom for the difference(s) by averaging neighboring or "equivalent" landmarks or by specifying one large triangle "to analyze first." This sort of ingenuity is acceptable as long as one corrects any *p*-values, Bonferroni-style, for the number of different ways in which one might have chosen to carry out that arbitrary reduction of degrees of freedom.

Significance levels computed by the usual tests are subject to two sorts of uncertainties in this context. There is, first of all, the usual matter of nonnormality, which may be handled for the shape coordinates by the same paraphernalia that apply in the general case: resampling schemes and permutation tests. For an example of the latter computation, see Sampson (1986). In addition, there is the aspect of nonlinearity of changes from one shape basis to another. An upper limit can be placed upon these effects by the non-Euclidean methods of Appendix A.2, or one may simply experiment with alternate expressions of findings to baselines that differ considerably in their levels of implied noise (Figure 5.4.3). For noise of large variance *known* to be circularly normally distributed a priori, the maximum-likelihood estimates of Mardia and Dryden are not susceptible to this nonlinearity; see Section 5.6.

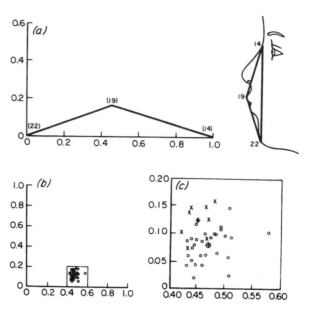

Figure 5.4.2. Comparison of two groups for a single triangle of landmarks. (*a*) The triangle. (*b*) The scatters. (*c*) A legible enlargement; X, exposed chil - dren; O, unexposed; symbols overwritten by +, centroids for the two groups.

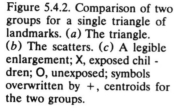

5.4.3. Examples of group mean comparisons

5.4.3.1. A single triangle. —

The Seattle Longitudinal Prospective Study of Alcohol and Pregnancy (Section 3.4.4) incorporates a small data set of familiar landmarks that we shall use in the course of several demonstrations in this book.

From Figure 3.4.13 we extract a triangle of landmarks spanning the front of the face: points #14 (Nasion), #19 (Upper vermilion), and #22 (Chin). The design of this comparison, contrasting the 28 children of relatively low prenatal alcohol exposure with the 8 children of relatively high exposure, was reviewed in Chapter 3, as was the provenance of the landmark locations. The analysis to follow is extracted from Bookstein and Sampson (1987, 1990).

In the empirical scatter (Figure 5.4.2) it can be seen that the two scatters for the groups separately are not far from circular, in spite of the considerable elongation of the triangle under study and the motley of different styles of landmark definition involved. There may be an outlying form in the unexposed group, one case with the lip point untypically far along the line from forehead to chin. The principal direction of group mean difference is perpendicular to this possible outlier, and so the computed value of T^2 for this pair of groups is not much affected. That T^2 is 23.8, $p \sim .00016$ on the normal assumption. Permutation tests support this conclusion. The effect could be reported as the relative motion of any vertex with respect to a baseline taken between the other two, or in several other ways. The general approach to a choice of report is our main concern in Chapter 6. This particular

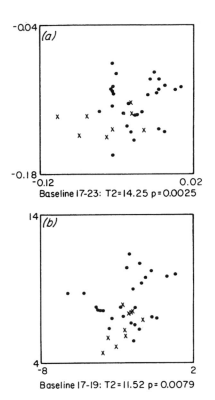

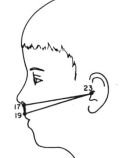

Baseline 17-23: T2=14.25 p=0.0025

Baseline 17-19: T2=11.52 p=0.0079

Figure 5.4.3. Effects of an extreme change in baseline. Landmarks are #17, #19, and #23 of Figure 3.4.13; symbols as in Figure 5.4.2. (*a*) Baseline #17–#23. (*b*) Baseline #17–#19. After Sampson (1986).

example has some unusual features; its interpretation is deferred to Section 7.3.3.4.

Another triangle from the same data set may be considered in isolation to indicate the effect of extreme changes in baseline. Sampson (1986) computed the three T^2-statistics for the same group comparison as applied to a triangle extremely wedge-shaped, that relating the earhole (#23) to the two points upon the upper lip (#17 and #19). The computed T^2-statistics for the comparison of groups to two different baselines (Figure 5.4.3), differing by a factor of about 8 in length, ranged from 11.5 to 14.2 only. The analysis to the shorter baseline, as expected, threw outlying points to distances that were greater fractions of the core variance of the scatter than did the analysis to longer baselines. That is, the reciprocal of the shorter baseline is longer-tailed, "less normally distributed."

5.4.3.2. A configuration of 10 landmarks. —

Section 7.5.5 will deal with features of the difference between the mean landmark configurations in a population of Apert patients and the locations of these landmarks in an age- and sex-matched normative population. The mean locations of the landmarks are shown in Figure 5.4.4 to a Sella–Nasion baseline.

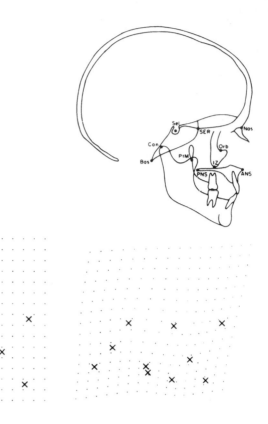

Figure 5.4.4. Mean locations of 10 craniofacial landmarks for 14 cases of Apert syndrome and the matched normative means, with the interpolating thin-plate spline.

bending energy 0.0864

We shall see in Chapter 7 that several aspects of this configuration show no difference from the normative mean at all: for instance, the shape of the cranial base, the landmark triangle Basion–Sella–Nasion. Nevertheless, there is much to describe. The T^2-test for difference in shape between this pair of configurations, using the shape coordinates of eight landmarks to a baseline from Sella to Nasion, has a value of 9,600, equivalent to an F-ratio of 240 on 16 and 10 degrees of freedom. The issue of shape difference is not in question.

5.4.3.3. Comparisons among multiple groups. —

The same generalizations of two-group to multiple-group comparisons that work for ordinary measurement vectors apply as well to the shape coordinates to any basis. The comparison of the between-group to the within-group variance-covariance matrix proceeds via the product Λ of all the nonzero relative eigenvalues, numbering more than one if the groups number more than two (Rao, 1973). In this example, we compute an overall significance level for the differences among configurations of four landmarks in the cranial bases of six patient groups. These data have been

162

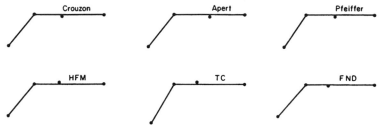

5.4.3. Examples

Figure 5.4.5. Mean configurations of four landmarks in six craniofacial syndromes. The landmarks are Basion, Sella, Spheno-ethmoid Registration, and Nasion (see Section 3.4.2): Apert syndrome ($N = 11$); Crouzon syndrome ($N = 24$); Pfeiffer syndrome ($N = 4$); HFM, hemifacial microsomia ($N = 78$); TC, Treacher Collins syndrome ($N = 9$); FND, frontonasal dysplasia ($N = 31$).

previously described in Grayson et al. (1985). Figure 5.4.5 presents the mean of two shape-coordinate pairs – those for Basion and for Spheno-ethmoid registration (SER) – to a baseline taken from Sella to Nasion. Table 5.4.1 presents the six-group MANOVA of these data, including all possible two-group comparisons. It will be seen that all groups differ significantly one from another except Crouzon from Pfeiffer. We now know the groups to be different in mean shape, but more work is required if we are to interpret those differences by some biological explanation. The differences are variously "at SER," "at Basion," or both; Chapter 7 will supply a language for correct reporting of such coordinate-dependent judgments.

5.4.3.4. Brizalina revisited. —

In Section 4.3.3 we introduced a small data set of four landmark locations for 10 specimens of *Brizalina* in each of two strata. We

Table 5.4.1. *MANOVA for two pairs of shape coordinates for six craniofacial syndromes*

Means (Sella– Nasion)	Crouzon ($N = 24$)	Apert ($N = 11$)	Pfeiffer ($N = 4$)	TC[a] ($N = 9$)	FND[a] ($N = 31$)	HFM[a] ($N = 78$)
$\nu_{1.Basion}$	−0.374	−0.363	−0.318	−0.321	−0.399	−0.380
$\nu_{2.Basion}$	−0.457	−0.463	−0.472	−0.544	−0.455	−0.456
$\nu_{1.SER}$	0.396	0.502	0.420	0.322	0.320	0.357
$\nu_{2.SER}$	−0.020	−0.028	−0.023	0.027	−0.007	0.022

Distances between strata (D^2 below diagonal, unadjusted significance of F above)

	Crouzon	Apert	Pfeiffer	TC	FND	HFM
Crouzon		.0000	.45	.0000	.0000	.0000
Apert	9.1		.0008	.0000	.0000	.0000
Pfeiffer	1.1	7.0		.0001	.0000	.0030
TC	6.8	28.5	9.1		.0026	.0002
FND	4.5	26.2	8.4	2.5		.0000
HFM	2.0	16.8	4.5	3.0	2.0	

[a]TC, Treacher Collins syndrome; FND, frontonasal dysplasia; HFM, hemifacial microsomia.

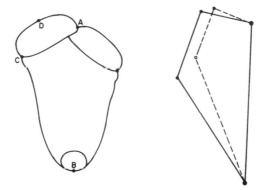

Figure 5.4.6. Mean shape coordinates to an aperture–proloculus baseline for the two proximal-chamber landmarks for two strata of *Brizalina*. Solid outline; stratum 4; dashed, stratum 2.

showed that the ordinary Fisherian linear discriminant function, though satisfactory for its intended purpose (which was discrimination), succeeded only at the cost of supplying coefficients that (1) confounded size difference and shape difference and (2) failed to indicate the biological meaning of differences among intercepts of the underlying allometric regressions.

Figure 5.4.6 represents the same comparison of strata as viewed purely in shape space by the construction of mean shape coordinates for the other two landmarks to a baseline from aperture to proloculus. (Even though the statistical analysis is independent of baseline, this is an appropriate choice, as it lies approximately along the growth axis of this organism.) We see that there is a substantial shape difference. The T^2 for this two-group comparison is 19.0, significant at $p \sim .02$ for the existence of a systematic group difference described wholly without reference to size. As the figure suggests, one of these landmarks contributes more to the discrimination than the other. The origin of the proximal chamber has been displaced relatively farther than the bulge point of that same chamber; also, you will recall that the latter is a geometric landmark, representing a curve but deficient in precision, whereas the former is an intersection of structures locatable with considerable precision both on the form and in drawings of the form. The T^2-statistic for the shape coordinates of the proximal point alone is 16.0, significant separately at $p \sim .004$. We shall return to this example yet again in Section 6.3.3 in order to interpret the meaning of this particular finding.

5.4.4. Mean differences in three dimensions

Landmark locations may be digitized in three dimensions with only moderately greater tedium than in two (Fink, 1990; Bookstein et al., 1991). Although the device of complex arithmetic does not transfer from two-dimensional analysis to three-dimensional,

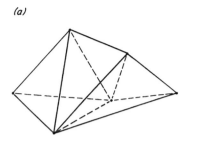

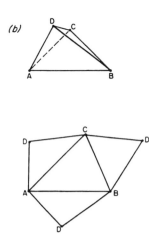

Figure 5.4.7. Basis for shape space in three dimensions. (*a*) Recoding landmark positions by a rigid set of tetrahedra. (*b*) Each tetrahedron may be expressed as the set of four shapes of its faces.

the machinery of shape space otherwise generalizes effectively. It remains true that all ratios of size variables measured between weighted combinations of landmarks are spanned by the set of shapes of triangles as long as the triangles form a rigid triangulation of the solid structure of landmarks. The manner in which this procedure goes forward is indicated schematically in Figure 5.4.7. A solid configuration of landmarks may be recorded exhaustively by the shapes of a number of **tetrahedra** into which it is divided. An octahedron, for instance, may sometimes be archived in the form of three tetrahedra, as in Figure 5.4.7*a*. Any tetrahedron, in turn, is fully, indeed redundantly, archived by the set of shapes of its four faces.

These four triangles involve a total of only five geometric degrees of freedom. There are six independent size measures (edge lengths), with one degree of freedom of net proportionality. Rather than take ratios to some composite size measure, it is better to build shape representations directly by accumulating the correct number of separate shape coordinates. The reassembly of the triangles into a three-dimensional structure is managed by constraints on the full set of these coordinates that represent the usual linear equivalence of different rigidly related subsets; hence (for small variations), again almost any basis for shape space is as good as any other. Symmetry may be a helpful guide to the choice of a particular representation.

As an alternative to this reduction of a tetrahedron to its faces, one can treat the set of four landmarks as the simple finite element in three dimensions, to be fitted by uniform transformations of space just as triangles of landmarks specify uniform transformations of the plane. The analysis of these strains as single 3×3 symmetric tensors results in sets of three principal strains – largest, smallest, and intermediate – along three direc-

165

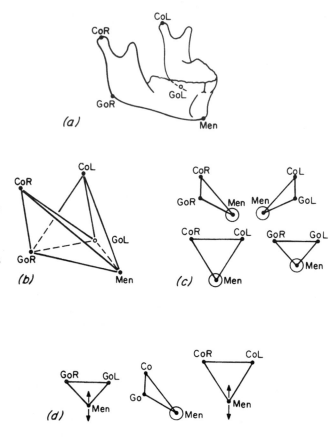

Figure 5.4.8. Five landmarks, two tetrahedra, and seven triangles for the analysis of the mandibu-lar-growth data. The data have a total of eight geometrical degrees of freedom. (*a*) Sketch of the landmarks in space. (*b*) Two te-trahedra sharing the face Go-nion–Gonion–Menton. (*c*) Full shape basis: shape coordinates for the four triangles shown. (*d*) Symmetric shape basis: ordi-nates for the isosceles triangles, averages of the two lateral trian-gles. CoL, CoR, left and right condylions; GoL, GoR, left and right gonions; Men, Menton.

tions mutually at 90°. For a pair of mean forms, the directions of these strains may be interesting. But the statistics of populations of these shapes requires five dimensions for its display (cf. Section 8.2.2), and I know no satisfactory means of visualizing this; hence the reduction to triangular shapes, with the associated two-dimen-sional data graphics, that I recommend here. Analysis of more than four landmarks in space by the method of finite elements is inappropriate for the same reason that the analysis of more than three landmarks in the plane by this method is inappropriate. There is an extended comment on this matter in Section 6.6.

5.4.4.1. Example: mandibular growth from age 8 to age 12. —

In preparation for an example to be worked in Section 6.5.4, we present here the overall T^2 for the difference in form of two samples of 5 three-dimensional landmark locations for 12 boys: the locations of their two condyles, two gonions, and menton at ages 8 and 12. These points were located by the photogrammetric methods of Grayson et al. (1988) from pairs of radiographs taken at 90° in the course of the University of Michigan University School Study.

166

An overall T^2-test may be applied to any eight ($= 3K - 7$ for $K = 5$ landmarks) independent "degrees of freedom" – directions in shape space – drawn from the full set of 14 shape coordinates. For instance, we can build the shape representation of this pentahedron out of four shape-coordinate pairs. One reasonable set is shown in Figure 5.4.8c. The matched T^2 for change over four years is 126, equivalent to an F-ratio of 5.75 on 8 and 4 degrees of freedom, and significant at the $p \sim .054$ level. However, the form we are studying is *symmetric*, maintained that way by normal function. There is hardly any variation of the abscissa of Menton in relation to the bilateral baselines Gonion–Gonion or Condylion–Condylion, and hardly any difference in changes for the two lateral triangles; inclusion of these redundant coordinates makes the full eight-coordinate variance-covariance matrix somewhat ill-conditioned. The appropriate T^2 computation is on changes in four shape coordinates only: the ordinate of Menton to the baselines Gonion–Gonion and Condylion–Condylion, and the average of the shape changes of the two lateral triangles. For that design, $T^2 = 41.6$, $F(4, 8) = 7.56$, $p \sim .008$. There is indeed a mean shape change with growth for the mandible in space (which, however, turns out not to involve the shape of the lateral triangle). It will be described in Section 6.5.4.

5.4.4.2. Asymmetry in three dimensions. —

When a scheme of landmarks incorporates locations paired by their approximate symmetry with respect to some midplane, then whether or not other, unpaired landmarks are presumed to lie near that midplane, there are generated extended structures (here, the two triangles Condylion left–Gonion left–Menton and Condylion right–Gonion right–Menton) the shapes of which may be compared by the method previously introduced for the general matched design. In that shape comparison, any mean difference between left and right antimeres corresponds to **directional asymmetry** (Van Valen, 1962), whereas variance of the shape-coordinate difference corresponds to **fluctuating asymmetry**.

5.5. COVARIANCES BETWEEN SIZE AND SHAPE

To this point the information about size discarded in the course of the two-point registration has remained excluded from the analysis. The information lost by this maneuver can be restored, in principle, by augmenting the shape coordinates with any size variable whatever. However, our interest will be principally in the detection and interpretation of correlations between size and shape. For this purpose, every size variable but one has a serious flaw: Every size variable but one is correlated with shape *even on the null model in which shape variation expresses no meaningful processes*. This point is a special case of a general observation due to Mosimann (1970) and explained at greater length in Bookstein et al. (1985:sect. 2.2). It is usually applied to lists of shape variables $X/g(X)$ derived from lists of size variables X by an arbitrary scaling g (recall the introduction to this chapter). In the present application, we need not measure any data; we can infer a frequently encountered structure of correlations between size and shape directly from the null model of circular perturbations. In this section of the chapter we first demonstrate how most size variables are meaninglessly correlated with some aspect of shape variation, then derive the formula for the single size variable that is not flawed in this way (the quantity called "Centroid Size" in Section 4.2), and finally indicate its power for two sorts of studies: those in which there is size allometry, and those in which there is not.

5.5.1. False allometries

As usual, we begin with the case of a single triangle, three landmarks. On the null model, the three vertices are displaced independently from their mean positions in both extent and direction. On this model, you will agree, size has no effect on shape – *nothing* has any effect on shape (there are no "factors"). Any statistical method we use to test allometry – perhaps the pattern of coefficients on a principal component (Section 4.3.2), perhaps the multiple correlation of size with shape space to be introduced later – *must* come up empty for data that were generated by this model. In this way we can reject most candidates for Size in advance of examining any data, by insisting that Size treat *shape noise* in a certain way.

Consider, for example, the perfectly legitimate size variable that is baseline length itself, the quantity specifically divided out in the rescaling underlying Figure 5.1.2. You might expect that as the resulting shape coordinates have somehow amalgamated this variable into their denominators, there should be some sort of problem with ratio correlation. In fact, there *is* such a correlation. Under the null model, baseline length correlates with the shape coordinates in a geometrically striking way *even though* those coordinates are uncorrelated with each other, as was shown in Section 5.3. This implies that we cannot conveniently use baseline length as a measure for testing the association of size and shape: It will not give us zero associations for the null model.

Let us borrow the notation of six perturbations ε – one each for each coordinate of each landmark – from Section 5.3.1.1, and, for simplicity, fix the quantity b, mean baseline length, at 1. For all ε small, the baseline length before the two-point registration is approximately $1 + \varepsilon_{2x} - \varepsilon_{1x}$, perturbation of the original length 1 by the x-displacements of the two endpoints separately, taken with opposite signs (Figure 5.5.1a).

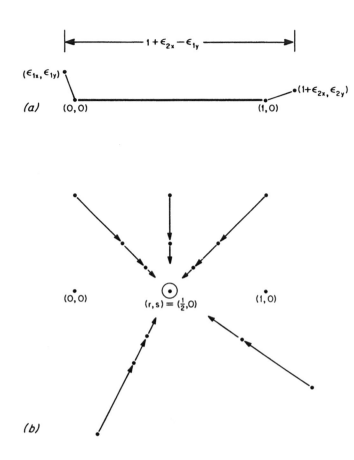

Figure 5.5.1. Correlations of shape coordinates with baseline size on the null model. (*a*) Approximation to baseline length. (*b*) According to equations (5.3.1), the covariances of the two components of shape with this size variable combine into a vector $\sigma^2(1 - 2r, -2s)$ pointing in the direction of the midpoint of the baseline. (The lengths of these vectors in the figure correspond to $\sigma = 0.5$.)

Equations (5.3.1) showed the shape coordinates as linear combinations of all six ε's:

$$\nu_1 = \varepsilon_{1x}(r - 1) + \varepsilon_{1y}(-s) + \varepsilon_{2x}(-r) + \varepsilon_{2y}(s) + \varepsilon_{3x},$$
$$\nu_2 = \varepsilon_{1x}(s) + \varepsilon_{1y}(r - 1) + \varepsilon_{2x}(-s) + \varepsilon_{2y}(-r) + \varepsilon_{3y}.$$

$$(5.3.1, b = 1)$$

[Here, (r, s) are the mean shape coordinates of third vertex of the triangle.] On the null model, all the ε's are independent normals with the same variance σ^2. In Section 5.3.1 we computed the variance-covariance matrix of the ν's as combinations of the coefficients of these ε's. There, all that mattered about r and s was the sum of square of the sides of the triangle with (r, s) as one vertex. In the present extension, we need a third linear combination,

$$(\text{baseline} - 1) \sim \varepsilon_{1x}(-1) + \varepsilon_{2x}(1).$$

Then the covariances of baseline length with the two shape coordinates are obtained by summing products of corresponding coefficients:

$$\sigma^{-2}\text{cov}(\text{baseline}, \nu_1) = -1(r-1) + 1(-r) = 1 - 2r,$$

$$\sigma^{-2}\text{cov}(\text{baseline}, \nu_2) = -1(s) + 1(-s) = -2s.$$

Hence, **the covariance of baseline length with shape is different for different mean shapes** (r, s). The two covariances $\sigma^2(1 - 2r)$ and $\sigma^2(-2s)$ may be organized into a single vector $\sigma^2(1 - 2r, -2s)$. But $(1 - 2r, 2s) = 2\{(\frac{1}{2}, 0) - (r, s)\}$; it lies along the vector pointing from the mean shape-coordinate pair (r, s) back toward the middle of the baseline. The larger is the mean s of the shape coordinate ν_2, the larger is the negative covariance $-2s$ of ν_2 with the baseline length – the ratio-correlation effect mentioned earlier. Other things being equal, the larger the baseline of the perturbed triangle, the lower the third landmark is dragged by division by that length. But its x-coordinate is "dragged" too. There is also a covariance with the horizontal shape coordinate ν_1, depending on r, the mean of ν_1, as $1 - 2r$. The pair of covariances is zero only for the "triangle" with third landmark fluctuating about the point $(\frac{1}{2}, 0)$ halfway along the baseline. For all other mean forms there is a covariance with size in the form of a "regression" toward that midpoint: Division by baseline length drags *both* coordinates toward this midpoint for larger baseline lengths.

Let us consider another example, not so obviously directional as the baseline. Recall that we are searching for a size variable that, regardless of the mean triangular shape (r, s), has zero covariance with both shape coordinates under the conditions of no allometry specified in the null model: identical random normal noise of small variance in each landmark coordinate separately. The size measure that is **area** surely has no directional bias–? From the textbooks (cf. Pedoe, 1970:5) we retrieve the formula for the area of a triangle with vertices at $(\varepsilon_{1x}, \varepsilon_{1y})$, $(1 + \varepsilon_{2x}, \varepsilon_{2y})$, and $(r + \varepsilon_{3x}, s + \varepsilon_{3y})$: the determinant

$$A = \frac{1}{2} \begin{vmatrix} 1 & \varepsilon_{1x} & \varepsilon_{1y} \\ 1 & 1 + \varepsilon_{2x} & \varepsilon_{2y} \\ 1 & r + \varepsilon_{3x} & s + \varepsilon_{3y} \end{vmatrix}.$$

(The formula comes from representing the area of the triangle as the sums and differences of triangles with sides parallel to the x- and y-axes.) Ignoring terms in the products of the ε's, much smaller than the effects we are studying, this expands to

$$A \sim \tfrac{1}{2}\big[s + \varepsilon_{1x}(-s) + \varepsilon_{1y}(r-1) + \varepsilon_{2x}(s) + \varepsilon_{2y}(-r) + \varepsilon_{3y}\big].$$

$$(5.5.1)$$

(Notice there is no contribution from ε_{3x}. Shearing the third vertex of this triangle parallel to the baseline does not change its area, up through terms linear in the amount of shear.)

Again, up to a factor of σ^2, because the ε's are independent and identically distributed, the covariances expected between this quantity and the shape coordinates (ν_1, ν_2) are just sums of products of corresponding coefficients of the ε's:

$$\sigma^{-2}\text{cov}(A, \nu_1) = (-s)(r-1) + (-s)(r-1) + s(-r) + (-r)s$$
$$= s(2 - 4r),$$
$$\sigma^{-2}\text{cov}(A, \nu_2) = r^2 + (r-1)^2 - 2s^2 + 1.$$

There is only one triangular shape for which these covariances are both zero: that for which $r = .5$ and $s^2 = \frac{3}{4}$. These are the equilateral triangles erected upon the baseline. For them, the symmetric shape measures, like perimeter^2/area, have no gradient direction (recall Section 5.1.3). Otherwise, *area* has covariances with shape, on the null model, for every other triangle. Notice that there is no relationship between these covariances and those for baseline length, even though area goes as baseline length times height; matters are not *that* simple.

5.5.2. The size measure we seek is Centroid Size

We could proceed in this vein to check other familiar measures (perimeter, height above baseline, etc.), but we would always discover the same phenomenon: Whatever familiar size measure you choose, under the null model of landmark variation by independent error on each original coordinate, its covariances with the shape coordinates (ν_1, ν_2) are both zero only for a very few mean triangular forms. That is, in the presence of circular normal landmark errors, most size measures cannot be used to test for dependence of shape on size or shape change on size change. In fact, the two covariances are guaranteed to be zero *regardless* of the mean form, and thus are guaranteed not to mislead about allometry, only for one somewhat unfamiliar measure of size. A geometric argument why this should be so (i.e., why there should be only one) may be found in Chapter 2 of Bookstein et al. (1985). [That there is *at most* one is already a consequence of Mosimann's theorem (1970) about independence of size $g(\mathbf{X})$ and shape vectors $\mathbf{X}/g(\mathbf{X})$.]

Here, for the sake of variety, we arrive at the same conclusion instead by an algebraic procedure counting degrees of freedom, as follows: I shall refer to "coefficients" for expansions of changes in size as the sum of multiples of the six ε's, the errors at the landmarks separately coordinate by coordinate. We begin with six degrees of freedom – all the sets of coefficients for the six ε's. Shifting each landmark horizontally by the same amount does not change size, so the net coefficient of $\varepsilon_{1x} + \varepsilon_{2x} + \varepsilon_{3x}$ must be zero; likewise that for $\varepsilon_{1y} + \varepsilon_{2y} + \varepsilon_{3y}$; likewise that for small *rotations* of the configuration, which may be taken to be the restriction $\varepsilon_{2y} - s\varepsilon_{3x} + r\varepsilon_{3y} = 0$ corresponding to rotation about $(0, 0)$. That leaves three degrees of freedom for the set of linear parts of size variables. Specifying zero covariance with (ν_1, ν_2), however, has placed two further independent homogeneous linear constraints upon these remaining dimensions – constraints whose coefficients are just those in equations (5.3.1). There is only one direction left, one pattern of coefficients; it represents the collection of multiples of some single size variable, essentially the only one meeting our requirements.

The single size variable that meets these requirements is, perhaps surprisingly, not a complicated function of the shape of the triangle. It has already been introduced, both for triangles of landmarks and for the general configuration of K landmarks, in Section 4.1. This is the variable called **Centroid Size**, which is the root-summed-squared set of interlandmark distances. That discussion presented three alternate characterizations of this same quantity: the root-summed-squared distance of all the landmarks from their center of gravity case by case; the sum of squares of the principal axes of the landmark scatter considered, again, for each configuration separately; and the average of the interlandmark distances when each is weighted by its own mean length.

> **On the null model, the size variable uncorrelated with all shape coordinates, and hence all ratios of homologously measured lengths, is Centroid Size.**

As usual, I shall supply multiple demonstrations of this crucial fact: one more geometric, the other more algebraic.

5.5.2.1. *Geometric derivation for a single triangle.* —

We saw that the covariance of shape coordinates with baseline length could be expressed as σ^{-2} times the vector $(1 - 2r, -2s)$ $= -2[(r, s) - (\frac{1}{2}, 0)]$ relating the third vertex to the midpoint of the baseline. If we could find some combination of side lengths for which the sum of the vectors corresponding to these covariances was zero, that would achieve our goal of zero covariance between that length measure and all the variables spanned by the shape-coordinate plane.

Now (Figure 5.5.2) each vector representing covariance of the shape coordinates (ν_1, ν_2) with baseline length corresponds to just double the **median vector** of the triangle from the movable vertex to the midpoint of the baseline. Written as ordinary vectors, these directions are $\frac{1}{2}(B + C) - A$, $\frac{1}{2}(C + A) - B$, and $\frac{1}{2}(A + B) - C$.

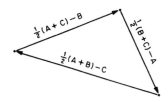

Figure 5.5.2. Diagram for the synthetic derivation of shape-free size (summed-squared edge lengths) for triangles under the null model. The vector covariance of shape with each side of the triangle is proportional to the median line to that side; but the vector sum of these is zero. That vector sum corresponds to the covariance of shape space with Centroid Size.

172

Clearly their sum is zero. To make these vectors into covariances, we had to normalize each baseline length to the same unit (we set $b = 1$ in Section 5.5.1). That is, the median vector is proportional to the covariance of edge length times that mean of that same edge length. Undoing the normalizations, then, so as to make the covariances back into median vectors, we have the following equation on 2-vectors:

$$\begin{bmatrix} 0 \\ 0 \end{bmatrix} = \left[\tfrac{1}{2}(B + C) - A\right] + \left[\tfrac{1}{2}(C + A) - B\right] + \left[\tfrac{1}{2}(A + B) - C\right]$$

$$= \tfrac{1}{2}\sigma^{-2}\left[|BC|\mathrm{cov}\left(|BC|, \begin{bmatrix} \nu_1 \\ \nu_2 \end{bmatrix}\right) + |AC|\mathrm{cov}\left(|AC|, \begin{bmatrix} \nu_1 \\ \nu_2 \end{bmatrix}\right)\right.$$

$$\left. + |AB|\mathrm{cov}\left(|AB|, \begin{bmatrix} \nu_1 \\ \nu_2 \end{bmatrix}\right)\right]$$

$$= \tfrac{1}{4}\sigma^{-2}\mathrm{cov}\left(|BC|^2 + |AC|^2 + |AB|^2, \begin{bmatrix} \nu_1 \\ \nu_2 \end{bmatrix}\right),$$

for small variations of $|AB|$, $|AC|$, and $|BC|$. (The notation $|AB|$ means "length of segment AB"; recall $\Delta|AB|^2 \sim 2|AB|\,\Delta|AB|$, etc.)

Hence the size variable we seek, the variable having zero covariance with both shape coordinates (and thus all shape variables) for triangles of any shape, is the sum of the sides of the triangle, each weighted by its own mean length. But this is equivalent to the sum of the squares of the sides of the triangle or any of its linearly equivalent reformulations (Section 4.1), of which Centroid Size is the simplest to phrase.

5.5.2.2. *Algebraic verification for a single triangle.* —

This result can be checked, somewhat tediously, by the linear algebra of the ε's that we used to show why other size variables did not work. Using that notation, by simple expansion of squares of sums we find the change in the length of a side corresponding to the perturbations of mean landmark positions $(0, 0)$, $(1, 0)$, and (r, s) by vectors $(\varepsilon_{1x}, \varepsilon_{1y})$, and so forth, to be (ignoring squares of ε's) the sum of terms

$$\Delta|AB|^2 + \Delta|AC|^2 + \Delta|BC|^2$$

$$= 2(\varepsilon_{2x} - \varepsilon_{1x}) + 2\left[r(\varepsilon_{3x} - \varepsilon_{1x}) + s(\varepsilon_{3y} - \varepsilon_{1y})\right]$$

$$+ 2\left[(r - 1)(\varepsilon_{3x} - \varepsilon_{2x}) + s(\varepsilon_{3y} - \varepsilon_{2y})\right].$$

Collecting terms, this is, up to a factor of 2, the form

$$\tfrac{1}{2}\Delta p^2 \sim \varepsilon_{1x}(-r - 1) + \varepsilon_{1y}(-s) + \varepsilon_{2x}(2 - r)$$

$$+ \varepsilon_{2y}(-s) + \varepsilon_{3x}(2r - 1) + \varepsilon_{3y}(2s). \qquad (5.5.2)$$

5.5. Size and shape

We may check that it is indeed a size variable – the coefficients of the three x-displacements total zero, as do those of the y-displacements, and the linear form corresponding to rotations – and that the summed product of its coefficients by those of the shape coordinates ν_1 and ν_2 [equations (5.3.1)] are exactly zero.

When the mean triangle is equilateral, all edges have the same weight in the formula for Centroid Size. In that case, and only in that case, is this preferred size variable equivalent to perimeter (and also to area and the other symmetric measures). The farther from equilateral is the triangle, the less symmetrically the landmarks contribute to Centroid Size, as each vertex is weighted by the vector sum of the two sides through it.

In 1984 I developed this theorem by a route much more difficult than either of these. I enumerated the five constraints on the coefficients of the six ε's, produced by straight matrix algebra the single linear combination (5.5.2) orthogonal to them all, and then recognized it as the combination of the edge lengths with each taken proportional to its own mean length. Surely it is much easier to verify this orthogonality than to discover it.

5.5.2.3. Proof in the general case. —

The foregoing proposition generalizes verbatim to the case of arbitrarily many landmarks; the generalization has already been set forth in the preceding text box. Because the space of shape variables is spanned by the linear projections of the shape-coordinate pairs dQ in various directions, it is sufficient to show that on the null model the covariance of Centroid Size with any shape-coordinate pair is the zero vector. The proof is a simple extension of the preceding development. We use the characterization of Centroid Size, for any configuration of landmarks, as the second moment of inertia about the centroid. Fixing one triangle the covariances of the shape coordinates of which are at issue, we decompose Centroid Size into three components (Figure 5.5.3): the moment of the triangle itself about its own centroid (its own quadratic Centroid Size), the moment of the other landmarks about their common centroid, and the moment of the two partial centroids (each weighted by its own landmark count) about each other. We know that the triangle's Centroid Size is uncorrelated with its own shape coordinates, and on the null model both the Centroid Size of the remaining landmarks and the separation of the two partial centroids are independent of the shape of the landmarks of the triangle; hence the shape coordinates of the triangle are independent of the Centroid Size of any number of landmarks, as was to be proved. A considerably longer proof of the same proposition using conventional algebraic notation may be found in Bookstein (1986a).

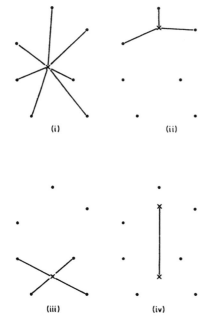

(i)   (ii)

(iii)   (iv)

Figure 5.5.3. Proof in a typical case of more than three landmarks. Centroid Size, the sum of the squared distances in (i), is equal to the sum of the squared distances in (ii) and (iii) together with 12 (3×4) times the squared distance in (iv). The only component of Centroid Size that could be correlated with the shape coordinates of a triangle of landmarks is the Centroid Size of the triangle itself (ii), but we just proved that that correlation was zero.

174

For sets of four or more landmarks, one can disentangle variances of noise imputed at the landmarks separately, still under the assumptions of independence and circularity (Section 5.3.1, last paragraph). The algebra of the preceding proof still goes through if Centroid Size is replaced by a new combination of summed-squared distances from the centroid after weighting each landmark inversely to its noise. Alternatively, one may take summed-squared distance with respect to a weighted centroid.

5.5.3. A single test for allometry

We now have a model generating a distribution for shape and a size measure uncorrelated with (indeed, independent of) shape. On the null model, there is no correlation between Centroid Size and the space of shape coordinates for arbitrarily many landmarks. But we can *observe* those covariances for any set of shape variables; they might or might not actually be zero. It is easy to convert this observation into a **test for allometry**: more specifically, a test capable of rejecting the null model in favor of one in which shape depends on size even in the presence of those independent errors around the mean landmark coordinates. The idea is to specify the effect of size as "something linear" in shape space, and allow measurement or developmental errors to be distributed around that linear "prediction." By the theorems earlier in this chapter, the meaning of "something linear" does not depend on the basis of shape coordinates we choose to use; thus the test avoids the need for specifying any particular shape variables in advance. Such a test is the ordinary multivariate statistical test for independence between the single variable that is Centroid Size and any basis vector for the space of shape variables – any set of sufficiently many shape variables. On the multivariate normal model, as is often appropriate for small variations in the range of sample shapes, a suitable test for this procedure is the usual F-test for the multiple regression of Centroid Size upon the list of shape coordinates. Hence:

> **On the assumption of circular landmark location errors, of the same variance at all landmarks, the existence of any aspect of shape depending allometrically upon size is tested unambiguously by the multiple regression of Centroid Size upon any basis of shape coordinates.** *Warning*: **Allometry found to be significant is not necessarily described by the coefficients of this regression!**

175

The demonstration of zero covariances between any of these size measures and the shape coordinates relies on the linearization of analytic relationships between the shape coordinates and the differential of size. Such a manipulation is less risky over substantial size ranges if Centroid Size is taken with linear dimension, using the value $\sqrt{p^2}$ (the root mean square of the axes of the second-order moment matrix case by case), or perhaps if it is rendered dimensionless by a transformation to the logarithm, as is suggested by Sampson (1986). But this is not the same variable as log General Size in Section 4.3.

Examples of the testing of size allometry by this procedure will be put off until Section 6.5, by which time the machinery will be in place for interpreting rejection of the null model.

5.5.4. Choosing a size variable for describing pure size change

The criterion of covariance between size and shape under the null model is relevant to the power of size variables for detecting group size differences even if the groups have the same mean shapes. That is, even in the absence of mean shape differences between groups, in the presence of shape noise it matters what size variable one chooses. Recourse to Centroid Size for such comparisons usually will increase the precision of the comparisons.

Let us suppose that the tests of group shape difference in Section 5.4 fail to reject the hypothesis of no mean difference in shape. Suppose, further, that this hypothesis remains rejected when mean differences are tested in a multivariate analysis of covariance that adjusts also for any shared allometry the data may show – that there is no shape difference between the groups even adjusting for any size differences between them. In that case, the statistics inform us, size change between the groups must be taken to be at the same ratio for whatever choice of a size variable we may adopt. But what size variable shall we choose in order to best estimate this ratio? Although there is no systematic shape *difference*, by supposition, there is nevertheless much shape *variation* within each group separately. Different size variables will tap this remaining within-group noise to different extents. Is there an optimal choice for the testing of size differences between groups under the assumption of no within-group factors, only independent, identically distributed (i.i.d.) normal noise at each landmark location?

To illustrate the comparative power of different choices of a size variable, it will be convenient to make reference to a simulated example (Figure 5.5.4). Consider two populations, each of $N = 17$ cases, shaped, on the average, like isosceles right triangles. Suppose the two populations differ by 10% in scale, and that within each population shape variation goes as our circular nor-

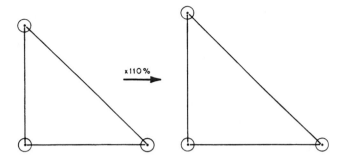

Figure 5.5.4. Simulation for computing the power of alternate size measures in the absence of shape change.

mal model of i.i.d. perturbations at each landmark separately, with standard deviation σ equal to 0.10 of the length of the equal sides of the smaller triangle.

Suppose we measure size as baseline length. The average on the left is 1.0, on the right, 1.1; the difference is 0.10. The standard error of this quantity is derived from the standard deviation of that length within groups by the ordinary one-dimensional formulas. In this simulation, using the notation of Section 5.3.1, the differential of baseline length is expressed in terms of the ε's as $\varepsilon_{2x} - \varepsilon_{1x}$, having standard deviation $\sigma\sqrt{2}$ within each sample and a net standard error for the difference between samples of

$$\left[2\sigma^2\left(\tfrac{1}{16} + \tfrac{1}{16}\right)\right]^{1/2} = 0.05.$$

Then the size difference between the populations is tested by a t-ratio of $0.10/0.05 = 2.0$ on 32 degrees of freedom.

Suppose, instead, we measure size by area. Ignoring contributions from terms in products of ε's, the mean area on the left is 0.50, on the right, 0.605; the difference is 0.105, just about the same as the difference in baseline length. Recall from Section 5.5.1 the expression for area in terms of the ε's:

$$A \sim \tfrac{1}{2}\left[s + \varepsilon_{1x}(-s) + \varepsilon_{1y}(r - 1) + \varepsilon_{2x}(s) + \varepsilon_{2y}(-r) + \varepsilon_{3y}\right].$$

In this simulation the mean shape (r, s) has been set to $(0, 1)$. Within samples, because the ε's are independent, the variance of A is σ^2 times the sum of squares of its coefficients: $\mathrm{var}(A) = [1^2 + 0^2 + 1^2 + (-1)^2 + 1^2]\sigma^2/4 = \sigma^2$. This is just *half* the variance $2\sigma^2$ of baseline length for the same mean change 0.10 of size, and so it will lead to a t-test for size change of 2.83, which is, of course, quite a bit more definitive.

We added information from two other pairs of ε's in the formula for area, but gained a factor of only 2 in the square of the t-ratio. This is because the size variable Area is still correlated with shape for this triangle, and so its test is inefficient by virtue of expressing that variation, which we know (by assumption) to be irrelevant.

177

Now suppose we measure size as Centroid Size p^2, the sum of the squares of the sides for this triangle. Ignoring terms in the squares of the ε's, the mean value of p^2 is 4 on the left, 4.84 on the right, for a difference of 0.84. The expression of the differential of p^2 in terms of the ε's, equation (5.5.3), had coefficients twice each of $-r-1$, $-s$, $2-r$, $-s$, $2r-1$, and $2s$. For $r = 0$, $s = 1$, the squares of these total 48. This t is larger than that for baseline length by a factor of $8/\sqrt{24}$, about 1.63; the test statistic is now about 3.25 for the same data set that previously showed a t of 2.0 *for the same size difference*. We are now exploiting the full power of the degree of freedom associated with size.

Not only in this instance, but in general, Centroid Size is the most powerful size variable to use for size comparisons on the null model for shape variation within group once the hypothesis of shape difference is rejected. The test using Centroid Size is the test of a mean difference adjusted for shape (a multiple-regression coefficient partialed on shape) rather than a test of mean size difference per se. Shape variation, *significant or not*, has been removed from Centroid Size before the testing; it has not been removed so from any edge length or from area. Thus the formula for Centroid Size combines the information from all the landmarks of the triangle, or more general configuration, with the greatest efficiency, on our null model, for the estimation of size change presuming the (previously tested) absence of shape change.

5.6. KENDALL'S SHAPE SPACE

A goodly proportion of the modern multivariate statistical method arose in response to questions about biological size and shape data. The *locus classicus* of discriminant-function analysis, for instance, is Fisher's study of four measurements upon irises, and Sewall Wright invented least-squares factor analysis for his studies of Leghorn chickens in the 1920s. The place of these analyses within the conventional multivariate tool kit is part of the standard textbook syllabus. There the apprentice biometrician is urged more or less automatically to consider size and shape as a matter of size variables such as measured distances, or shape variables such as size ratios, and to write down models for their joint distribution. In this spirit, Chapter 4 began with the space of homologous distances for a set of landmarks, and the earlier sections of this chapter characterized the corresponding shape variables via their ratios. The shape coordinates serve as a device for making this particular style of multivariate analysis as efficient as possible.

There is another statistical embedding of morphometric questions relating them to a remarkably different set of cousins. A set of landmark locations has a shape that the shape coordinates describe by a variety of ratios. But the set of locations is also a single configuration with respect to which other configurations are more or less "nearby." In this alternative statistical context, any shape of a set of landmarks is a single point in a shape space of appropriate structure. Analysis could proceed by direct reference to natural descriptions of such a space, such as "shape distance," rather than by recourse to any set of shape variables undergoing multivariate maneuvers of the more familiar biometric form.

The principal initiatives in this area have been David Kendall's. Beginning in the middle 1970s, he has systematically pursued problems in the global statistical geometry of shapes generated by data that typically are not landmark-related at all: locations of "standing stones" near Land's End, Cornwall, for instance, or quasars on astronomical photographs. Of such shapes of point sets, usually not consisting of landmarks, one can ask questions quite different from those to which we are accustomed. For example, are there "too many collinearities" of the points in sets of three? And do points appear to have been located independently of their neighbors, or is there some evidence of local patterning?

The two approaches to shape, via variables and via equivalence classes, came into contact when Kendall commented on my construction of the tie between the multivariate and the deformational approaches (Kendall, 1986). He pointed out that my coordinates in effect lived in a tangent plane touching his shape space in the vicinity of the mean form. Since the publication of that comment there has emerged a collection of statistical developments tying landmark data to this rather distinctive alternative to "conventional" multivariate biometrics.

In this section I shall attempt to explain this newer statistical approach to landmark data and its relation to the biometric themes emphasized in this book. There is less convergence than most of us in the field would wish. While there are some intriguing similarities of approach, notably in the matter of tests for group differences in form, the two contexts do not really support analyses in the same spirit. The approach in Kendall's style is far more elegant mathematically and is geometrically "global," concerned with differential geometry, whereas the methods of this book are all "flat." But approaches after the style of Kendall are too restricted in their choice of distance metric to match many reasonable biological questions and, at present, offer no equivalent to the features of shape comparison, culmination of the shape-coordinate praxis, that will be presented in Chapter 7. Instead, the analyses of these shape manifolds seem tailor-made for applications to large bodies of existing data about point processes having nothing to do with biological landmarks – points on maps, on the celestial sphere, and the like. Small (1988) reviews the Kendall approach with an eye toward its breadth of applications outside biometrics, concluding, as I do, that the incompatibility with research into what determines landmark locations is profound and worrisome. Goodall and Lange (1990) seem more optimistic.

The discussion that follows is no substitute for studying Goodall (1991), Kendall (1984, 1986, 1989), or Mardia and Dryden (1989*a,b*). The Kendall approach to shape studies is substantially more mathematical than are biometric techniques; I have not contributed to it; and I am not capable of explaining it in words that are solely my own. The following comments derive in great part from the papers presented by Ian Dryden, Colin Goodall, John Kent, and Kanti Mardia at the Workshop on Shape Theory organized by Goodall at Princeton in April of 1990. These four should be considered unindicted coauthors of this section, responsible (along with David Kendall) for everything that might be correct here. The discussion to follow is needed later in this book in connection with the discussion of Procrustes superpositions (Section 7.1) and in the course of explaining and justifying the principal warps and relative warps (Sections 7.5 and 7.6).

5.6.1. Shapes as equivalence classes

In the introduction to this chapter I mentioned two feasible approaches to the statistical characterization of shape. One approach adumbrates shape via its direct measurements, which (for landmark data) are essentially ratios of size variables; the other approach, encountered more often in geometrical than in statistical argument, defines shape as the information remaining in a configuration of landmarks once information about position, orientation, and scale is discarded. The shape-coordinate formalism presented thus far in this chapter is a systematic attempt to realize the statistics of landmark shapes according to the *former* definition. Kendall's approach begins instead with the latter characterization.

Consider any set of K points $\{X_i\}$ in m-dimensional Euclidean space. (In our applications, these will of course be the landmarks.) This discussion will be restricted to the case $m = 2$, the Euclidean plane, where the mathematical similarities between the two approaches are greatest. To construct the classes of $\{X_i\}$ equivalent up to position, scale, and rotation, it is sufficient (though not necessary) to produce representatives of each class for which the requisite transformations have been undone. Standardizing position is easy: Put the centroid at $(0, 0)$. Rescaling is likewise simple: Put Centroid Size equal to 1. (Section 5.5 argued a preference for Centroid Size based on its orthogonality to shape under a certain model; in the Kendall approach its choice is predicated instead on a certain crucial metric to be introduced presently.) There results what Kendall, Goodall, and others call a "pre-shape," a point on what may be imagined a "sphere" of $m \times (K - 1)$ matrices all having unit "length." Finally, we must correct for the *rotation* of forms (for two-dimensional data, this is just one circle's worth of ambiguity). The space that the rest of us call "Kendall's shape space," which he denotes Σ_2^K, is the set of equivalence classes on

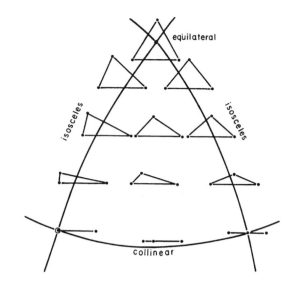

Figure 5.6.1. Kendall's spherical blackboard for the shape manifold Σ_2^3, with some typical triangular shapes.

the preshape sphere with respect to these rotations. Because for $m = 2$ these spaces have no singularities, they have also been called shape *manifolds*.

The resulting construction is most legible for $K = 3$, the case of triangles of points in the plane. This space Σ_2^3 of triangular shapes is mathematically equivalent to an ordinary sphere. [This might have been guessed already, as the set of ratios $(Z_3 - Z_1)/(Z_2 - Z_1)$ represents the complex projective line $\mathbf{CP}^1$, which maps onto a sphere stereographically; but there was really no reason to suspect it had the correct metric geometry.] Figure 5.6.1 shows one-twelfth of this sphere, which Kendall calls his "spherical blackboard." The tie between this sphere and the plane of shape coordinates is quite direct: My shape coordinates represent the tangent plane to this sphere in the vicinity of the mean form. Restricting the sphere to the part covered by this blackboard presumes that we are free to relabel the vertices of the triangle or replace it by its mirror image as appropriate. Shape coordinates for the same triangle to different baselines represent different bases spanning this same tangent plane at the same point of the blackboard.

As I explained, Kendall typically refers to this sphere not to ask questions about mean forms but for more general investigations into distributions of triangular (and higher-order) shapes. One can ask, for instance, if point sets are more nearly collinear than might be expected on a suitable null model, as well as whether or not they concentrate at a mean shape, and so on. To ask such questions, one must begin with a suitable reference distribution for what is "expected." Kendall noted early on the happy property that if points are generated independently and identically on the Euclidean plane according to a circular normal distribution (of any variance), then the induced distribution of shapes on the

181

shape sphere is *uniform*! (Of course, our landmarks are not identically distributed in this sense; they have different means.) Hence visible clusters of points on the spherical blackboard represent modal types of shapes, visible concentration upon the "equator" represents a preponderance of collinearities, and the like.

5.6.2. The metric geometry of shape space

In Kendall's shape space, the mention of Centroid Size is not accidental. It was chosen to scale representatives of shape classes because it serves as denominator for an important construction, *geodesic distance*. For any set of landmarks $\{X_i\}$ in the original Euclidean plane, we can imagine the set of shapes derived by holding all but one of the X's at fixed position and varying that one in a circle about its original position. We would like the metric assigned to shape space (the set of "shapes" of all such sets of X's, correcting for centroid, orientation, and scale, all of which usually change whenever one of the X's moves) to be such that the shapes generated by circles in the original landmark plane are all at the same distance from the original shape $\{X_i\}$ in the shape space. That is, to a circle around one landmark in data space should correspond something very nearly a circle in shape space. In this way, the geometry of shape space will be a "Riemannian submersion" of the original Euclidean geometry. In particular, "shortest distances" between pairs of shapes, *as long as they do not involve recentering, rotation, or rescaling*, will be shortest whether viewed in shape space or in the original Euclidean data plane; these are often referred to as "horizontal geodesics." Kendall (1984) showed (it is not so simple) that if distance ρ is taken as a sort of complex correlation between centered shapes $\{w_i\}$ and $\{z_i\}$ according to

$$\cos^2\rho = \frac{\Sigma w_i z_i^C \Sigma w_i^C z_i}{\Sigma w_i w_i^C \Sigma z_i z_i^C}, \qquad (5.6.1)$$

then the shape space is an appropriate submersion of the original Euclidean geometry. (The notation ^{C} here stands for complex conjugation, reflection in the real axis.) The denominator of this formula is the product of the two Centroid Sizes of the landmark configurations separately. That is, Centroid Size is the size variable geometrically "orthogonal" to shape distance in Kendall's space, just as it was the size variable statistically "orthogonal" to shape variation in the shape-coordinate plane. We shall encounter this measure of distance again in discussions of Procrustes superposition (Section 7.1). It is often called *Procrustes distance*, after the Greek robber who modified the sizes of his "guests" to fit his bed (which, of course, had unit Centroid Size). The advantage of formula (5.6.1) is that the requisite rotation that must be partialed from the landmark configurations in order to get to shape actually cancels out of the formula. Written in terms of centered landmarks, it actually applies to their equivalence classes – their shapes – explicitly. Put another way: It is unnecessary to superimpose two forms to compute how far apart they are at closest superposition.

A crucial property of the shape spaces Σ_2^K, unfortunately not true of shape on point sets in three or more dimensions, is their **homogeneity**. Whatever the number of landmarks in two dimensions, the geometry of shape variation is the same at every shape, just like the symmetry of the "spherical blackboard" Σ_2^3 in the figure. This is equivalent to stating that the technology of shape statistics for group differences in two dimensions does not depend on the shape of the mean form. I am indebted for my understanding of this point to John Kent.

5.6.3. The Mardia–Dryden distribution of Bookstein shape coordinates

The distribution of the shape coordinates for triangles under a null model of circular normal noise at each vertex (Section 5.3) was an approximation only, ignoring all terms of order greater than 1 in the ε's. The dependence of this approximation upon baseline is the topic of Appendix A.2.2. But nowhere in that presentation is there any estimate of the "error" of the approximation for a fixed baseline; I was not able to calibrate that error. Almost as soon as my 1986 article came to his attention, Kanti Mardia and his student Ian Dryden realized that certain tricks familiar to the more mathematical multivariate statistician (but not to me) could be wielded to produce that distribution *in closed form*, indeed, as an almost simple formula. The answer, with an associated method of maximum-likelihood estimation, appeared in Mardia and Dryden (1989a,b). The only change of notation from that in this book is the subtraction of 0.5 from the first shape coordinate, v_1, in order to render the baseline symmetric around the y-axis. This corresponds to using a baseline from $(-0.5, 0)$ to $(0.5, 0)$, or, equivalently, to shape coordinates

$$(U_k, V_k) = \frac{Z_k - (Z_1 + Z_2)/2}{Z_2 - Z_1}$$

for multiple landmarks $k = 3, \ldots, K$. These are called the **Bookstein shape coordinates** (Mardia and Dryden named them, not me!); their distribution, the **Mardia–Dryden distribution** for landmark locations varying by noise of variance σ^2 about a mean shape Θ with baseline length 1 in the Euclidean plane, is written $\mathcal{B}_{2K-4}(\Theta, \sigma^2)$. The character $\mathcal{B}$, I acknowledge with some astonishment, stands for "Bookstein." The following exegesis of the Mardia–Dryden distribution is taken from Goodall (1991).

183

5.6. Kendall's shape space

The homogeneity of the shape spaces Σ_2^K, already referred to, means that one can "rotate" the whole shape space to a configuration in which one of the landmarks has expected position $(1, 0)$ while all the others vary about $(0, 0)$. This "rotation," an *isometry of the shape sphere*, is not related to the rotation of landmark locations partialed out in the course of constructing a single shape; instead, it "rotates" the landmark means in such a way as to change apparent shape without changing Procrustes distance between shapes. For a single triangle of landmarks, for instance, this means that we can carry out our shape statistics perfectly well by proceeding as if the mean position of the third landmark lay exactly atop either of the baseline points (Figure 5.6.2). The assertion is closely analogous to the Fisher–Cochran theorem for real-valued sums of squares (Rao, 1973:185), a maneuver that can be used to derive the F-distributions of linear-regression theory. Basically, if a set of landmark coordinates are identically and independently normally distributed, then so is any orthogonal rotation of them. Here, "orthogonality" is in the space $\mathbf{C}^K$ of the full vector of landmarks, not in the plane $\mathbf{R}^2$ of the landmarks separately. There is always a rotation that takes one mean to $(1, 0)$ and the rest to $(0, 0)$. The distribution of the shapes of the null model, after this rotation, can be written as a list of "new" landmarks with independent entries

$$t_1 \sim \mathbf{N}\left(\begin{bmatrix} 1 \\ 0 \end{bmatrix}, \sigma^2\right),$$

$$t_i \sim \mathbf{N}\left(\begin{bmatrix} 0 \\ 0 \end{bmatrix}, \sigma^2\right), \qquad \text{for } i > 1.$$

The centroid has already been partialed out by the first column of the rotation [i.e., the rotation is a Helmert matrix (Mardia et al., 1979)].

There remains the question of what distribution this yields in shape space. The Procrustes distance of this shape $\{t_i\}$ from the mean is, by formula (5.6.1), $\cos^2\rho = t_{11}^2 / \Sigma\Sigma t_{ij}^2$. On the null model this quantity has a marginal distribution derivable from the original Gaussian circles. Here t_{11}^2, the squared x-coordinate of the first rotated "landmark," is $\chi_1^2(1)$, a noncentral χ^2; all the other terms are ordinary χ_1^2. Then $\cot^2\rho$ has numerator and denominator independent and can be recognized as a noncentral F. Because the Riemannian submersion is homogeneous, and because of the original symmetries of the model, this converts to an expression for the distribution of the shape coordinates per se as this probability is distributed uniformly over circular shells of varying Procrustes radius on Kendall's spherical blackboard (the case $K = 3$) or its generalization to more than three landmarks. Goodall and Mardia (1990) assure the reader that its expansion in

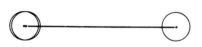

Figure 5.6.2. The "standard triangle" for representing the exact distribution of the shape coordinates about any mean form on the null model of i.i.d. Gaussian noise at each landmark; see Goodall and Mardia (1990). The distribution of shapes around any mean triangle is the same as the distribution around this mean triangle. On the null model it is a function of Procrustes distance alone.

184

more familiar functions (cf. Rao, 1973:216) yields the hypergeometric form published in Mardia and Dryden (1989*a*).

5.6.4. Contrast of the two approaches to shape space

In this way the locally linearized geometry of the shape coordinates introduced in this chapter may be viewed as an approximation to the exact analysis of data under the same model (identically distributed circular normal errors at each landmark separately). The preferred role of Centroid Size is unchanged. Then in the limit of either small errors or large samples, all the approximations of this chapter converge to the maximum-likelihood estimates. This entails the asymptotic efficiency of the approximate tests for differences among group mean shapes, to any baseline, and also of the tests for allometry (because Centroid Size preserves its characterization in the linearization of the shape-coordinate statistics).

But the testing of mean differences, and the computation of regressions of size upon shape, is not all of morphometrics. I therefore close this discussion of the ties between Kendall's shape space and mine with a **warning**: The Procrustes geometry of Kendall's space, which seems indeed natural for questions about unlabeled point configurations, is not necessarily appropriate to process-oriented biometrical questions.

The mathematical elegance of Kendall's space arises from its homogeneity, the fact that at a certain level the statistics of all mean landmark configurations are "the same": not the *methods*, mind you, but the actual *statistics*. It is that very homogeneity of Kendall's space, the presence of a sphere of equivalent directions of shape variation at every point of the space, that is the crux of the biometrical difficulty. Chapter 7 of this volume will be devoted to "features of shape comparison," preferred subspaces of shape space that house biological explanations of different types. One subspace, for instance, includes only the uniform transformations, those that are the same for every landmark triangle; others include particular sorts of gradients of change. These spaces have metrics of their own that arise from natural aspects of the explanations to which findings there are put; *and these metrics are not the same as the Procrustes metric, equation (5.6.1), that applies isotropically everywhere in Kendall's space.* For the computation of means, the difference between these metrics does not matter, at least asymptotically. But for the computation of regressions, principal components, factors, and other aspects of the *variability* of shape, different metrics lead to different findings. We shall see, in fact, that to extract biologically meaningful features of shape difference or shape change from a landmark data set requires reference to two completely different metrics, anisotropy and bending energy, and these are not only separate (applying to

185

complementary subspaces of shape space) but also formally incommensurate, not interconvertible by any sort of ratio.

Chapter 6, for instance, will derive one of these "natural" metrics, the one for comparing nondegenerate triangles (and, by extension, for comparing the uniform parts of nonuniform changes) in which distance is proportional to the logarithm of the greatest ratio of strains required to change one form into the other by a uniform shear. In a small vicinity of a mean form, this distance is approximately proportional to Kendall's; but over larger regions it "bends" the geometry. (The relation between these two "distances" is discussed at length in Appendix A.2.) The results of regression or principal-component analysis involving the shape of a configuration of landmarks will depend on the distance criterion (of an observed configuration from the configuration predicted by the regression or by the first-component score) for which the sum of squares is to be a minimum. It is the very elegance of the geometry of Kendall's space that interferes with the pursuit of biological explanations whenever those explanations would require a breaking of the strong symmetries underlying the geometry. This is no criticism of Kendall's own work, which has studiously avoided biological applications. The notion of uniform transformations, for instance, seems irrelevant to questions about standing stones in Cornwall. But in morphometric applications, wherein biological processes exist and account for landmark changes at different scales, it is proper to be somewhat suspicious of a statistical distribution that (Figure 5.6.2) permits us to rearrange our mean landmarks arbitrarily on the page without changing the structure by which the findings are reported.

Kendall (1984:98), in the course of introducing his spherical blackboard, claims that "for most practical and theoretical purposes the labeling of the vertices is unimportant." This unintentionally parochial statement may be read instead as the equivalent of my warning: If the labeling of vertices is important, Kendall's methods may not be helpful. For biological applications, it *does* matter what the spacing of the landmarks is, and it *does* matter where structures start and end and where forces, real or metaphorical, impinge. When the structure of Kendall's spaces is extended to incorporate the requisite degree of identity of landmarks, correlation between displacements at different landmarks, and differences in landmark-specific variability (Goodall, 1991; Mardia and Dryden, 1990), the gains in elegance (such as the language of "geodesics") are lost. In biometrics, the elegance of Kendall's shape spaces is likely to contribute far more to mathematical foundations than to practical analysis of real data for the discovery of real explanations. The spaces encompass one of the most beautiful matches of pure geometry to problems in applied statistics that I have ever seen. Alas, they are other problems than mine.

6
Principal axes of shape change for triangles

The preceding chapter set forth statistical machinery for unambiguously detecting effects upon shape – group difference, size allometry, covariances with exogenous variables. We showed how a space of shape variables apparently based on an arbitrary choice of triangles and baselines supported multivariate statistical analyses independent of those choices and equivalent to the study of all ratios of size variables as the latter were defined in Chapter 4. But the analysis so far has been carried out in purely statistical language, unrelated to biology and related only weakly even to the geometry that drives this practice. The coefficients in which findings are embodied remain functions of the baseline (or baselines) chosen for shape coordinates even as the statistical testing of those findings is invariant against changes of basis (Section 5.2.3).

This chapter and the next introduce methods for describing shape change in a manner having this same invariance against changes in choices of triangles and shape coordinates. This chapter concentrates on the simplest context of landmark morphometrics, the case of a single triangle. We shall be introducing the reporting of shape change by **symmetric tensors**, a report having precisely the requisite independence. We shall emphasize routines by which hints of underlying biological process may be gleaned from its geometry in diverse typical cases. The use of the symmetric tensor as a *universal* preliminary report of change in a single noncollinear triangle is the most important geometric formalism in morphometrics. I shall derive it in two independent languages, the "algebraic version" and the "geometric version," in the hope that the reader will be enlightened first by one or the other derivation and then by their interplay.

Because the next two sections are mostly analytic, it may be useful to precede them by a summary of their biometric implications. The shape coordinates, as the preceding chapter emphasized, make it unnecessary to specify further particular shape variables for landmark analyses. Augmented by only a single size variable, they make unnecessary any explicit reference to the space of homologous distances as well. If this be granted, then we are free to make the specification of particularly useful or suggestive measurements wait upon completion of the statistical analysis. We can generate variables a posteriori by reference to the explanations or effects with which they are aligned (e.g., the invariants and covariants of a mean shape change or size allometry, or the long axis of a shape scatter). This chapter shows how to manage this transition for triangles of landmarks. For instance, to any change of mean position in the shape-coordinate plane corresponds one specific ratio of size variables defined on the three landmarks of the pair of triangles. In most cases, this ratio is "close to" (within 15° of, correlated more than .96 with) an even simpler report, an angle, ratio of sides, or aspect ratio of the triangle. Thus the same technology that calibrates the statistical assessment of findings generates a variety of suggestive interpretations.

The core of the argument connecting deformations to variables is found in Section 6.3, on the "naming" of directions in shape space. The argument there depends heavily on the analytic geometry worked out in Sections 6.1 and 6.2. Section 6.4 proves that the technique is "sufficient" (in a useful technical sense) for any number of landmarks. In Section 6.5 this most important style of analysis is demonstrated, as is its application to biological understanding, in several examples drawn from studies in two- and three-dimensional craniofacial growth, in craniofacial anomalies, and in micropaleontology.

6.1. ALGEBRAIC VERSION

This section will show how a uniform mapping of a square into a parallelogram may be reported by a particular pair, usually a unique pair, of directions that are perpendicular both before and after transformation. One of these directions bears the greatest ratio of lengths of corresponding segments from square to parallelogram, the other, the least ratio. These directions are called the principal axes or biorthogonal directions, and the ratios are called principal strains. In this section, all the derivations are by formulas involving Cartesian coordinates of the vertices of the parallelogram.

6.1.1. Square into parallelogram

Consider the transformation (Figure 6.1.1) that takes a square of landmarks on one form into a parallelogram on another. (Landmarks do not usually come in exact squares. In Section 6.2 we shall see that this objection is of no consequence.) As in Section 2.2, we treat this set of four pairs of points as a sample from a homology function to be extended as smoothly as possible, first to

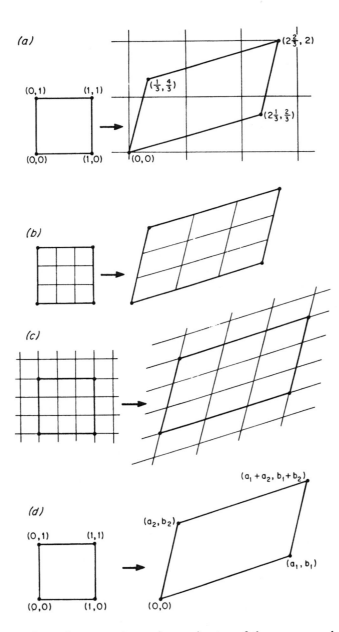

Figure 6.1.1. Mapping of square into parallelogram. (*a*) Landmarks. (*b*) Computed homology. (*c*) Linear extrapolation. (*d*) Cartesian coordinates.

a correspondence between the entire perimeter of the square and that of the parallelogram, then to a *linear* (or *affine*, or *uniform*) mapping of the entire interior of the square onto that of the parallelogram (Figure 6.1.1*b*). To say that the mapping is linear is to assert that it leaves straight lines straight and parallel lines parallel, and preserves proportions along lines. Because of this uniformity, we can extend the mapping unambiguously outside the limits of the original data – **extrapolate** it, in other words, so as to relate the whole plane of the square to that of the parallelogram (Figure 6.1.1*c*).

189

Let us now assign Cartesian coordinates on both planes (Figure 6.1.1*d*) so that the square has sides of length 1. The transformation can then be written linearly, with or without matrix notation:

$$(x, y) = x(1, 0) + y(0, 1) \rightarrow x(a_1, b_1) + y(a_2, b_2)$$
$$= (a_1 x + a_2 y, b_1 x + b_2 y)$$

or

$$(x, y) \rightarrow (x, y) \begin{bmatrix} a_1 & b_1 \\ a_2 & b_2 \end{bmatrix}. \qquad (6.1.1)$$

Explicitly reading the graph paper of Figure 6.1.2*a*, we have, for this example, $a_1 = \frac{7}{3}$, $b_1 = \frac{2}{3}$, $a_2 = \frac{1}{3}$, $b_2 = \frac{4}{3}$.

6.1.2. A parameter for directions

We shall mostly be interested in the effect of this transformation upon distances in different directions. Specifically, we want to be able to write down a formula for the ratio by which distances change under the transformation, direction by direction; we need that formula so that we can set its derivative to zero and so determine the directions in which the ratio is largest or smallest. To handle all this analytically, we need to assign a letter (an algebraic parameter) for directions. One obvious choice is some trigonometric function of the angle between the direction under consideration and the horizontal. (Trig functions are easier to handle than the angles themselves; recall the discussion at the start of Chapter 5.) We shall use the **tangent** of this angle, and denote it by α. The value α can be viewed as the height at which a line passing through the origin $(0, 0)$ and making an angle $\tan^{-1}\alpha$ with the horizontal crosses the vertical line $x = 1$ (Figure 6.1.2*a*). It is also equal to the **slope** of the line in question. The vertical direction gives us the "value" $\alpha = \infty$. We shall recognize this as a special case as necessary. (For instance, it is the value of α with $1/\alpha = 0$.)

Directions that do not cut the right-hand edge of the starting square may be assigned values of α according to the linear extrapolation of Figure 6.1.1*b*. For instance, the direction exiting the square at the point $(\beta, 1)$ of the top edge is assigned the value $\alpha = 1/\beta$ corresponding to the point $(1, 1/\beta)$ at which the extension of that segment cuts the line $x = 1$. The alternate parameter $\beta = 1/\alpha$ is **slope with respect to the (positive) y-axis**.

Using this construction, we can easily determine the relation between the values of α for pairs of lines that are perpendicular. As can be seen in Figure 6.1.2*c*, the perpendicular to the line of parameter α, which leaves the square at the point $(1, \alpha)$, connects the origin to the point $(-\alpha, 1)$, which, extended, intersects the

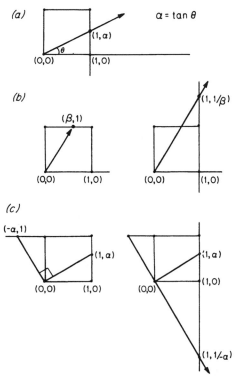

Figure 6.1.2. Describing directions through a point. (*a*) $\alpha = \tan \theta$ is the height at which a line through $(0, 0)$ making an angle θ with the horizontal cuts the vertical $x = 1$. (*b*) Lines that cut $x = 1$ outside the starting square are assigned values of α according to the linear extrapolation of Figure 6.1.1c. (*c*) Perpendicular lines have α's that are negative reciprocals.

vertical $x = 1$ at the point $(1, \gamma)$, with $\gamma = -1/\alpha$. The dot product of these two directions is

$$(1, \alpha) \cdot (1, -1/\alpha) = 1 \cdot 1 + \alpha \cdot (-1/\alpha) = 1 - 1 = 0.$$

[This is a version of the trigonometric identity $\tan(\theta + 90°) = -1/\tan \theta$.]

6.1.3. Extremes of strain: the principal axes

What does the transformation we are talking about do to lengths in the direction associated with α? *Before* transformation, the vector $(1, \alpha)$ had squared length $1 + \alpha^2$. *After* transformation, it is the vector $(a_1 x + a_2 y, b_1 x + b_2 y)$, with $x = 1$ and $y = \alpha$ – the vector $(a_1 + a_2\alpha, b_1 + b_2\alpha)$ having squared length $(a_1 + a_2\alpha)^2 + (b_1 + b_2\alpha)^2$. We wish to investigate the ratio of these, the expression

$$\frac{(a_1 + a_2\alpha)^2 + (b_1 + b_2\alpha)^2}{1 + \alpha^2}. \tag{6.1.2}$$

It is a typical mathematical ploy to characterize a function by locating its *extrema* (maxima and minima). These are among the values of α for which the derivative of the expression (6.1.2) with

191

respect to α is zero. The numerator of this derivative is

$$(1 + \alpha^2)\frac{d}{d\alpha}\Big[(a_1 + a_2\alpha)^2 + (b_1 + b_2\alpha)^2\Big]$$

$$-\Big[(a_1 + a_2\alpha)^2 + (b_1 + b_2\alpha)^2\Big]\frac{d}{d\alpha}(1 + \alpha^2)$$

$$= (1 + \alpha^2)\big[2a_2(a_1 + a_2\alpha) + 2b_2(b_1 + b_2\alpha)\big]$$

$$- 2\alpha\Big[(a_1 + a_2\alpha)^2 + (b_1 + b_2\alpha)^2\Big]$$

$$= \alpha^3\big(2a_2^2 + 2b_2^2 - 2a_2^2 - 2b_2^2\big)$$

$$+ \alpha^2\big[2a_1a_2 + 2b_1b_2 - 2(2a_1a_2 + 2b_1b_2)\big]$$

$$+ \alpha\big(2a_2^2 + 2b_2^2 - 2a_1^2 - 2b_1^2\big) + (2a_1a_2 + 2b_1b_2).$$

The coefficient of the cubic term is zero. Dividing through by -2, we see that the derivative of expression (6.1.2) is zero for α such that

$$\alpha^2(a_1a_2 + b_1b_2) + \alpha\big(a_1^2 - a_2^2 + b_1^2 - b_2^2\big) - (a_1a_2 + b_1b_2) = 0.$$

The quantity (6.1.2) for which we are finding the extrema is called the squared **strain ratio**, ratio of lengths in the parallelogram to the corresponding lengths in the square. The directions along which it is maximized or minimized are called the **principal directions, principal axes,** or **biorthogonal directions** of the strain. We keep the strain ratio squared only to avoid having to take square roots in expressions like (6.1.2); it is easier just to take the square roots of the particular values of strain in which we are interested – these are typically only two.

This is a quadratic equation in α, of a special form: an equation $A\alpha^2 + B\alpha - A = 0$ with the first and the third coefficients opposite. All of the coefficients represent quantities that may be familiar to you. The coefficient B of the linear term is the difference of the squared lengths of the images of adjacent sides of the starting square: the difference between the length $L_1^2 = a_1^2 + b_1^2$ of the image of $(1,0)$ under the transformation, and the length $L_2^2 = a_2^2 + b_2^2$ of the image of $(0,1)$ under the transformation. The coefficients $\pm A$ of the other two terms are plus and minus the dot product of the same two vectors: $(a_1, b_1) \cdot (a_2, b_2) = (a_1a_2 + b_1b_2)$. Call this D. The quadratic equation for α is then

$$D\alpha^2 + \big(L_1^2 - L_2^2\big)\alpha - D = 0. \tag{6.1.3}$$

The product of the two roots of this equation is $-D/D = -1$. The directions the α's of which multiply to -1 are *perpendicular*; so the two principal axes of the strain lie at 90°. Tuck this fact away for a moment.

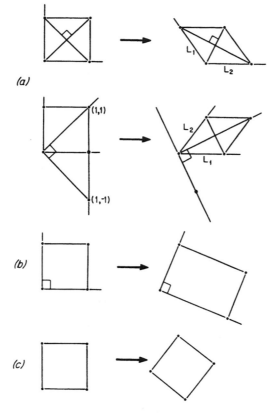

(a)

(b)

(c)

Figure 6.1.3. Special cases of the strain equation. (*a*) $L_1^2 = L_2^2$: square to rhombus. (*b*) $D = 0$: square to rectangle. (*c*) $L_1^2 = L_2^2$ *and* $D = 0$: square to square.

6.1.3.1. Special cases.—

Let us consider some special cases of this scenario.

(*a*) $L_1^2 = L_2^2$ (Figure 6.1.3*a*). The vectors into which the sides of our starting square are taken have equal lengths, so that the transform of a square is a rhombus. The equation for α becomes $D\alpha^2 + 0\alpha - D = 0$, or $\alpha^2 = 1$, $\alpha = \pm 1$. Hence whatever the angle between the sides of the rhombus, and whatever their length, the principal strains are along the vectors $(1, 1)$ and $(1, -1)$, which are the diagonals of the square. The transforms of these segments are the diagonals of the rhombus, which are perpendicular also.

(*b*) $D = 0$ (Figure 6.1.3*b*). The vectors into which the sides of our starting square are taken have dot product zero. In other words, they are perpendicular; the sides of the square are transformed onto the sides of the rectangle. The equation for α becomes $(L_1^2 - L_2^2)\alpha = 0$, which is *linear* and has only the one root $\alpha = 0$ (as long as $L_1^2 \neq L_2^2$).

But if we had use $1/\alpha$ (slope with respect to the *y*-axis) as our parameter instead of α, we would have gotten the quadratic

$$D(1/\alpha)^2 + \left(L_1^2 - L_2^2\right)(1/\alpha) - D = 0,$$

193

which, for $D = 0$, has the root $1/\alpha = 0$ or $\alpha = \infty$. That is, interchanging the role of the x- and y-axes, we see that there are still two principal directions $\alpha = 0$ and $1/\alpha = 0$ corresponding to the x- and y-axes of the square. The mapping transforms them onto the sides of the rectangle, which are themselves perpendicular also.

(c) $D = 0$ *and* $L_1^2 = L_2^2$ (Figure 6.1.3c). In this case the square is transformed into another square. The equation for α becomes

$$0 = 0,$$

so that *all* directions α are extrema of the strain ratio. The transformation has merely rotated and rescaled the original square, leaving it square, without change of shape; change of length in all directions is by the same ratio. We have investigated the statistics of this sort of shape change in Section 5.5.4.

6.1.4. Preservation of perpendiculars

We noticed that the principal axes for the special cases $D = 0$ and $L_1^2 = L_2^2$ are perpendicular after transformation, and we saw that in all cases they were perpendicular *before* transformation (first and last coefficients of the quadratic for α equal and opposite.) Let us ask an ostensibly different question:

> For what sets of perpendicular directions on the square are the image directions likewise perpendicular?

We can write the perpendicular directions on the square by using the pair of directions with parameters α and $-1/\alpha$. These correspond to directions $(a_1 + a_2\alpha, b_1 + b_2\alpha)$ and $(a_1 - a_2/\alpha, b_1 - b_2/\alpha)$ on the parallelogram. We want this pair of directions to be perpendicular: There results the equation

$$(a_1 + a_2\alpha, b_1 + b_2\alpha) \cdot (a_1 - a_2/\alpha, b_1 - b_2/\alpha) = 0$$

or

$$\alpha(a_1 a_2 + b_1 b_2) + (a_1^2 + a_2^2 - b_1^2 - b_2^2) - \alpha^{-1}(a_1 a_2 + b_1 b_2) = 0.$$

Multiplying through by α, we arrive at

$$D\alpha^2 + (L_1^2 - L_2^2)\alpha - D = 0,$$

the same equation we had before. Hence:

> The *principal axes* of greatest and least rate of strain are the same as the *biorthogonal directions* that both start and finish at 90°.

This is the **one crucial fact** of morphometrics. All else (to quote Rabbi Hillel) is commentary.

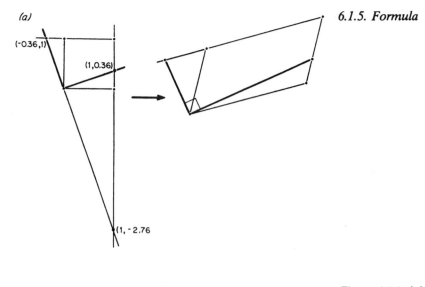

(a)

(-0.36,1)

(1,0.36)

(1, -2.76

6.1.5. Formula

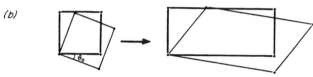

(b)

θ_0

Figure 6.1.4. (*a*) Principal directions of the strain in Figure 6.1.1. (*b*) Interpretation in terms of a new α that is slope to a different "horizontal" (one of the principal strains).

6.1.4.1. Example: Figure 6.1.1.—

In the case of Figure 6.1.1, we had $(a_1, b_1) = (\frac{7}{3}, \frac{2}{3})$ and $(a_2, b_2) = (\frac{1}{3}, \frac{4}{3})$. Then $L_1^2 = \frac{53}{9}$, $L_2^2 = \frac{17}{9}$, and $D = \frac{15}{9} = \frac{5}{3}$. The quadratic for α becomes

$$\tfrac{5}{3}\alpha^2 + \left(\tfrac{53}{9} - \tfrac{17}{9}\right)\alpha - \tfrac{5}{3} = 0$$

or

$$5\alpha^2 + 12\alpha - 5 = 0.$$

Its roots are

$$\frac{-12 \pm \sqrt{12^2 - 4 \cdot 5 \cdot (-5)}}{2 \cdot 5} \sim -2.76, 0.36.$$

These lie upon the square and its image as shown in Figure 6.1.4*a*.

6.1.5. A simpler expression for strain

Because there always exist these **biorthogonal directions**, by changing our parameter from $\alpha = \tan \theta$ to $\alpha = \tan(\theta - \theta_0)$ (where θ_0 is one of these directions), we can guarantee that we are always in special case (*b*) of Section 6.1.3.1: the case $D = 0$. Figure 6.1.4*b* shows the same shape change using this new starting square.

195

From equation (6.1.2), the squared strain in terms of the new α is

$$\left[(a_1 + a_2\alpha)^2 + (b_1 + b_2\alpha)^2\right]/(1 + \alpha^2)$$
$$= \left[(a_1^2 + b_1^2) + 2(a_1a_2 + b_1b_2)\alpha + (a_2^2 + b_2^2)\alpha^2\right]/(1 + \alpha^2)$$
$$= (L_1^2 + 2D\alpha + L_2^2\alpha^2)/(1 + \alpha^2).$$

In this universal "special case," we have $D = 0$. The squared strain is then $(L_1^2 + L_2^2\alpha^2)/(1 + \alpha^2)$. Recalling that $\alpha = \tan(\theta - \theta_0) = \sin(\theta - \theta_0)/\cos(\theta - \theta_0)$, and further recalling that $\sin^2 + \cos^2 = 1$, we see that this simplifies to

$$\left(L_1^2 + L_2^2\frac{\sin^2(\theta - \theta_0)}{\cos^2(\theta - \theta_0)}\right)\Bigg/\left(1 + \frac{\sin^2(\theta - \theta_0)}{\cos^2(\theta - \theta_0)}\right)$$
$$= \left[L_1^2\cos^2(\theta - \theta_0) + L_2^2\sin^2(\theta - \theta_0)\right]/$$
$$\left[\cos^2(\theta - \theta_0) + \sin^2(\theta - \theta_0)\right]$$
$$= L_1^2\cos^2(\theta - \theta_0) + L_2^2\sin^2(\theta - \theta_0). \tag{6.1.4}$$

That is, the squared strain in an arbitrary direction is a simple trig-weighted function of the strains in the principal directions. It follows immediately, if we did not know it already from Section 6.1.2, that one of the principal directions (θ_0 or $\theta_0 + 90°$) bears the maximum strain, and the other the minimum.

6.1.6. Equation for the principal strains

We have identified the principal directions as those of maximum or minimum ratio of length in the parallelogram to corresponding length in the square; but we have not determined the actual values of these extreme ratios. The algebra of this computation is simplest if we go about it indirectly, as follows. Instead of computing the strains as a function of direction, let us compute direction as a function of strain along it. In general, as we rotate from the direction of minimum strain (in this example, $\tan^{-1}0.36$ west of north, Figure 6.1.4a) to the direction of maximum strain (here, $\tan^{-1}0.36$ north of east), the strain must smoothly rise. (It cannot overshoot, because the latter direction was the maximum of strain; and cannot go up, then down, then up again, or else it would bear other directions along which the derivative is zero – but our algebra found a total of just two such directions.) As we rotate further, from $\tan^{-1}0.36$ north of east around to $\tan^{-1}0.36$ east of south (which is the same direction along which we began, but measured with the ruler upside down), the strain ratio must similarly *fall* smoothly from this maximum back down to the minimum again. Then (see Figure 6.1.5) every strain in between the maximum and

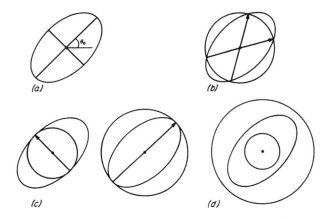

6.1.6. Principal strains

Figure 6.1.5. Direction as a function of strain. (*a*) Sketch of the strain ellipse, formula (6.1.4). (*b*) Strains between the maximum and the minimum correspond to two directions. (*c*) The maximum and minimum strains are attained at only one direction each. (*d*) Circles outside the extrema of strain correspond to no directions.

the minimum should be encountered along *two* directions, the first passed as we rise from minimum to maximum, the second passed as we fell back to the minimum; but strains equal to the maximum or the minimum should be encountered along one direction only.

We could convert this property of the principal strains into a formula for them if we could devise a quadratic equation in α for which the roots would be the directions having a particular strain. The strains we seek would then be the values for which that equation has only one root rather than the usual two. If the strain in a particular direction is λ and we write $\mu = \lambda^2$, then we have

$$\mu = \frac{(a_1 + a_2\alpha)^2 + (b_1 + b_2\alpha)^2}{1 + \alpha^2},$$

as before. For any strain $\sqrt{\mu}$, the directions α for which the strain is $\sqrt{\mu}$ are the roots of

$$\mu(1 + \alpha^2) = (a_1 + a_2\alpha)^2 + (b_1 + b_2\alpha)^2$$

or

$$\left(a_2^2 + b_2^2 - \mu\right)\alpha^2 + 2(a_1a_2 + b_1b_2)\alpha + \left(a_1^2 + b_1^2 - \mu\right) = 0.$$

These are familiar coefficients [recall the development of equation (6.1.3)]: This is

$$\left(L_2^2 - \mu\right)\alpha^2 + 2D\alpha + \left(L_1^2 - \mu\right) = 0.$$

Along the principal directions, which are extrema of λ and hence of μ, this equation must have only a single root for α, and so its *discriminant*, the expression under the square-root sign in the quadratic formula, must be zero:

$$(2D)^2 - 4\left(L_1^2 - \mu\right)\left(L_2^2 - \mu\right) = 0. \qquad (6.1.5)$$

197

But this is just a quadratic equation for μ. After dividing by 4, it is

$$\mu^2 - \left(L_1^2 + L_2^2 \right)\mu + \left(L_1^2 L_2^2 - D^2 \right) = 0.$$

The constant term is

$$\left(a_1^2 + b_1^2 \right)\left(a_2^2 + b_2^2 \right) - \left(a_1 a_2 + b_1 b_2 \right)^2 = \left(a_1 b_2 - a_2 b_1 \right)^2,$$

the squared area A^2 of the parallelogram that is the image of the square. So our equation for μ becomes

$$\mu^2 - \left(L_1^2 + L_2^2 \right)\mu + A^2 = 0. \tag{6.1.6}$$

If $D = 0$, we have $A^2 = L_1^2 L_2^2$; the solutions for μ are $\mu = L_1^2$ or $\mu = L_2^2$. This was the case of principal axes along the sides of the square, so that the principal strains were just the lengths of the sides of the parallelogram (here a rectangle). If D is not zero, one root is less than the minimum of L_1^2 and L_2^2, and the other is greater than the maximum. If $L_1^2 = L_2^2$, the case of the rhombus, we have $L^2 - \mu = \pm D$, $\mu = L^2 \pm D$, from equation (6.1.5).

Continuing with the example in Figure 6.1.1, we have $L_1^2 = \frac{53}{9}$, $L_2^2 = \frac{17}{9}$, $A^2 = L_1^2 L_2^2 - D^2 = \frac{676}{81}$, $A = \frac{26}{9}$. The equation for μ becomes $81\mu^2 - 630\mu + 676 = 0$, whence $\mu \sim 6.49$ or 1.29. The strain ratios $\lambda = \sqrt{\mu}$ are thus about 2.55 and 1.13. These can be verified in Figure 6.1.4.

Most statisticians will recognize the equation for μ as the determinantal criterion

$$\begin{vmatrix} L_1^2 - \mu & D \\ D & L_2^2 - \mu \end{vmatrix} = 0,$$

the characteristic equation of

$$\begin{bmatrix} L_1^2 & L_1 \cdot L_2 \\ L_1 \cdot L_2 & L_2^2 \end{bmatrix} = \begin{bmatrix} a_1 & b_1 \\ a_2 & b_2 \end{bmatrix}\begin{bmatrix} a_1 & a_2 \\ b_1 & b_2 \end{bmatrix},$$

the symmetrization of our transformation matrix

$$\begin{bmatrix} a_1 & b_1 \\ a_2 & b_2 \end{bmatrix}.$$

We have thus expressed the change of shape in Figure 6.1.1, originally presented in an arbitrary coordinate system, in terms of one pair of perpendicular directions, the principal axes, and two numbers, the strains in these directions. The effects of the shape change upon lengths in every direction can be computed from its effects in these directions by equation (6.1.4). In this way we eliminate all traces of the origin and orientation of the coordinate system of either form separately, that in which the square was digitized or that in which the parallelogram was digitized. This is the representation of uniform strain by a **symmetric tensor**, which you may think of, for now, as just this sort of algebraic quantity: a pair of directions and two strain ratios, the purpose of which is to report changes of length without further reference to Cartesian coordinates. The coordinate system computed here pertains only to the representation of the shape change, and it is different, in general, whenever either form changes. We shall have more to say about this concept in Section 6.2.5.

6.1.7. Effect of scale changes

It is important to check that principal axes do not change when the scale of the square or the parallelogram is changed. The equation for α, $D\alpha^2 + (L_1^2 - L_2^2)\alpha - D = 0$, is homogeneous in the scale of (a_1, b_1) and (a_2, b_2). This means that if the scale of the right-hand parallelogram, image of the square, is suddenly changed by a factor s, each of a_1, a_2, b_1, and b_2 is multiplied by the same factor s; D and the two L_i^2 are each multiplied by s^2; and the equation for α becomes

$$s^2 D\alpha^2 + \left(s^2 L_1^2 - s^2 L_2^2\right)\alpha - s^2 D = 0,$$

which has the same roots as before. **Principal axes are invariant under change of scale.**

The equation (6.1.6) for μ is not homogeneous in this way. If the scale of the parallelogram is changed by a factor s, the coefficient $(L_1^2 + L_2^2)$ is multiplied by s^2, and the coefficient A^2 by s^4. The roots of the new equation are thus s^2 times the roots of the old. Because μ is the square of the strain ratio, it follows that the strains λ are increased by the same factor s by which the scale was changed. All this is, of course, just as it should be, because the strains are ratios of lengths in the parallelogram to corresponding lengths in the square.

6.2. GEOMETRIC VERSION

This section will show how the principal axes introduced in the preceding section may be constructed on paper by ruler and compass as they describe the transformation of one triangle of landmarks onto another homologous triangle. The construction proceeds using the shape coordinates of the triangles to any baseline. Crucial features of the statistical description of small-to-moderate shape changes are shown much more clearly in this way than by the algebra of the preceding section. These features include the approximate directions of the principal strains as a function of the direction of change of the shape coordinates, as well as the approximate ratio of those strains as a simple multiple of the distance the shape has "moved" in the shape-coordinate plane.

6.2.1. The circle construction for the principal axes

As landmarks do not come in squares, like chocolate, the foregoing constructions are of no direct relevance yet to analysis of landmark data. The little patches of tissue were simply *declared* to correspond, square to parallelogram, like the little patches in the thin-plate spline figures scattered throughout this book. The computation of the principal axes and principal strains was an algebraic unfolding of that assumption. In fact, only three landmarks were involved: The position of the image of the upper right corner $(1, 1)$ of the square in Figure 6.2.1a is computed as the vector sum of the images of the corners $(0, 1)$ and $(1, 0)$. So the analysis is really of a right-isosceles triangle of landmarks and their homologues.

But except for algebraic convenience, nothing about the analysis makes reference to that right-isosceles shape of the starting form. Then there ought to be possible another approach to this same computation in which abstract square patches of tissue (and those "bloodless little vectors," Bookstein et al., 1985) would be replaced by a configuration of real landmark locations, three of them, forming a triangle. Because principal axes do not change when either of a pair of figures is rescaled (Section 6.1.7), we shall assume that one pair of these landmarks is found at the same distance in a pair of forms. Then we can draw the triangles as if that pair of landmarks were at the same *locations on the paper* in the drawings of both forms: the two-point registration to that baseline (Figure 6.2.1a), as we have already seen it in the course of constructing the shape coordinates (Figure 5.1.1). There are four points involved in this construction: landmarks A and B, at the same locations in both forms, and point C in one form homologous to point C' in the other. The algebraic approach of the preceding section can be adapted easily to this new setting (cf. Goodall, 1986). But ultimately it will be much more useful for morphometric interpretations and biological understanding if we eschew algebra for geometry and explicitly *construct* principal axes with ruler and compass instead of computing them decimally. For instance, the Fortran program for the principal axes published in Bookstein et al. (1985) simulates this construction.

The construction that seems simplest is based (Figure 6.2.1b) on the circle through C and C' with its center on AB. That center is located where the **perpendicular bisector** of the segment CC' intersects the extended line AB. Whether that intersection is between A and B or outside the interval they form does not matter. (The case in which this intersection does not exist is dealt with in Section 6.2.1.1.) The circle centered at that intersection

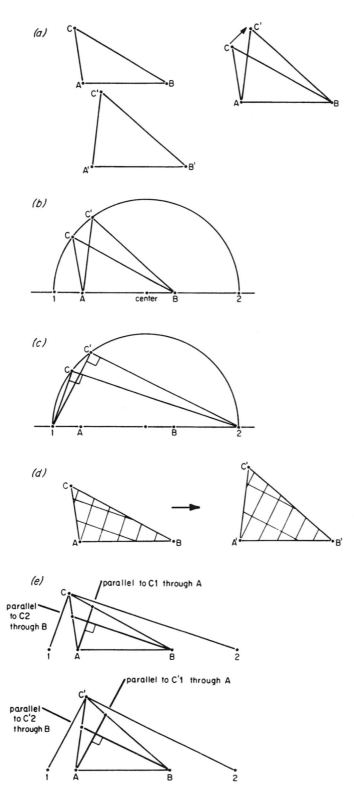

Figure 6.2.1. Circle construction for the principal axes. (*a*) When a pair of landmarks is at the same distance in a pair of forms, the comparison reduces to a comparison of the two positions C and C' of the third vertex when the triangles are superimposed. (*b*) There is (usually) a circle through both points C centered on the baseline AB where the perpendicular bisector of CC' intersects the baseline. (*c*) The angles $1C2$ and $1C'2$ are both right angles. (*d*) These directions are thus the biorthogonal directions for the uniform transformation relating the interiors of the triangles. (*e*) They can always be interpreted by vectors connecting one vertex of the triangle to a point dividing the opposite side in a fixed fraction.

201

and passing through both positions C and C' of the third land-mark will intersect the baseline (perpendicularly) in two auxiliary points – call them 1 and 2. The angles $1C2$ and $1C'2$ are each inscribed in a semicircle; hence, from a theorem of Euclid, each measures 90° (Figure 6.2.1c).

Now let us reinterpret the scene of two points and a baseline as the change of shape that we originally had in mind, between the two triangles ABC and ABC'. *If we assume that this change is uniform along the segments joining the landmarks*, then we may conclude that the points 1 and 2, like the baseline points A and B, are left unmoved by the transformation. (A uniform transformation leaving two points of a line fixed leaves every point of the line fixed.) *If we assume further that the transformation is uniform throughout the interiors of the triangles, and throughout their planes beyond* (Figure 6.2.1d), then the direction $1C$ is transformed into the direction $1C'$, and likewise $2C$ into $2C'$. (A uniform transformation takes straight lines into straight lines.) Thus we have found a pair of directions that (1) correspond under the implied uniform transformation of Figure 6.2.1d and (2) are at 90° both before and after transformation. By the algebra of Section 6.1, these **must** be the principal axes, directions bearing the maximum and minimum strains. In this example the strains are 1.414 ($1C$ to $1C'$) and 0.943 ($2C$ to $2C'$). (These must be multiplied by whatever scale change was imposed to match the distances AB in the first step of the construction.) The principal axes are the same for the transformation $ABC' \rightarrow ABC$, as they are aligned with the intersections of the same circle with AB. This invariance is not at all obvious from the algebraic development in the preceding section.

In the construction the principal axes often will be drawn outside the triangles to which they apply. There is no need to express the principal axes as directions with reference to point C and its homologue C' whenever point 1 or point 2 is outside the triangular form; we can easily redraw the same directions inside the triangles. If point 1 is outside the triangle, for instance, then a line parallel to $1C$ through one of the other vertices, A or B, must pass inside the triangle to intersect the opposite side. Likewise, if point 2 is outside the triangle, a line parallel to $2C$ through one of the remaining vertices must intersect the opposite edge properly. We can thus express each principal direction as a segment relating one of the vertices of the triangle – A, B, or C – to a point dividing the edge opposite in a fraction less than 1 (Figure 6.2.1e). By the linearity of the assumed transformation, the transform of each of these transects divides the appropriate edge of ABC' in the same fraction. The ratios of length of sides of the crosses inside the triangles are the same as the principal strains: 1.414 for the segments from A to a point 22% of the way from C to B, and 0.943 for the segments from B to a point 38% of the way from C

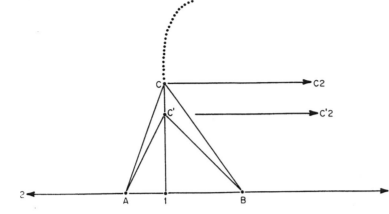

Figure 6.2.2. Circle construction for infinite radius. The point 2 is at infinity along the baseline "in both directions." The principal directions 1C and 2C are nevertheless well defined.

to *A*. If points 1 and 2 are both between *A* and *B*, then both of these transects pass through vertex *C*: There is nothing wrong with such a case.

6.2.1.1. Special case. —

In some special cases the circle we drew in Figure 6.2.1*b* cannot be drawn. Suppose that point *C'* is displaced from point *C* directly toward or away from the line *AB*. Then, as the line *CC'* is perpendicular to the line *AB*, the perpendicular bisector of *CC'* is parallel to *AB* and does not intersect it anywhere (Figure 6.2.2). The center of the "circle" is infinitely far away. Its intersections with the baseline are then the point 1 directly underneath the segment *CC'* and the point 2 at infinity along the baseline. The directions 1*C* and 1*C'* are then the same, namely, the direction *CC'*, and the directions 2*C* and 2*C'* are likewise the same, namely, the direction of the baseline itself, which is always an acceptable transect of the triangle. This will be one of the special cases in Table 6.3.1.

The strain along 2*C* is the same as the strain along *AB*, which is 1.0 (because the length *AB* does not change over the transformation). The strain along 1*C* is just the ratio of distances 1*C'* : 1*C*, which is the ratio of heights of the two triangles. This configuration is analogous to special case (*b*) of Section 6.1.3.1: One of the principal strains is along a side of the form. In all other cases, as we noted algebraically in Section 6.1.5, one principal strain is usually *greater* than all the strains observed between pairs of the three landmarks involved, and the other is usually *less*. This is most clearly shown in Figure 6.2.1*c* for the general construction: Relative to the change of length between any pair of landmarks *A* and *B* as baseline, one of the segments 1*C*, 2*C* is becoming relatively *longer* as the point *C* "moves" to *C'*, and the other is becoming relatively *shorter*.

203

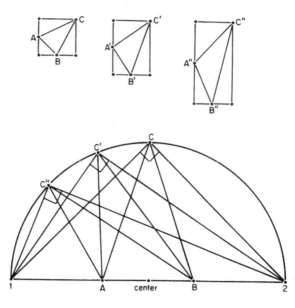

Figure 6.2.3. Three shapes equally spaced along a "straight line": iteration of the same shape change (increase of the vertical axis of the square by 50%) twice.

6.2.1.2. An even more special case. —

The points C and C' may coincide. In this case the triangle ABC has not changed its shape; this corresponds to special case (c) of Section 6.1.3.1. As there is then no perpendicular bisector of CC', the construction fails. In this case, *all* directions are principal directions, as the rate of change of length (in the assumed uniform transformation) is the same in every direction.

6.2.1.3. Using the same circle more than once. —

One can pass from consideration of two triangles on the same baseline AB to consideration of three, ABC, ABC', ABC'' (Figure 6.2.3). When the three points C lie on a single circle centered on AB, as drawn, then the points 1 and 2 are the same for all comparisons of two of the triangles ABC. That is, the change from ABC to ABC' has the same principal axes as the change from either to ABC'', and so on. This turns out to be the most sensible criterion for declaring that the three triangular forms ABC, ABC' and ABC'' **lie on a line** in shape space. The geometry in which these semicircles are the "straight lines" is the so-called **Poincaré model of the hyperbolic plane.** It is developed in Appendix A.2.

6.2.2. Change of baseline

A change of baseline does not affect the outcome of the circle construction when it is interpreted as producing a pair of directions upon the form – that is, when it is interpreted as a symmetric

204

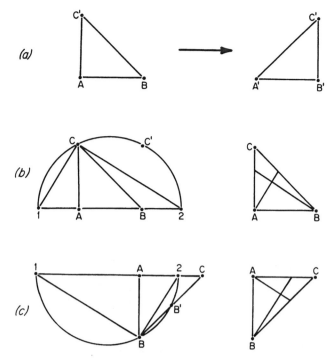

Figure 6.2.4. Change of baseline does not affect the outcome of the circle construction. (*a*) Left-isosceles right triangle deforming into right-isosceles version. (Not a reflection!) (*b*) Construction of principal axes to baseline *AB*, "moving" points *C* and *C'*. (*c*) The same to baseline *AC*, "moving" points *B* and *B'*. The axes lie in the same positions with respect to the triangle, regardless of their orientation upon the printed page.

tensor. The circle construction of Section 6.2.1 appears to require that one arbitrarily fix the length of one interlandmark distance (there *AB*) in preparation for the two-point registration that reduces the analysis to the consideration of two points with respect to one line. We saw at the end of Section 6.1 that the rescaling necessary to enforce this assumption does not alter the axes (the extremal values of α). But what about the fact that we chose one particular pair of landmarks to serve as baseline? Because the construction results in some pair of directions that are at 90° both before and after the uniform transformation, and because this pair of directions is unique, **it cannot matter what baseline we choose.** See, for example, Figure 6.2.4. We saw a similar invariance for shapes of scatters in Section 5.1.2, but it was approximate; the invariance of the constructed principal axes and principal strains here is exact.

In fact, because we are modeling the transformation as linear, we could register on points in between the landmarks rather on the landmarks themselves and still arrive at the same directions for the principal axes. In Figure 6.2.5 we demonstrate this using a computed point in place of the "moving" landmark, point *B*. But we can do even better than this, at least in hindsight. If we use as a baseline one of the principal axes themselves, we can arrange that each of the two remaining landmarks will appear to be undergoing displacement at the same rate toward or away from a line through a third landmark, as shown by the following demonstration.

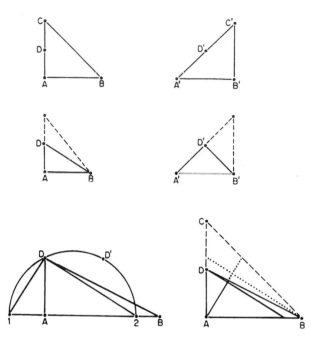

Figure 6.2.5. The circle construction can use points other than the original landmarks. Replacing point *B* with a computed point *D* halfway between *A* and *B* results in the same axes.

Let us choose as baseline the direction of larger principal strain, *AE* in Figure 6.2.6. As the strain along *AE* (i.e., the ratio *AE′* : *AE*) is the *larger*, the remaining two landmarks *B* and *C* appear to move *toward* the axis. Had we chosen the baseline *BF* for the construction, bearing the smaller principal strain, it would appear that the little vectors representing apparent displacements

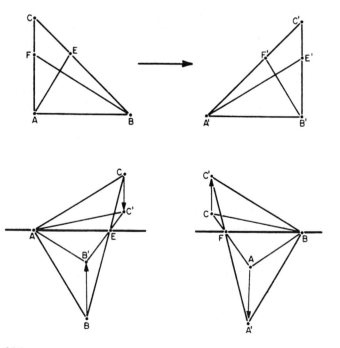

Figure 6.2.6. The circle construction "reduces" to the case of infinite radius. [Compare the discussion of the "universal special case," *D* = 0, Section 6.1.3.1(*b*).] The same shape change as in the preceding two figures is shown as the imputed motion of two landmarks perpendicularly and proportionately toward (or away from) a baseline through the third.

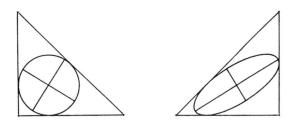

Figure 6.2.7. Origin of the ellipse in Figure 6.1.5, strain as a function of direction. The ellipse is the image of a circle under the uniform deformation.

of the remaining landmarks *A* and *C* would then point *away* from the baseline. A rotation of 90° in the baseline has induced a rotation of 180° in that vector as diagrammed. Of this 180°, 90° is the rotation of the paper of this book required to being *BF* to the orientation previously occupied by *AE*, but the remaining 90° is actual rotation upon the triangle. The little vectors that connect two positions of the same landmark in a two-point registration are not engraved upon the biological forms even if the connection represents "growth" or some other intrinsically biological process. Vectors like *CC'* rotate *upon the forms* as a function of our choice of baseline. It is the principal axes that do not rotate, not the direction *CC'*, which does. We saw this before in Section 5.1.2, in connection with rotation of scatters of shape coordinates. Of course, the change to this new basis leaves circular the distribution expected on the null model (Section 5.3.1) of independent circular noise at each landmark.

6.2.3. Another proof of the existence of principal axes

To derive the equation for μ, the squared strain ratio, in Section 6.1.6, I sketched a figure of an oval (Figure 6.1.5a) labeled "strain as a function of direction." We can arrive at this same figure geometrically by imagining a circle drawn inside the left-hand form, the starting triangle (Figure 6.2.7). It is deformed as its points are transformed along with every other point inside the triangle. Even the ancient Greeks knew that the curve into which a circle is taken by such a transformation is an ellipse (cf. the discussion of sectioning a cylinder by a plane, Hilbert and Cohn-Vossen, 1952:7–8).

You know than an ellipse has two **axes**, which lie at 90° and about each of which it is symmetric. One of these is the longest diameter of the ellipse, and one the shortest. In this application, the diameters of the ellipse directly embody the strain ratios pertaining to the diameters of the circle that mapped into them. Hence, one axis lies along the direction of greatest strain, the other along that of least strain. An extension of this reasoning shows without any algebra that the two diameters of the circle that are transformed into the principal axes are likewise perpendicular upon the circle. In this way the geometric approach of this section can be shown to be completely equivalent to the algebraic approach of the preceding section.

207

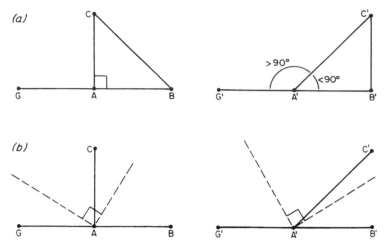

Figure 6.2.8. Alternate proof that there exists a pair of biorthogonal directions.

We can likewise work with the other property of the principal axes, their biorthogonality, and prove without algebra that there must be a pair of directions that lie at 90° both before and after transformation. Let us simply choose an arbitrary perpendicular pair of directions in the left-hand (starting) form and see what angle they make in the right-hand form. If that angle is likewise 90°, fine – we have our pair. Otherwise (Figure 6.2.8*a*), of the two supplementary angles at A', one is less than 90° and one greater. Let us imagine rotating our perpendicular pair from (AB, AC) to (AC, AG) on the left, keeping them always perpendicular. Then the lines on the right rotate from ($A'B'$, $A'C'$) to ($A'C'$, $A'G'$). In this rotation their angle passes from a value less than 90° to a value greater than 90°. At some position in between these extremes (Figure 6.2.8*b*), the angle on the right must pass exactly through the value of 90°, the same as the value on the left. A compact argument indeed!

In this form, the argument makes no essential reference to landmarks. My shape nonmonotonicity theorem (Bookstein, 1980*a*) extends this same logic to show that in any series of three distinct shapes, linked howsoever by a differentiable homology function, and for any ordering of those three shapes, there are shape measures agreeing with that ordering. This buttresses the argument that "ordination" in terms of biological shape is not a promising line of biometric inquiry (Section 2.4.2).

6.2.4. Approximations for small changes

Let us return to the circle construction of Figure 6.2.1. If the points C and C' are sufficiently close together (after superposition on fixed AB), we can approximate the circle through C and C' by a circle through C tangent there to the direction CC' (Figure 6.2.9). The center of this circle is located at the point P where the perpendicular to CC' through C crosses the baseline. (If the

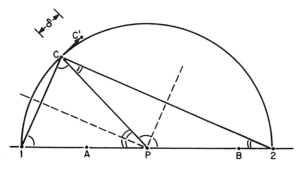

Figure 6.2.9. Approximation to the principal axes for small shape changes. The angle $C'CP$ is 90°. The principal directions $C1$ and $C2$ nearly bisect the angles at P between the direction perpendicular to the apparent motion of point C and the baseline.

change were not small we would be obliged to use the perpendicular bisector of CC' instead.)

Because all radii of a circle are equal, triangles $PC1$ and $PC2$ in Figure 6.2.9 are both isosceles; we mark equal angles as shown in the figure. Because angle $2C1$ is 90°, and the angles of triangle $2PC$ total 180°, we must have angle $2PC$ equal to twice angle $P1C$. Then the direction $1C$ is a bisector of the angle $2PC$. Similarly, the direction $2C$ is a bisector of the angle $1PC$. Hence:

> **For small changes of shape, in a registration on two points the principal axes bisect the angles between the perpendicular to the apparent trajectory of the third point and the baseline.**

If we rotate baselines, the true axes will of course rotate with the tissue at the same rate; because they are *bisectors* of an angle involving the apparent motion of the third landmark, that "vector" must rotate twice as fast as the baseline. As we are here pretending to hold that baseline fixed in a horizontal orientation on the page, the pseudovector will appear to rotate twice as fast in the direction opposite from that in which the baseline is rotated upon the form. We saw an example of this in Section 6.2.2: The apparent displacement rotated by 180° when we switched baselines by 90°, from one principal direction to the other. As another example, the standard error of the direction in shape space of a mean difference between two samples of triangular forms, as approximated by the standard error of the difference of mean shape coordinates in the direction perpendicular to that mean difference, is just double the standard error of direction of the principal axes that summarize this comparison (see also Section 6.5.1.4).

We can do better than approximating the axes for small changes; we can also approximate the strains along them. Write δ for the distance between C and C', as indicated in Figure 6.2.10, and write h for the height of point C above its baseline. The increase from distance $1C$ to distance $1C'$ is very nearly the projection of

209

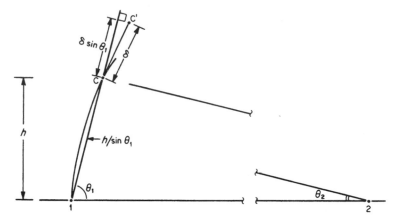

Figure 6.2.10. Approximation to the principal strains. The anisotropy of this transformation is nearly δ/h.

the vector CC', of length δ, in the direction of $1C$; this projection is just $\delta \sin \theta_1$, where θ_1 is the angle at point 1, as shown. (Remember that the sum of the angles at 1 and 2 is 90°.) The strain in this direction differs from 1.0 by this increment divided by the starting length of the segment, which is $h/\cos \theta_2 = h/\sin \theta_1$. Hence the strain is very nearly

$$1 + \left[\delta \sin \theta_1 / (h/\sin \theta_1)\right] = 1 + \frac{\delta}{h} \sin^2 \theta_1. \qquad (6.2.1)$$

Similarly, the strain along $2C$ is

$$1 - \frac{\delta}{h} \sin^2 \theta_2 = 1 - \frac{\delta}{h} \cos^2 \theta_1.$$

Hence the ratio between the principal strains is

$$\left(1 + \frac{\delta}{h} \sin^2 \theta_1\right) \Big/ \left(1 - \frac{\delta}{h} \cos^2 \theta_1\right) \sim 1 + \frac{\delta}{h}\left[\sin^2 \theta_1 - (-\cos^2 \theta_1)\right]$$

$$= 1 + \frac{\delta}{h},$$

independent of the direction CC'. This ratio is called the **anisotropy** of the uniform transformation. It is the ratio of axes of the ellipse into which the circle is deformed – a measure of the extent to which the transformation "does different things in different directions": the extent to which it is a shape change. A discussion of measuring anisotropy for transformations that are not uniform will be found in Section 6.6. The standard error of δ for any mean comparison (as approximated by the standard error of the mean difference of shape coordinates along its own direction) is thus the same (up to a factor h) as the standard error of the anisotropy of that mean change, independent of any uncertainty of direction, as long as the change *has* a direction to whatever level of statistical significance one prefers. See also Section 6.5.1.4.

In this way, we see that the anisotropy of the shape change – the ratio of the principal strains – is closely related to the ordinary Euclidean distance measure as applied to the half-plane of points "moving" to fixed baseline. This particular distance metric, in the form of its logarithm, is, in fact, the natural hyperbolic metric associated with the geometry for which circles perpendicular to the baseline are "straight lines," as we hinted at the end of Section 6.2.1. For further development of this geometry of triangles, see Appendix A.2. The accuracy of this approximation, like that of the rotational invariance of the scatter of shape coordinates, relates to the "diameter" of the scatter in this same non-Euclidean geometry. By comparison (Section 7.1), distance in Kendall's shape manifold (Procrustes distance) goes as $\delta / \sqrt{p^2}$; the factor h has been replaced by the square root of Centroid Size, which does not go to zero with h, and so permits triangular shapes to cross the locus of collinearity.

In Figure 6.2.1, the anisotropy is 1.414 divided by 0.943, or 1.500. The approximation using the mean scaled height 0.7 of the triangles yields $\delta / h = 0.283 / 0.7 = 0.404$, which is the logarithm of 1.498. Thus the error in the approximation is almost entirely the error of taking $\log(1 + x)$ as equal to x.

6.2.5. This is the tensor description of shape change

The preceding is the representation of biological shape change by a **symmetric tensor**. In general (Lanczos, 1970), a tensor is a mathematical operator upon one or several vectors that supplies the same answer regardless of the coordinate system in which the vectors are measured. Misner, Thorne, and Wheeler (1973) offer the effective metaphor of the "geometric machine" that is fed a scheme of vectors in an arbitrary coordinate system and produces numerical values (scalar quantities) that are independent of that coordinate system. In this implementation, the tensor in question is a *relative metric tensor* or *strain tensor* that accepts two vectors as arguments.

Directions like *AB* and *AC* are vectors: They have directions that rotate with coordinate systems and lengths that do not change under those rotations. The construction of strain here is a tensor because it corrects for rotations of the vectors in either image. The invariant numbers that the tensor puts out are lengths and dot products (cosines of angles, in effect) in the "after" triangle corresponding to unit vectors in the "before" triangle. In the notation of Section 6.1, the scalars are $L_1 \cdot L_1$, $L_2 \cdot L_2$, and $L_1 \cdot L_2$. These are just the entries of the matrix in Section 6.1.6.

6.2.6. Direct observations of anisotropy

In studies of biological and geological microstructures, one often encounters data about **textures** that have shape and orientation but no information about homology. For instance, the shapes of cells within an epithelium or across a section may show systematic trends of elongation or directionality with respect to some biologically meaningful polarity (craniocaudal, proximodistal, dorsoventral, mediolateral); geological inclusions may show alignment with respect to a physical orientation (axis of strike, river flow).

Often these features can be modeled by ellipses. For instance, they may be blobs with centroids and moments about those centroids; then each second-order moment matrix corresponds to a particular ellipse with the same axis directions and lengths. Or outlines might be extracted, then fit as ellipses directly. It is tempting to "measure" these inclusions in the same way one measures triangles by axes of ellipses; in this case we can treat the ellipses as "representing" deformed circles. There are three parameters characterizing ellipses in this way, two axis lengths and an angle. We choose two of these, anisotropy (the axis ratio) and this angle, to present in the shape-coordinate plane. "Size" (perhaps the product of the axes) is reserved as an exogenous scalar correlate, just as it was for landmark data.

The statistical methods of this section for testing mean differences in shape space apply directly to such orientation data. One can check for mean shape differences, size allometry, covariance with exogenous quantities, and so on, provided that all ellipses are viewed in a consistent coordinate system. The reduction of the shape and orientation of a single ellipse to a pair of shape coordinates is via the construction indicated in Figure 6.2.11. One treats the ellipse as a representation of finite strain and assigns it the shape coordinates of the triangular shape to which a standard triangle (of any arbitrary shape) is taken by the strain in question. This will be seen to be precisely the inverse of the construction of principal axes from finite strains of triangles, as explained in this section. The choice of that standard triangle determines the usual nuisance variables of orientation and position of the corresponding scatter in shape space. These bear no serious consequences for statistical analysis. "Baseline length" is now not a homologous distance but a representation of the diameter of each ellipse in one particular direction. The treatment of size allometry must therefore by somewhat careful; size should be measured by the area of the ellipse, not by the size (baseline length, Centroid Size, or otherwise) of the transformed "standard" triangle.

One can standardize this construction against the choice of the starting triangle by assigning each ellipse the polar coordinates (r, θ), with r being 1.0 less than the anisotropy, or better, the logarithm of the anisotropy, and θ set to *twice* the angle between the major principal axes of the ellipse and the (arbitrary) horizon-

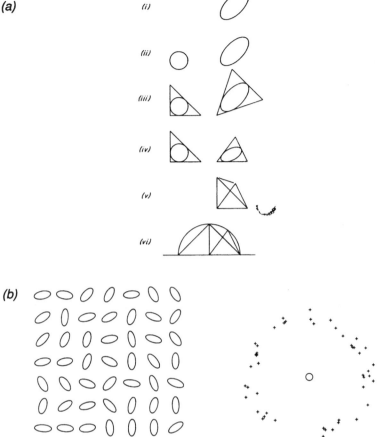

(a)

(i)

(ii)

(iii)

(iv)

(v)

(vi)

(b)

Figure 6.2.11. Representation of unlabeled ellipses by a shape-coordinate pair. (*a*) Any ellipse, interpreted as a strain ellipse, may be represented by the shape of the triangle into which that strain transforms some standard triangle. (i) Ellipse (datum). (ii) Circle to ellipse. (iii) Circumscribed triangles corresponding under the implied transformation. (iv) Rotate, rescale to standardize the "baseline." (v) Superimpose. (vi) The principal axes of the circle construction are the axes of the original ellipse. (*b*) A population of ellipses (left) is thus represented by a scatter of shape coordinates (right) in the polar approximation given in the text. There is no correlation between orientation and shape in this little simulation. A uniform shear of the left-hand scene would lead to a shift of centroid in the right-hand scatter and thus would be detected statistically with considerable power (Bookstein, 1986*c*).

tal of the imposed coordinate system. This scatter is shown in Figure 6.2.11*b* for the ellipses from Figure 6.2.11*a*. (This is the appropriate linearization of the geometry of Appendix A.2.)

There result statistical tests for differences in texture, covariates of texture, and so forth, that ought to be more efficient than either tests of the anisotropy alone – those tests reduce to consideration of the polar radius r only – or conventional multivariate tests of that radius together with the angle of the axis per se (as the precision of that angle is highly variable over cases, being inversely proportional to the anisotropy, Section 6.5.1.4).

6.2.6.1. In three dimensions. —

In the same way that landmark-free oriented structures in two dimensions may be subjected to the statistical tests of shape space by considering them as strain tensors for an arbitrary landmark "standard" (Section 6.2.4), one might execute statistical tests of effects upon the shape of ellipsoidal features of texture in three dimensions by the reduction to the shape spaces of the four triangular faces of the tetrahedron into which the data, treated as strain ellipsoids, transform an arbitrary standard form. I have no examples of this procedure to show at this time.

6.3. FROM TENSORS TO VARIABLES: MEASURING A SHAPE COMPARISON

All the figures of the preceding section can be reinterpreted in terms of the space of **shape coordinates**, as set forth in Chapter 5. The construction of the principal axes is a manipulation of a *pair* of triangular forms – a *pair* of points in shape-coordinate space; but the approximations of Section 6.2.4 demonstrate that the geometry of this construction makes reference mainly to **directions** in this space. It then becomes possible to integrate the preceding discussion of comparisons of triangles with the discussion of the preceding chapter dealing with shape variables in their more familiar statistical form. That tie and a surprising duality between angles and distance ratios that underlies it are the subjects of this section. Some of this material has appeared in Bookstein (1983).

6.3.1. Naming directions in shape space

Although the statistics of Chapter 5 were essentially complete, most of the language of biology was excluded. Group differences were reported as "directions in shape space"; they need to be named biologically instead. Often this necessary next step proceeds by identifying familiar variables, ratios or angles, that have nearly the same gradients as the changes in shape coordinates observed between groups or induced by covariates. For triangles of landmarks, and as a first step for more complex configurations, the features of the shape-change tensor are most helpful in this regard.

We saw in Section 5.1.3 that ordinary shape variables – ratios of distances, angles, and the like – have directions in the plane of shape coordinates. For small shape variation, each variable corresponds to a direction running through a small patch of that space. The tensors of the preceding section are thereby a language for describing directions in shape space as well as they describe pairs of points there.

In one direction this correspondence is straightforward (Figure 6.3.1, top). For any shape variable in the vicinity of a mean form, there is a line element in shape space, to which there usually corresponds, by the construction in Figure 6.2.9, essentially one particular deformation tensor. That is, there is a uniform deformation corresponding to the gradient of any shape variable measured on a nondegenerate triangle of landmarks. (We do not know

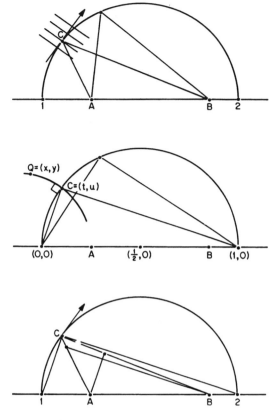

Figure 6.3.1. Interpretation of shape changes by shape variables. Top: Any direction in shape space is interpretable as (some power of) a deformation tensor (that corresponding to any two triangles with shape coordinates on the circle shown). Middle: The gradient of the ratio of sides of a rectangle is normal to the circle of the construction in Figure 6.2.1. Bottom: One shape variable with gradient along an observed displacement is the ratio of lengths in the principal directions of that displacement interpreted as a deformation.

"how much deformation" corresponds to a particular shape variable – how much anisotropy for this particular pair of principal axes – until we specify how far to move a point of shape space along the direction in question. We stretch one axis by a ratio $e^{\delta/h}$, then rescale to suit the baseline of the data.) It is of more interest, however, to execute the inverse of this reinterpretation: given a deformation, to find a variable that corresponds. That is, we wish to determine, for any particular displacement in shape space (i.e., any observed deformation), one of the class of shape variables that "catches" that deformation – one of the shape variables having a gradient precisely along the observed shape displacement. (The language of the "catcher" is from modern data analysis: Mosteller and Tukey, 1977.) In this way we have "named" the shape displacement in a biologically suggestive way.

As usual, the geometry is simplest if we begin with a special case. In the middle panel of Figure 6.3.1 we examine the change in shape of one right triangle into another. If we use as baseline the two endpoints of the hypotenuse, then the other sides of the triangle serve the function of the distances $1C$ and $2C$ in Figure 6.2.1. Consider now the ordinary shape variable that is the ratio between these lengths. Place point 1 at $(0, 0)$ and point 2 at $(1, 0)$,

215

and assign the third landmark C its shape coordinates (t, u). The circle in the construction of principal axes is $(t - \frac{1}{2})^2 + u^2 = \frac{1}{4}$ or $t^2 + u^2 = t$. The normal to this circle at C is then the vector from C to the center of the circle, the vector $(t, u) - (\frac{1}{2}, 0) = (t - \frac{1}{2}, u)$. Consider now the points $Q = (x, y)$ having the same ratio of distances to 1 and 2. This criterion, that $1Q : 2Q = 1C : 2C$, corresponds to the equation $(2C)(1Q) = (1C)(2Q)$ or

$$\left[(t - 1)^2 + u^2 \right](x^2 + y^2) = (t^2 + u^2)\left[(x - 1)^2 + y^2 \right],$$

or, recalling that $t^2 + u^2 = t$ for points C on the circle,

$$(1 - 2t)(x^2 + y^2) + 2tx = t.$$

This is another circle (Pedoe, 1970: sect. 18.3). It center lies at the point $(-t/(1 - 2t), 0)$. The normal through C to *this* circle, which is the direction of fastest change in the ratio $1C : 2C$, is thus $(t, u) - (-t/(1 - 2t), 0) = (t(2 - 2t)/(1 - 2t), u)$.

But these two normals are perpendicular, because their dot product is $(t - \frac{1}{2}, u) \cdot (t(2 - 2t)/(1 - 2t), u) = u^2 + t^2 - t = 0$. It follows that (for distances $1C, 2C$ along principal axes of the shape change) the *gradient* of the ratio of sides $1C : 2C$ is *along the direction in shape space in which point C is moving*. In fact, this was proved (in a quite different way) in Section 5.1.3, where we showed that the gradient of the angle at C was perpendicular to the gradient of the ratio of sides at C by observing that to be true at either end of the baseline, then invoking the invariance of the invariant-covariant duality.

But, as shown at the bottom of Figure 6.3.1, this construction applies to *any* shape change of triangles. (Recall from Section 6.2.2 that we can replace any landmark by a linear combination in the construction of the principal axes. One simply replaces landmarks A and B of the baseline by points 1 and 2 of the circle construction, leaving point C alone.) Hence:

> **For any direction of change in the space of a pair of shape coordinates, one shape variable having that direction as its gradient is the ratio of lengths measured along the principal axes when that shape change is interpreted as a uniform deformation.**

We have thus arrived at a formal proof of what may have seemed intuitively almost obvious in the development of Section

216

6.2. If lengths along one of the principal axes (say $1C$) are growing most rapidly over a change, and lengths along $2C$ most slowly, then the ratio $1C:2C$ "ought to be" the shape variable most sensitive to the observed change. We have just proved that, indeed, its gradient is precisely along the shape trajectory observed. The ratio of the principal axes is the shape variable we would like to have measured: It is the *shape-change factor* that underlies that change of shape as measured in any other way. Yet we need neither have measured it nor guessed at its identity – it falls neatly out of the tensor analysis.

It is this happy coincidence that permits the morphometrician to switch back and forth between tensors and shape coordinates, between vectors of shape change and their biological interpretations. In practice, statistical computations proceed using shape coordinates, and findings are given potentially biological interpretations by means of the tensors corresponding to these mean changes, covariates, and so forth, when reinterpreted as deformations.

6.3.2. Invariants and covariants expressed using the principal axes

In Section 5.1.3 we saw that shape variables in the vicinity of a mean form come in pairs having gradients at 90° in shape-coordinate space. Each variable's gradient (direction of maximum rate of change) lies along the level lines (direction of no change) of the other. By a simple extension of language, we may refer to the *invariants* and *covariants* of particular deformations. The *covariant* of a particular displacement in shape space, we have just seen, is the ratio of lengths measured in the principal directions. The *invariant* must be the (essentially unique) shape variable having gradient at 90° to this direction. Alternatively, it is the variable whose *level lines* lie along the assigned displacement vector in shape space. From Figure 6.3.1 we can see that one variable having the appropriate direction for its level curves is the **angle between the principal axes**: They remain at 90° over the transformation, which is exactly what one wants an invariant to do. Conversely, in changes along the gradient of the *angle* between a pair of directions beginning at 90°, for instance, rotation of the diagonals of a square, the *ratio* of distances in those directions is unchanging (diagonals of a rectangle are equal).

A certain symmetry seems to be emerging here. The difference between invariants and covariants of a shape change, which was associated with rotation of the shape-space gradient by 90°, seems to be associated with the interchange of "ratio" and "angle" in the naming of the variables. Angles as invariants go with ratios as covariants, and vice versa. We can take this one step further by recalling (Figure 6.2.9) the relation between directions of small

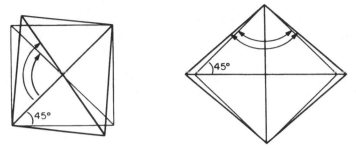

Figure 6.3.2. Duality of sets of principal axes at 45°. Left: As a square begins to be deformed into a rectangle, the angle changing most rapidly lies between the diagonals the ratio of which is not changing and which lie at 45° to the ratio of lengths changing most rapidly (ratio of sides). Right: As the square begins to be deformed into a rhombus, the angle changing most rapidly lies between the sides the ratio of which is not changing and which lie at 45° to the lengths the ratio of which is changing most rapidly (the diagonals).

changes in shape space and the directions of the principal axes of the corresponding deformations. The principal axes rotate half as fast as directions in shape space – their construction involves angle bisectors. Then rotation of shape-change vectors by 90°, such as is required to interchange "ratio" and "angle" as invariant/covariant, represents *rotation of the principal axes by 45°*.

For instance (Figure 6.3.2, left), in the change from square to rectangle, we already know (see Section 6.1.3.1) that the ratio of lengths changing fastest is that of the sides of the square. Then (1) the ratio of lengths of the *diagonals* of the square is unchanging, as is the angle between the sides, and (2) the *angle* between those diagonals is a covariant of the deformation, changing neither more nor less sensitively than the ratio of the sides, to which they lie at $\pm 45°$. The situation at the right in the figure, square to rhombus, is exactly the reverse.

Distance ratios and angles, although each dimensionless, appear to be incommensurate (cm/cm versus degrees – how many degrees in a ratio of 2:1?). They are made commensurate in the geometry of the shape-coordinate plane itself: We measure either by reference to the log anisotropy δ/h of the equivalent deformation. Section 7.6 will be devoted to explaining a similar method of making shape measures commensurate when they involve four or more landmarks, a method that requires recourse to two different "distances."

6.3.3. A table of shape variables for reporting differences

These ratios of sides at 90°, in two sets (along the principal axes, or at 45° to the principal axes), or, equivalently, the angles between the same pairs of directions (at 45° to the principal axes, or along the principal axes), provide a canonical set of shape-variable names for reporting any observed shape change. But it is difficult to comprehend reports about the effect of a shape change in which one is interested as "change by a factor of 1.08 in the ratio between [or: change by 4° in the angle between] the length from landmark *A* to a point 0.28 of the way from *B* to *C*

218

and the length from landmark B to a point 0.71 of the way from A to C." (These are as boring and difficult to follow as the geodetic descriptions of plots of land in the proceedings of the zoning boards of small American towns.) We need a way of reporting approximations to these in ordinary language whenever possible. Naturally, if the optimal shape variable is equivalent to a simple familiar measure of the form – if "ratio of the length AB to the distance from C to a point 0.45 of the way from A to B" is actually the ratio of height to width – we should report using ordinary language instead. Now nine shape variables lie conveniently at hand to use for labeling shape changes: the three angles of the triangle, the three ratios of sides, and the three aspect ratios (height to each of three baselines). This suggests a systematic search over the alternate interpretations of any shape effect to see if any of these simple descriptions may apply. If one does, the way in which it lies on an organism usually will suggest one or more biological interpretations directly. The interpretations may invoke the invariant, the covariant, or both.

Ratio of sides and angle between sides, we have seen, are duals: Deformations having the one as covariant have the other as invariant. We are a bit less familiar with the dual for the third sort of vernacular shape-change report, change of aspect ratio. As the gradient of that ratio represents displacement of the third landmark directly toward (or away from) the baseline, the dual transformation, encountered in Section 5.1.3, must displace it at a direction 90° removed, which is to say, directly *along* the baseline. The axes of this transformation, which is called a **simple shear**, must be at 45° to those of the dual: Then they must lie at ±45° to the baseline. We have seen this already in the transformation of square to rhombus [Section 6.1.3.1(*a*) or Figure 6.3.2].

Now we can set up a table of shape-change reports in the form of a two-by-two scheme of alignments. For each of the three sides of the triangle, the principal directions may align nearly along it, or nearly at 45° to it; for each of the three angles of the triangle, the principal directions may align with the bisector or at 45° to the bisector. In each of these 12 canonical cases (four configurations times three sides or angles) there is a conveniently described *covariant*, a conveniently described *invariant*, and a conveniently suggestive interpretation of the (biological) process that may underlie the observed change.

6.3.3.1. *Brizalina, again.* —

We return to the running example of four landmarks in two strata of *Brizalina*, a little data set previously considered by multivariate analyses of distance measures (Section 4.3.2) and later by T^2-test (Section 5.4.3.4). In the shape-coordinate analysis we noted that to a baseline from aperture to proloculus point, one shape-coordi-

6.3.3. Table of variables

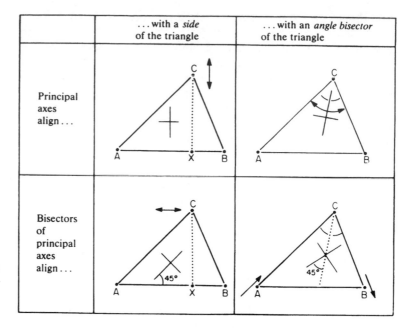

	... with a *side* of the triangle	... with an *angle bisector* of the triangle
Principal axes align ...		
Bisectors of principal axes align ...		

Figure 6.3.3. The four alignments of principal axes with simpler elements of a triangle, to be used in conjunction with Table 6.3.1.

nate pair, that for the proximal origin of the ultimate chamber, accounted for most of the T^2. The construction of principal axes corresponding to the mean shape change for that coordinate is shown in Figure 6.3.4. We find ourselves in the upper left cell of Table 6.3.1: One principal axis is nearly aligned with the segment from proximal point to proloculus point. The shape change may therefore be described as alteration in the relative height of the triangle measured to that edge. Equivalently, we may refer to the change as an *opening of the vertex angle* of this spiral form. Or we may refer as well to the evolutionary implications of the invariant of the transformation: the angle at landmark C, maintained at 90°.

The alignment of the principal directions corresponds quite precisely to the algebraic dominance of two particular loadings in the group discrimination factor of Section 4.3.2: The distance from proximal point to aperture has the most negative loading, and that from proximal point to proloculus the most positive. Hence the ratio of those two distances is likely to approximate an "optimal" descriptor of the shape discriminator. As the distances in question lie at nearly 90°, they are indeed the natural descriptor as generated by the tensor methods. (That is, the case in the upper left cell of Table 6.3.1 actually applies here to two sides: Triangle ABC is a right triangle.) Recall that there was no hint whatever of this biological feature in the discriminant function for the same pair of strata in terms of six distance measures: Those contrasted the distance $|BC|$ with the distance $|BD|$, but the contrast expressed only noise around size allometry. The canonical loadings weighted measures of the ultimate chamber almost

220

	...with a *side* of the triangle	...with an *angle bisector* of the triangle
Principal axes align...	*Covariant*: ratio of altitude CX to baseline AB – aspect ratio of triangle ABC to this baseline	*Covariant*: angle at C (the closer this angle is to 90°, the greater its statistical power)
	Invariant: ratio $AX : XB$ in which the foot of the perpendicular to side AB from vertex C divides that side	*Invariant*: ratio of edges $AC : BC$ (if this is 1 : 1, refer to case at left)
	Interpretation (arrow): C is moving *toward* (or away from) baseline AB, up to scale change	*Interpretation* (arrow): the angle at C is opening (or closing)
Bisectors of principal axes align...	*Covariant*: ratio $AX : XB$	*Covariant*: ratio of edges $AC : BC$
	Invariant: ratio $CX : AB$	*Invariant* (approximate): angle at C (if 90°, use scheme at upper left)
	Interpretation (arrow): point C is moving *along* baseline AB, up to scale change	*Interpretation* (arrow): edge AB is rotating with respect to angle C, up to scale

Table 6.3.1. *Familiar shape variables for particular alignments of the principal axes (to be used in conjunction with Figure 6.3.3 for the purpose of turning shape-coordinate findings into English)*

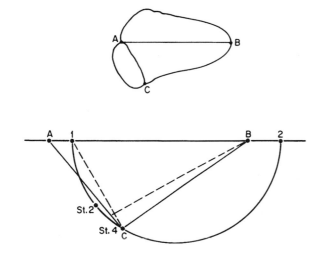

Figure 6.3.4. Principal axes corresponding to the mean difference between strata of *Brizalina* for the shape coordinates of the proximal boundary of the ultimate chamber to a baseline from aperture to proloculus. Mean shape coordinates are $(0.233, -0.330)$ and $(0.360, -0.442)$. Both principal axes nearly connect two landmarks. For the scatters, see Bookstein and Reyment (1989:669).

equally, and pretended to ignore the distance $|BC|$ as "not chang-ing" between the groups. In fact, it participates equally *and oppositely* in the two principal features of this shape change: an increase in General Size, and a decrease in the ratio of length $|BC|$ to that size.

6.4. ANALYSES OF MORE THAN THREE LANDMARKS

This section explains the role of distances between constructed landmarks in describing changes of any number of landmarks by extremes of ratios. The contribution of these ratios to description of the change is not complicated, but it is limited to the language of triangles already introduced. To go beyond descriptions of triangles requires a different set of descriptors than distance ratios.

6.4.1. The transect theorem (strain ratios for any number of landmarks)

It might be imagined that for configurations of four or more landmarks the extraction of the largest and smallest mean strains (ratios of distances between a pair of mean forms) would lead to geometrical constructions distinctly more complicated than these. Surprisingly, no further complexity is necessary. For any set of landmarks, the constructed distances $|c_i Z_i|$ (the size variables of Section 4.1) showing the maximum or minimum mean ratio be-tween two groups are lengths of segments from one landmark to some weighted average of two others – transects of triangles as we have been studying them all along. However many landmarks we have observed, all the distances we need to use in reports of shape change in *this* style are either direct length measurements between landmarks or else principal axes for the change of some triangle. Then the complexity of the search for largest and small-est ratios in the $(2K - 4)$-dimensional space of distance ratios for K landmarks is limited to the combinatorial search through a set of triangles, numbering at most $K(K - 1)(K - 2)/6$. (In practice, one does not consider all possible triangles, of course, but begins with those not too skinny. There are no problems of multiple comparison in connection with this approach, as the whole is under the control of the single global T^2-test for *any* shape change reviewed in Section 5.4.) Because the analysis of deforma-tion for triangles is a simple matter for ruler and compass, or the equivalent quadratic formula, the search for extremes of ratios of distances does not require any empirical numerical optimization at all: Not even a single continuous parameter is involved. (Other sorts of descriptors, optimal in other senses, will be introduced in Chapter 7.)

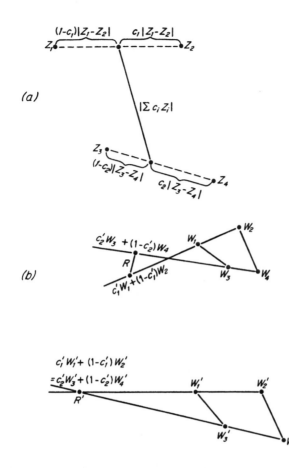

Figure 6.4.1. Strain for a proper transect of a quadrilateral. (*a*) Join of the point c_1 of the way along the top edge to the point c_2 of the way along the bottom edge. The theorem under review states that no such segment can bear a proper maximum or minimum of strain between two mean landmark configurations. (*b*) The global extrema of the strain ratio lie well outside the intended limits of these data. Here, the minimum strain (zero, up to statistical fluctuations) corresponds to the intersection of the edges of the second form, which is "homologous" (using the algebra of constructed landmarks, Section 4.1) to a finite distance on the first form as shown.

The assertions of the preceding paragraph, slightly sharpened, are the gist of Theorem 2 in Bookstein (1986*a*). I shall call it the transect theorem, because the distances involved usually transect ("cut across") triangles. The basic points of the demonstration are two. Supposing that a ratio of distances between two constructed landmarks (weighted combinations of landmark locations) is largest or smallest, one can first show that the ratio does not involve more than four landmarks; then one can show that at least one of the landmarks is redundant, so that the extremal distance is from one landmark to a combination of two others. But these are just the transects of triangles, as studied exhaustively in the preceding three sections. This second step includes some ideas that will be relevant to the study of inhomogeneous transformations (Section 7.4), and so I shall enlarge here upon its import.

6.4.2. Part of the proof

Distances measured using four landmarks come in two varieties: distances relating two weighted averages of two (Figure 6.4.1), and distances from one landmark to the weighted average of three others (Bookstein, 1986a: Appendix Lemma 3). The set of segments linking two points, one on each of two opposite edges of a quadrilateral of landmarks, can be considered a function of two variables, c_1 and c_2, each specifying the proportion in which one of the ends of the distance measure cuts one of the edges (Figure 6.4.1a). The squared *length* of any such segment will be a quadratic form in these two parameters together with coordinates of the four corner landmarks. Specifically, it will be the sum

$$[c_1 P_{1x} + (1 - c_1)P_{2x} - c_2 P_{3x} - (1 - c_2)P_{4x}]^2$$
$$+ [c_1 P_{1y} + (1 - c_1)P_{2y} - c_2 P_{3y} - (1 - c_2)P_{4y}]^2$$

of terms for the squared x- and y-differences between the endpoints of the segment. The squared *strain ratio* for this length between the two mean landmark configurations will be a ratio of two such quadratic forms in the same parameters c_1 and c_2.

The geometry of this ratio is exactly analogous to the geometry of the principal axes of an ellipsoid in three dimensions. (The establishment of this analogy and the method of **relative eigenanalysis** it supports are the concerns of Section 7.6.1.) The principal axes of an ellipsoid are just the stationary points of the "strain ratio" by which the ellipsoid is deformed from a sphere. [In the present case, there is no "sphere," but instead the formula for length of the segment using (c_1, c_2) in the first form.] Of the three axes of the ellipsoid, one is the longest diameter, one is the shortest, and one is a so-called saddle point around which diameters are increasing in two quadrants and decreasing in two others. Exactly the same is true of our problem in c_1 and c_2: There will be three combinations of these two parameters corresponding to the three axes of our "ellipsoid."

But we can construct two of these axes (eigenvectors) by hand. One is shown in Figure 6.4.1b: the "segment" corresponding to the intersection of the edges of one quadrilateral, and its homologue in the other form. The "strain ratio" for this pair (c_1, c_2) is zero – a positive length has been shrunk to zero. (Do not worry that this intersection is far outside the data. The conclusion of the theorem deals only with interior transects, those of potential biological meaning; the figure merely illustrates the algebra.) Likewise, the *maximum* "strain ratio" falls outside the limits of the quadrilaterals. The strain corresponding to the intersection of edges of the *first* quadrilateral is infinite, clearly corresponding to the "long axis" of the ellipsoid in your mind. As there are no remaining extrema of strain, the third axis of the quadric comparison, even if it were found to lie properly inside the quadrilaterals (i.e., to pertain to weighted combinations with $0 < c_1,\ c_2 < 1$), would have to be the stationary axis, that for which the ratio tends upward in two quadrants and downward in two others. It follows that whatever the configuration of mean landmarks in a pair of forms, no transect of the quadrilateral like that in Figure 6.4.1*a* can bear a proper extremum of the strain ratio. Therefore, not all of the four landmarks are necessary: Those homologous distance ratios that are largest or smallest for a particular mean comparison can be characterized using at most three landmarks.

6.4.3. Implications of the transect theorem for studies of distance ratios

This theorem, although valuable and reassuring, is somewhat limited in application. Much of the work of reporting shape change deals with the issue of the *patterns* of these strain ratios, not their absolute extrema. The description of these patterns is the primary concern of Chapter 7.

Unless one's landmarks all lie nearly in one line, the set of all the distances between them in pairs contains all the biological shape information of the original locations, so that shape coordinates, in particular, are encrypted there. But it does not follow that arbitrary statistical manipulations, such as principal-component analysis of all those interlandmark distances, will yield the same information as does analysis of the shape coordinates. The transect theorem states that ratios of interlandmark distances need not (and, in practice, usually do not) serve as the variables of greatest utility for contrasting mean shapes. Some analyses of these variables fail to detect effects on shape, such as group differences, as efficiently as would a suitable analysis of the shape coordinates; other analyses of distance ratios, though statistically equivalent to the analyses of the shape coordinates, cannot be as clearly reported. Let us reconsider the inspection of cross-ratios of simple interlandmark distances, as sketched in Section 4.3.3, and show precisely what information it ignores. The following critique applies explicitly to any method that scans the $K(K-1)/2$ ratios of interlandmark distances between a pair of samples to find the largest and smallest – analogues to the rightmost column of Table 4.3.2 – and then tests this contrast for significance (e.g., the method of "Euclidean distance matrix analysis" introduced by Lele, 1989). Methods of this class incorporate two fatal morphometric errors that I shall demonstrate using a pair of simulated shape changes.

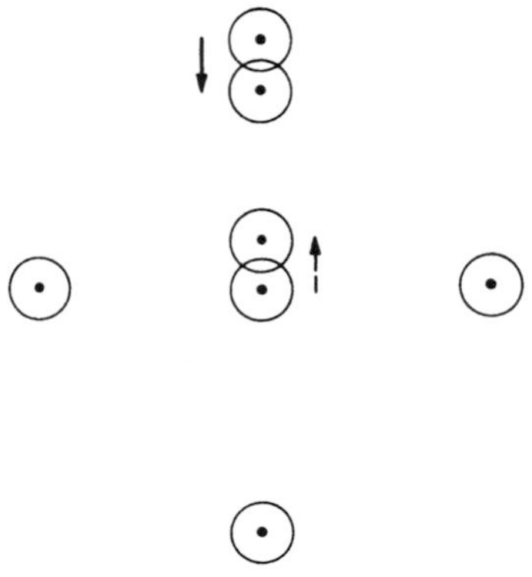

Figure 6.4.2 shows the usual complex-normal model for variation among five landmarks roughly in the form of a quincunx. The method of shape coordinates and the methods of Kendall's shape space arrive at nearly the same statistical test for relative movement of any one of these landmarks by a fixed distance in any direction (this is the property of "Riemannian submersion" mentioned in Section 5.6). I shall show that a temptingly simple method of cross-ratios is inefficient for detecting this sort of

Figure 6.4.2. Simulation for the argument about efficiency of the cross-ratio method. Dashed arrow: First shape change. Solid arrow: Second shape change.

225

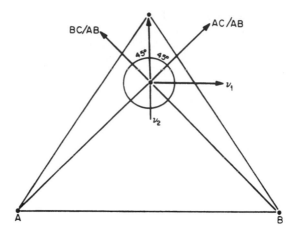

Figure 6.4.3. Simple distance ratios are inefficient for the detection of most of the transects described in Section 6.4.1.

change. Compare a shape change by displacement of the central point toward the north landmark with a change by displacement of the north point toward the central point. If we are comparing mean distances, that between the central and the north landmarks will drop by some 10% in both cases. In the former simulation, but not the latter, the distance from the center to the south landmark will increase by 10% correspondingly. Thus the extreme change of cross-ratio will tend to be about 20% for the former change, versus only somewhat more than 10% for the latter change (we can expect some of the distances among the lower four landmarks to have become smaller, but not by as much as 10% if samples are of reasonable size). As computations easily verify, the efficiency of the method of cross-ratios for detecting changes of the latter geometry is thereby quite a bit lower than for detecting the former sort: There are "too many" possible denominators whose random shrinking has to be ruled out, as it were, before we can credit the numerator with expanding.

Furthermore, this simulation shows the method of cross-ratios at its best, applied to changes that are precisely aligned with the vectors between mean landmark locations. Figure 6.4.3 shows a case to which the conditions of the transect theorem apply with more bite: a simple change of mean shape between two isosceles triangles. The discrimination is borne by the vertical shape coordinate ν_2, changes in which can be expressed by changes in the distance ratio $(|CA| + |CB|)/4|BA|\sqrt{2}$. The simple ratio best reporting this change will be the ratio of one of the equal sides, $|CA|$ or $|CB|$, to the baseline. On the shape-coordinate plane, where (on the null model) correlation is approximated by cosine (Section 5.3.1.1), we see that either of these simple ratios makes an angle of 45° with the optimal discriminator, and thus has efficiency $1/\sqrt{2} \sim 71\%$ for the detection of this change.

Thus the cross-ratios of simple edges are effective neither for the detection of shape change against digitizing noise nor, according to the transect theorem, for its description in biologically interpretable terms whenever it *is* detected. The theorems of this and the preceding chapter provide a useful tool, in fact, for critiques of many newly proposed methods for landmark analysis. In general, methods that do not detect group differences as efficiently as do the shape coordinates waste data and require excessively large samples to show the same effect to a specified precision or significance level. (The simple edge ratio requires twice as large a sample as the transect to achieve significance in Figure 6.4.3). There are no offsetting advantages in light of the corresponding simplicity of the shape coordinates. The less efficient methods are irrecoverably defective, then, and should never be used for testing. Section 6.6 will turn to another system of shape analysis, the so-called finite-element method, which *can* be fully efficient, and will indicate what pains must be taken to achieve that end.

6.5. BIOMETRIC ANALYSIS OF TRIANGLES OF LANDMARKS: EXAMPLES

This section will use triangles of landmarks to demonstrate a wide variety of multivariate statistical strategies. Study these examples thoroughly: Many important general remarks are embedded here near specific instances of the features of shape analysis to which they apply.

The formalism of shape coordinates permits the interpretation of effects upon shape as vectors of mean difference or mean expected difference. These, in turn, support all of the usual maneuvers of multivariate statistics: the testing of such effects as group membership, size allometry, correlation with exogenous covariates, autocorrelation, factor structure, and so forth. The same reinterpretation of these vectors as deformations that permitted us to compute the principal axes of single changes permits, as well, the computation of principal axes for any of these other sorts of covariances with triangular shape. Any multivariate procedure that arrives at a vector of coefficients for the shape coordinates may be reinterpreted by way of the principal axes of that vector when it is taken to describe a deformation of the triangle. In this way, not only group mean differences but also correlations with various other factors may be assigned principal axes and strains that ease us toward biological interpretations. Chapter 7 will introduce descriptive tools other than principal strains that apply to configurations more complex than triangles. But often the tensor description of change in a single or typical triangle is sufficient for reporting considerably more complex configurations; and many of the more advanced descriptions begin by presuming that the best-fitting description by a pair of principal axes has already been reported and "partialed out."

In this respect, landmark data are much more congenial to multivariate statistical analysis than are the data of other subject

227

areas. Elsewhere the statistical organization of the variables is not accompanied by this spatial organization. In no other field, for instance, do variables come in pairs of invariant and covariant in involution (Section 5.1.3). Furthermore, within morphometrics the analysis of shape coordinates represents a more profound exploitation of multivariate analysis than is found in the more classic analyses of suites of distances and angle or ratio measures (cf. Reyment et al., 1984), in the course of which this spatial organization of alternate measurement schemes is not referenced. This point was touched on in Section 4.3.3, where it was noted that the limitations of multivariate morphometrics ultimately owed to its concentration upon covariances only, rather than being able to make reference to mean forms. It is in the means of distances, of course, that the positions of the landmarks are encoded. Analyses of the shape coordinates by the methods of this and the next chapter all use that information extensively to add power and redundancy to the reporting of statistical findings.

6.5.1. Human cranial growth, ages 8 to 14 years

As a first example of the systematic exploitation of the tensor interpretation of findings based in the shape coordinates, I shall turn to the longitudinal University School Study (Section 3.4.2) and, for now, examine one single triangle, the largest that can be formed out of these data. This is the triangle Basion–Nasion–Menton joining the two endpoints of the *cranial base* – Nasion, at the bridge of the nose, and Basion, at the front of the foramen magnum – to Menton, the landmark at the bottom of the chin. These are landmarks #30, #35, and #38 in Figure 3.4.3.

In order to illustrate a diversity of biometrical designs in the same data set, I have chosen a serial subsample of this data base: 36 males and 26 females for whom there are usable films taken at age 8 years $\pm$ 6 months and at age 14 years $\pm$ 6 months. There results a two-group (male/female) two-wave (age 8/age 14) longitudinal design that permits many different comparisons. Each of these will be computed in one or another space of shape coordinates, tested there for statistical significance, and then given a tentative biological interpretation by reexpression in terms of principal axes of deformation tensors. Because the design is longitudinally matched, changes between the ages can legitimately be called "growth"; in this section I shall use the words "growth" and "change" interchangeably. A complete listing of this small data base can be found in Appendix A.4.1. Many of the analyses to follow were published in Bookstein (1984b).

For data sets this compact, it is often possible to devise a graphic that presents nearly all of the data in readable form. As the design is longitudinally matched, the object of display might be the pair of shapes corresponding to the two ages observed for each case in the subsample. These pairs should be drawn as

228

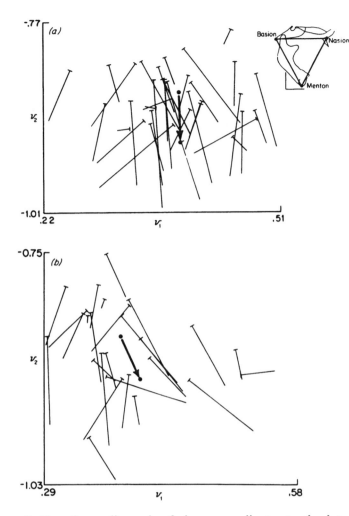

Figure 6.5.1. Data for the University School Study example. These diagrams incorporate all of the information available in this analysis except for size (which is retained for subsequent computations: cf. Figure 6.5.7). In these scatters, each case is represented by one pair of shape coordinates at age 8 and another pair at age 14. This pair of points is connected by a "pin" having its "head" at the location corresponding to the earlier shape. The means of the pinheads and pinpoints are drawn in large dots upon each scatter and are connected by the vector that is the mean shape change. (*a*) 36 males. (*b*) 26 females. Shape coordinates are those of Menton to the Basion–Nasion baseline. After Bookstein (1984*b*: Figure 9).

vectors linking the earlier pair of shape coordinates to the later pair, child by child. In Figure 6.5.1 I have chosen to indicate the sense of these vectors by a pin with head at the earlier observation. The baseline for construction of shape coordinates is taken along the cranial base itself, from Basion to Nasion; of course, this choice will not affect the findings as long as they are reported in the proper baseline-independent way.

6.5.1.1. *Difference between boys and girls at age 8.* —

The simplest question we might ask deals with sexual dimorphism between the groups at the earlier age. The mean shape coordinates of Menton to this baseline (Figure 6.5.2*a*) are, for the 8-year-old boys, (0.380, −0.858), and for the girls, (0.391, −0.856). The difference between these two means is insignificant by Hotelling's T^2($p \sim .74$). Significant or not, this mean shape difference corresponds to an interpretation in terms of principal axes

229

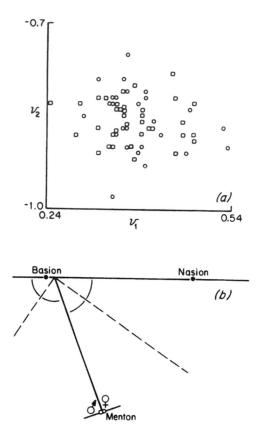

Figure 6.5.2. Dimorphism of form between boys and girls at age 8. The mean difference between these two groups is insignificant by T^2. (a) Scatter. (b) Principal axes.

as sketched in Figure 6.5.2b. The observed significance level of the T^2 states that the orientation of this optimal shape variable is wholly unreliable given the within-group scatter in the data: There is not enough intergroup shape difference to identify with confidence the principal strains along the ratio of which it lies. The insignificance of the T^2 does not assert the absence of *size* differences between the groups (Table 6.5.1). Nor does it assert (see Section 6.5.1.3) that the mean difference between groups would be insignificant if tested with one degree of freedom by shape variables (such as the ratio of lengths in the principal directions) aligned with this observed difference. We shall see, though, that that significance level is biased. In this instance, the simple two-group t-test using the optimal ratio of distance measures indicated is likewise insignificant. (The anisotropy of the mean difference is only 1.3%.) In the sequel we shall encounter an example that is not so consistent.

The shape coordinates omit precisely one further morphometric fact about each of these triangles: size. One version of size, baseline length, has been divided out in the construction of the coordinates. Nevertheless (see Section 5.5), the appropriate examination of potential effects of size upon these shapes proceeds using a suitable version of Centroid Size: $\sqrt{p^2}$, root-summed-squared edge length. If there were only one group under study, a test for allometry would proceed using the ordinary multiple regression of size upon the shape coordinates, as explained in Section 5.5. In this two-group design, we should instead exploit the comparable analysis of covariance. The statistical analysis is the same whether we consider the multivariate (here, bivariate) dependence of the shape-coordinate vector upon one single covariate, size, or instead consider the univariate dependence of size upon the vector of shape coordinates. Table 6.5.1 presents the usual decomposition of covariance for the latter design: a test for so-called **static allometry** at either age. Predictions of size are by multiple regression of $\sqrt{p^2}$ on the two shape coordinates separately by age and by sex. There is no size allometry – no change of shape with size – within either sex or pooled across the sexes, at either age.

The structure of Table 6.5.1 may be viewed as the remodeling of Table 4.3.1 appropriate to the investigations of allometry using Centroid Size and the shape coordinates in place of General Size and the space of distance measures. When General Size (allometric size) is replaced by Centroid Size (geometric size), the same allometry that was to be seen in the variation of "size loadings" (regression coefficients of the log distances on General Size) is seen instead in the dependence of Centroid Size upon these shape coordinates. (Recall from Section 5.5.3 that the multiple regression of Centroid Size upon shape is merely a device for arriving at the correct statistical test – independence of Centroid Size from all the dimensions of shape space. The multiple regression coefficients have no particular meaning for the description of allometry even should the null hypothesis of isometry be rejected.) Whether or not allometry is found, the test of size-adjusted group shape differences by comparison of individual intercepts in the

6.5.1. Human cranial growth

Table 6.5.1. *Static allometry, Basion–Nasion–Menton, by sex, separately at ages 8 and 14 years (36 boys, 26 girls)*

Group	Adjusted mean size $\sqrt{p^2}$	"Prediction" of size		Significance of regression
		Intercept	Coefficients	
Age 8 (net significance of covariates .70)				
Boys	7.302	7.482	$-1.164, -0.309$	n.s.
Girls	7.054	7.736	$+0.997, +1.255$	n.s.
Diff. sig.@	.0004		0.162	
Age 14 (net significance of covariates .30)				
Boys	8.263	7.906	$-1.527, -1.029$	n.s.
Girls	7.914	7.804	$+0.117, -0.052$	n.s.
Diff. sig.@	.0001		0.031	

log-covariance analysis, Table 4.3.1, is less powerful than the corresponding test of mean shape coordinates adjusted for regression on Centroid Size (a mean comparison not demonstrated here). For a longer discussion of the interactions between these two approaches to the same phenomenon (allometry) in the same data (landmark locations), see Bookstein (1989c).

6.5.1.2. Mean growth, age 8 to age 14. —

The general direction of the pins in Figure 6.5.2 is clearly downward in both samples. In addition, there appears to be a component of growth "toward the right" (in this registration) for the girls. We shall first test these changes for significance, in two different ways, and then interpret them, and also the difference between them, by recourse to the principal axes of the corresponding tensors.

The most straightforward approach to testing these differences is by ordinary two-group T^2 applied to the scatters at ages 8 and 14 separately. There result T^2-statistics of 49.3 for the boys and 14.6 for the girls, corresponding to p-levels of less than .0001 and .0019, respectively. Such a computation, however, ignores the longitudinal aspect of the data. We do better to exploit this matching by testing the mean of the explicitly observed individual shape changes against zero. These changes may be given a scatter in their own right (Figure 6.5.3). We have, in effect, gathered all the pinheads of Figure 6.5.1 at the same point, which now has coordinates $(0, 0)$ rather than those of the mean age-8 shape-coordinate pair. Notice that their distribution is not far from circular (but see Section 6.5.1.6). A matched T^2 for these changes separately by sex could be computed as in Section 5.4.3: one test for the significance of the mean shape change for the boys, and another for the girls. But in reality there was no need to compute any statistic for testing these change scores. For the subsample of boys, all pins (vectors of change scores) point downward, an event having a probability of perhaps 2^{-34} on a sensible null hypothesis. That is, every boy's Menton grows farther away from the Basion–Nasion baseline as a multiple of the length of that baseline. For the girls, all the pins point downward except one, an event of probability $26 \cdot 2^{-24}$. Both of these probabilities are satisfactorily small.

In matched studies such as these, an alternative statistic to Hotelling's T^2 is available that can speed graphical computations. One can compare the length of the mean vector to the mean of the lengths of the individual vectors that make up the sample. These lengths are taken directly in shape-coordinate space (i.e., directly upon Figure 6.5.3). Recall (Section 6.2.4) that the ratio of this length to the height of the starting form measures the anisotropy (directionality) of the shape change. Thus, up to this shared factor of the relative height of the mean form, the length

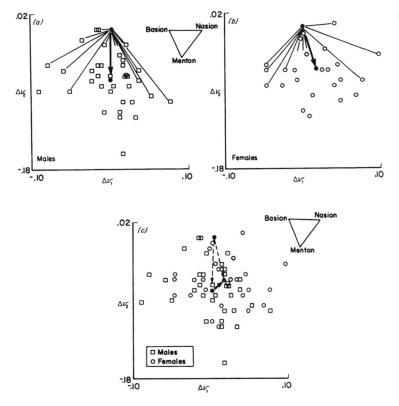

Figure 6.5.3. Explicit display of change scores for the shape-coordinate pairs in Figure 6.5.1, by displacement of all age-8 shapes to a common point. (*a*) Boys. (*b*) Girls. (*c*) Both sexes, indicating means of change by sex and also the vector difference between these means. After Bookstein (1984*b*: Figure 10).

of the mean vector in Figure 6.5.3 represents the anisotropy of the mean deformation, whereas the mean length of the individual change vectors in the same figure represents the mean of the anisotropies for the sample of shape changes child by child. Values of this ratio greater than about $2/\sqrt{N}$ are significant for mean shape change at about the conventional .05 level (Bookstein, 1984*a*). In this example, the ratio is about .892 for boys, .865 for girls; there is no doubt that these values exceed the appropriate .05 thresholds (about .33 and .39).

In addition to the matched T^2 for the mean changes separately by sex, there is also the ordinary two-group T^2 testing the difference between the mean changes in the two sexes, the little stubby vector in Figure 6.5.3. The T^2 for this test of growth dimorphism is 4.31, $p \sim .13$.

Thus far we have been examining only probability levels and vectors in shape-coordinate space. The values of T^2 are already independent of baseline. To render the report of the geometry of these changes likewise independent of our choice of baseline, which has no biological reality, we must reinterpret all these differences in terms of principal axes and principal strains – in **tensor** terms. That is, we want to find the pair of directions on the face – the pair of transects of this triangle – whose ratio is the covariant of the age difference or group difference in the figures.

233

6.5. Examples: triangles

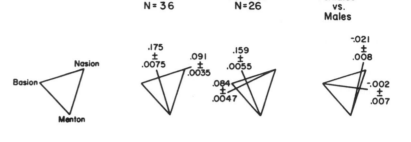

Figure 6.5.4. Tensor interpretation of the three mean differences of shape coordinates in Figure 6.5.3. Differences in baseline length have been restored to the computation of mean strain ratios; then their standard errors can be computed. Left to right: Growth, boys; growth, girls; growth dimorphism. The directions of these principal axes are interpreted in the text. After Bookstein (1984*b*: Figure 10).

Application of the circle construction to the three vectors in Figure 6.5.3 results in the three sets of principal axes (two mean changes and their difference) shown in Figure 6.5.4. Each of these is now a transect of the triangle, a length that might have been measured with a ruler directly on the original x-rays. Notice that rotation (from boys to girls) of the mean difference vector by 14° in the shape-coordinate plane (the angle between the vectors in Figures 6.5.3*a* and 6.5.3*b*) has resulted in a rotation of the principal axes by precisely half that much upon the form (the angle between the axes in Figures 6.5.4*a* and 6.5.4*b*).

In the graphical presentation of these strains, to aid the interpretation we have restored the information about size (i.e., the distance from Basion to Nasion) that was divided out when we constructed the shape coordinates. This restoration can proceed in one of two ways. The approach I prefer (Bookstein, 1982*b*) takes the shape-coordinate findings as instructions for measurements to be carried out back in the space of the original digitized data at its actual scale. Interpreting the principal directions as vectors connecting one landmark to a weighted average of two others, one computes these lengths explicitly triangle by triangle, and then their ratios (the growth strains); these are then averaged. This permits the computation of standard deviations for the strains in the principal directions case by case, and thus standard errors for the means of those strains, as indicated in the figure. Alternatively, one may compute the strains to fixed baseline length using the formula in equation (6.2.1), and then multiply each of these by the average fraction by which baseline length has changed between the age-8 and age-14 samples for each sex. These two approaches result in the same means to two significant figures, but the latter does not supply estimates of the standard errors of these means.

The interpretation of these pairs of principal axes is straightforward. That for mean growth in boys (Figure 6.5.4) may be described as Menton's "moving straight away from" the Basion–Nasion baseline. (This is the upper left cell of Figure 6.3.3 or Table 6.3.1.) For boys, growth of distances in this direction was at a mean of 17.5% over the six years of study, versus 9.1% for growth in the perpendicular direction, directly along the cranial-base baseline. (The ratio $1.175:1.091$ represents an anisotropy of 7.7%. According to Section 6.2.4, this quantity estimates δ/h, where δ is the mean distance moved and h is the mean "vertical" shape coordinate v_2. To recover δ, multiply the anisotropy by h, which is about 0.86; the result is consistent with the length $\delta = 0.065$ of the mean vector in Figure 6.5.3a.) There is no doubt that these mean strains are significantly different from zero and from each other. In their directions they correspond to well-known aspects of normal craniofacial growth. Growth at the cranial base is paced by growth of the brain, which is substantially complete by the starting age of these data. The average composite of the various processes intervening between there and the chin – enlargement of the jaws, eruption of additional permanent teeth, and so on – has the effect of moving the apparent position of the chin along a "growth axis" perpendicular to the cranial base. The classic cephalometricians knew that the growth axis was perpendicular to the cranial base and that the cranial-base axis was the direction of least growth over this range; but they did not realize that these two propositions entail one another. Their equivalence is a matter for geometry, not for biology. The mean observed shape change for girls (Figure 6.5.4) differs only slightly from that for boys. Principal directions and mean principal strains are almost the same and merit no separate interpretation.

6.5.1.3. Cost of T^2. —

The question of growth dimorphism is a little more interesting. Recall that the T^2 for the difference of this pair of growth changes was significant at $p \sim .13$ only. The tensor interpretation of this change (Figure 6.5.4) indicates that it is *wholly directional*. Growth dimorphism is expressed in only one aspect of this triangle, distance from Nasion to Menton; perpendicular to that direction (along what the orthodontist calls "facial depth"), there is no dimorphism whatever. In the figure, each principal strain is accompanied by its own sample standard error (which is computed by the usual pooling formulas, as there is no matching between these samples of boys and girls). These standard errors are approximately equal because the triangle is approximately equilateral. The formulas that apply under the null model have been published in Bookstein (1984a). The T^2 of the shape coordinates tested the difference of these two mean strains *from each other*; but we see also that the larger of them is different from zero when considered as an ordinary t-ratio.

The idea behind Hotelling's T^2 is a variant of the notion underlying Student's t. T^2, like $(t)^2$, is the squared ratio of an observed mean difference to *its own* standard error. For student's t, this ratio is significant at the conventional 5% level above about 2.0 (a little more for small samples, a little less for larger ones).

The equivalent threshold for $\sqrt{T^2}$ on *two degrees of freedom* – the appropriate number for a pair of coordinates, as we have here – is about 2.54 instead of 2.0. The ratio of thresholds, $2.54 : 2.0 \sim 1.27$, is attempting to approximate $\sqrt{\pi/2}$, the expected value of $\sqrt{\chi^2}$ on two degrees of freedom.

T^2 is the correct statistic for the question of whether or not there is any sexual dimorphism in shape. The test corrects for the fact that chance differences could have arisen in any direction of the shape-coordinate plane. The best single discriminator of triangular shape between groups needs to be a 25% better discriminator than if we had known in advance that discrimination was to be precisely in its direction, and so had measured that shape variable alone. Hence the use of the T^2 rather than Student's t costs us about as much as a 25% increase in precision of estimate would gain us: It demands an increase, in other words, of $(\pi/2) - 1 \sim 57\%$ in sample size. In exchange for this payment, we have gained the ability to check for shape difference in the directions of all shape gradients, whether we anticipated them or not. Notice that the variable that best discriminates old from young boys is different from that appropriate for girls, and both are different from that best describing the growth dimorphism.

It follows in our example that the algebraically larger of the principal strains, $2.1 \pm 0.8\%$, **must not** be tested for significance separately against zero. The appropriate test, rather, first determines the significance of its difference from the *other* principal strain – this is another way of phrasing the T^2-test under discussion. In this instance, that difference is significant at only the 13% level. As the principal strains cannot be distinguished with confidence, all that remains is to test their average (which is an estimate of net size change) against zero. For these data, that test rejects the null hypothesis of no dimorphism between these two samples of youngsters in regard to the triangle Basion–Nasion–Menton at $p \sim .01$. The boys have grown a mean of 0.97 inch of $\sqrt{p^2}$, and the girls, 0.84. The difference in growth rates in the principal directions of this comparison (equivalent to the aspect ratio to the Nasion–Menton baseline) seems to show a dimorphism significant by ordinary one-dimensional Student's t at about 4%. But this is the wrong significance level, because the t is the wrong test: The replacement of 4% by 13% is another way of demonstrating the cost of the proper statistical procedure, the T^2.

6.5.1.4. Standard error of the principal axes. —

When an observed shape difference or shape change is statistically significant by the T^2-test, one infers that the principal directions exist in the sense that it it unlikely that the data were generated by changes of lengths at the same rate in all directions. The question naturally arises of the standard error of the estimate of

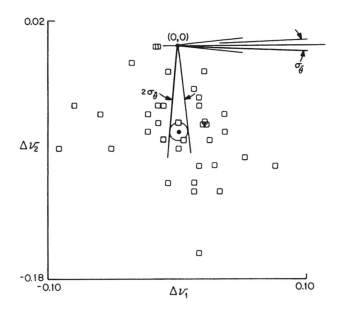

Figure 6.5.5. Standard error of the principal directions. The standard error of the direction of the mean shape-change vector (here exemplified by the scatter for boys from Figure 6.5.3) is, for nearly circular shape scatters, just the angle whose tangent is the ratio of the standard error of the scatter to the length of the mean vector. The little circle around the mean change has radius the average of the two standard errors of the mean for the shape coordinates plotted (in this example, these are shape-change scores). The standard error of direction of the principal cross is exactly half of this angle, owing to the step of angle bisection in the approximation to the circle construction.

that pair of directions. These are easily generated from the confidence interval for the mean vector underlying these axes. Figure 6.5.5, for instance, shows the usual scatter of shape-change vectors for the 36 boys of this study and indicates by a circle the standard error of that mean in a typical direction. (The radius plotted is actually the mean of the computation for the two shape coordinates separately.) The standard error of the direction of this vector is very nearly the arctangent of the ratio between this radius and the length of the mean vector, and the standard error of direction of the principal axes is half that arctangent. The longer this mean vector (i.e., the sharper the distinction between the principal strains – the larger the anisotropy of the mean change), the more precisely are these principal directions determined.

The test for growth dimorphism by T^2 incorporates a test for this difference of directions as one of its degrees of freedom. The other is a sum of squares for differences in the mean anisotropy of growth in the two sexes as estimated along their pooled "growth axis." As can be seen in Figure 6.5.3*c*, these two contributions to the net T^2 are of approximately the same magnitude in this example.

6.5.1.5. *Correlates of shape.* —

We have seen that there is no statistically significant difference in mean shape changes for these two groups of children. This might be phrased as a finding of "no correlation" between shape change (over these years, for these data) and sex. But there is the possibility of other correlations involving these shapes. In this

6.5. Examples: triangles

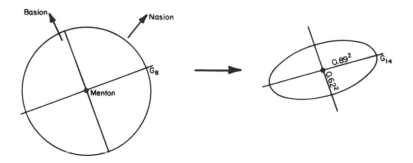

Figure 6.5.6. Shape autocorrelation (boys, age 8 to age 14, Menton to the Basion–Nasion baseline) analyzed by canonical correlation.

section we review two: shape extrapolation (the prediction of age-14 shape from age-8 shape) and size allometry (the prediction of shape change from size change).

In Figure 6.5.1a, for instance, the vector of mean change does not seem to enlighten us about most of the observed variation in shapes. Rather, pins that start at the left tend to end at the left, and likewise the right. In the flesh, faces that begin with Menton relatively far backward (along the cranial base) appear to end up in a similar predicament six years later, and similarly those that begin with Menton relatively far forward. Faces that begin with Menton relatively *high* appear to end up that way, but perhaps not so consistently. It is not clear if there is a similar pattern for the girls' data (Figure 6.5.1b).

The manner in which the entire set of shape variables at age 14 may be predicted by the age-8 set is embodied in the ordinary **canonical correlation analysis** relating the two two-dimensional shape spaces. In general, canonical correlation analysis applies to two sets of variables measured upon the same cases. The technique constructs the pair of linear combinations (one involving the variables of the first set, and the other those of the second) that have the highest correlation, then the pair having the highest correlation subject to the constraint of being uncorrelated with both members of the first pair, and so on. In the present context, this familiar multivariate technique computes two pairs of axes: one bearing the highest correlation across the ages of analysis, and the other the lowest.

For the boys' data (Figure 6.5.6), the canonical analysis indicates an ellipse of shape predictability with axes of lengths $.890^2$ and $.620^2$ along vectors $(.958, .237)$ and $(-.291, .973)$. These predict nearly parallel variables in the shape-coordinate plane: shape variables for the 14-year-olds with directions $(.951, .362)$ and $(-.312, .933)$. The direction of greatest predictability at age 14 is nearly perpendicular to the line Basion–Menton. Because the gradient of the angle Nasion–Basion–Menton is very nearly along this vector, that angle is a very stable measure of shape. Its expected value is not constant – over these six years it increases in mean by about $1.6°$ – but the variance of its change score is smallest, as a fraction of population variance, out of all shape

238

variables defined using these three landmarks. Perpendicular to this gradient of best forecast is the gradient corresponding to shape variables that change most noisily over these six years. Here that direction seems to be along the gradient of the distance from Menton to Basion divided by the length of the baseline: that is, the ratio of Basion's distances to Menton and to Nasion. In this cranial-base registration, the direction of Menton is the stablest shape measure, and the scaled position of Menton along that direction the least stable.

Bookstein (1990c, but written in 1984) analyzed these same data by the Partial Least Squares (PLS) method of Section 2.3.2, replacing the multiple regressions underlying canonical correlations by sums of simple regressions (the direct singular-value decomposition of the cross-correlation matrix). Correlations of the shape coordinates within the ages separately are $\pm.05$, indicating that there should be little effect of this substitution upon the coefficients, but, of course, considerable adjustment to the interpretation of those numbers. The correlation reported by the PLS between the estimated latent-variable scores has "dropped" from .890 to .889; the vector of saliences at age 8 is (.961, .276) and at age 14, (.961, .277). This identity of the PLS coefficients across the two ages reinforces the decision to ignore the within-age correlations that is embedded in the computational logic of PLS. In other examples of PLS analysis of shape coordinates (cf. Tabachnick and Bookstein, 1990a), PLS makes a great deal more difference for the coefficients. This is partly because, unlike either canonical coefficients or canonical loadings, they are not affected by intentional multicollinearity of exogenous variables (Sampson et al., 1989) when that multicollinearity expresses good measurement design. Recall, also, that those coefficients can be interpreted separately as covariances with latent variables – we shall do exactly that in a moment – whereas canonical-variates coefficients cannot be interpreted in this way (Section 2.3.2.2).

By either technique, the finding of this growth-prediction study is that the "vertical" position of Menton, its relative distance away from the Basion–Nasion line, is the most unstable over time. An explanation of this instability of vertical extent is available by exploiting the variable omitted from all these computations: the measure of triangular size. Figure 6.5.7 repeats the usual scatter of shape change for these boys and indicates over each point the change in size (in units of $\Delta\sqrt{p^2}$, change in root-mean-squared edge length in hundredths of inches) over the six years of observation. The regression equation corresponding to this scatter is

$$\Delta\sqrt{p^2} \sim 0.75 - 0.27\Delta\nu_1 - 3.3\Delta\nu_2,$$

having an R^2 of .295, significant at $p \sim .003$. The standard error of each regression coefficient is 0.90. The separate covariances of

6.5. Examples: triangles

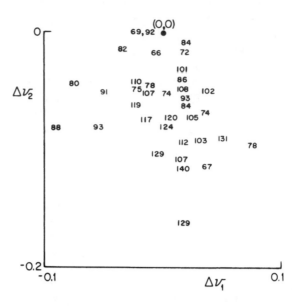

Figure 6.5.7. Size allometry in boys. Size change, in units of $100\sqrt{p^2}$ inches, is indicated at the endpoint of each of the shape-coordinate change vectors from Figure 6.5.3a. The allometry is apparent in the increase of the size-change measurement down the scatter.

Figure 6.5.8. Factor structure of the residual of Menton's shape coordinates after correction for size allometry. Apparently there is a direction of greater variation aligned with the anatomical ambiguity of Menton, the poorly defined point "at the bottom of the chin."

the $\Delta\nu$'s with $\Delta\sqrt{p^2}$ (the correct coefficients of the size-change effect, according to the logic of Section 2.3.2) are -0.0007 and -0.0038, the latter (like the corresponding regression coefficient) significant at about three times its standard error. For males, at least, the changes in shape that are more nearly vertical (as referred to the Basion–Nasion horizontal) are associated with the larger increases in size. In fact, the cranial base is a quite conservative structure; as far as this triangle is concerned, size-related variation in individual facial growth is expressed mostly along the growth axis in the lower face. Because we cannot predict size change from age-8 shape, the size loading of shape change in this gradient direction will be expressed as directional noise in the size-free analysis: the lower predictability $(.62^2)$ of changes along

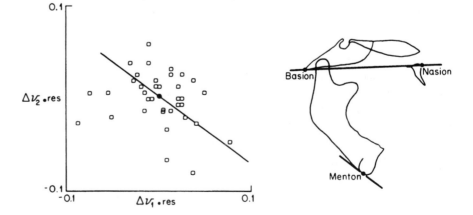

240

the growth axis. This correlation was not manifest in the static allometry of the 14-year-old males considered separately; only the analysis of change detects it.

6.5.1.6. *Factor structure of Menton.* —

The shape-change scatter for the boys (Figure 6.5.3*a*) is not quite circular. It has a long axis of variation pointing somewhat to the lower right, along the direction of the margin of the lower jaw. Some of this shape is not noise, but the allometry we just identified. To pursue the structure of what is left after allometry, we proceed just as in conventional regression, by constructing residuals: deviations of the changes of shape coordinates from age 8 to age 14 from the deviations that would be predicted from knowledge of the concurrent size change. In effect, this adjusts for our inability to predict the pubescent growth spurt in these boys, by consideration of the facial bones or by any other source of information known to the auxologist. When we carry out this adjustment, there results the scatter of shape-change residuals in Figure 6.5.8. (The gradient we corrected lay nearly at 90° to the long axis, and its partialing sharpened the apparent anisotropy.) In this residual scatter there seems to be a long axis of otherwise unexplained shape variation along the direction of uncertainty in the localization of the point Menton, the "bottom" of the chin. It is quite difficult to see just where the "bottom" of this curve is (cf. the diagram accompanying the definition, Figure 3.4.3). This excess of digitizing noise in one direction is typical of landmarks of Type 3 (Section 3.3.3).

There is a comparable failure of circularity in the scatter of starting forms, the pinheads in Figure 6.5.1. This extension of direction, however, is stable over the six years of this little substudy. My guess is that it is expressing real variation in the position of the upper jaw as it affects the rotation of the lower about the hinge at the condyle.

6.5.2. Size allometry and ecophenotypy for a microfossil

Section 3.4.3.4 introduced the features of eigenshape "averages" of samples of *Globorotalia truncatulinoides*. The averages bore three fairly clear extrema of curvature, which suggested themselves as landmarks for the "corners" of this approximately triangular form. We noticed as well variation in the curving of these forms between landmarks and suggested that it be archived to a certain extent by "pseudolandmarks" halfway between pairs of landmarks as measured by arc length. In this section we analyze only the three corners of the form; Section 7.3.3.3 will proceed with the exploitation of the further information about curving. In contrast to the preceding example, which involved two bipolar comparisons (boys versus girls, age 8 versus age 14), the current data set is from a single-group design with a continuous covariate (latitude). I shall use these data to demonstrate additional analyses of correlations with shape. The examples here will include principal-component analysis, another, more striking instance of size allometry, and *ecophenotypy* (correlations of shape with environment, the latter aspect measured here by latitude core by core). The data for this example are presented in their entirety in Appendix A.4.3.

To measure size differences, Lohmann's original analysis (1983) included average areas inside the entire curvilinear outline of the specimen, regardless of landmark triangles. Our morphometric method (Section 5.5) instructs us instead to use some version of Centroid Size, the summed-squared edge length. On the model of circular landmark noise, area is the optimal measure of size only in the vicinity of a mean form that is an equilateral triangle. For these forms, which are neither rectilinearly triangular nor quite equilateral, the correlation of area with p^2 is nevertheless .988. Had Lohmann located these landmarks (see Section 3.4.3.4), there would have been no need to measure area.

6.5.2.1. A principal component correlated with size and latitude. —

Clearly the scatter of these mean shapes (Figure 6.5.9) is not circular. In fact, the first principal component of the covariance matrix of these coordinates explains 93% of their summed variance by a vector along the direction (.978, −.211), the obvious major axis of the "ellipse" in the figure. Shape variation in this direction may be measured by the ratio of distances along the two principal axes constructed in Figure 6.5.9c. The measure of shape involved here is apparently the aspect ratio of triangular shape to the edge #3#1 (Table 6.3.1). This seems to match Lohmann's characterization (1983) of the corresponding eigenshape as the transformation from conical to compressed. (This is the second eigenshape; the first represents the pooled mean shape of all 20 samples.) Variation in this ratio correlates .901 with latitude: a pretty demonstration of ecophenotypy.

But the ν_1 coordinate of these points, all by itself, correlates .914 with latitude! In fact, it is mere accident that this direction of shape variation, whether our principal component or Lohmann's, is so neatly correlated with latitude; it was computed to explain variance, not this covariance.

Likewise, it is clear from the scatter in Figure 6.5.9b that this component of the data is correlated with size; but it is not obvious that it is a proper characterization of the effect of size on these average forms – that it is the covariant of size allometry within the shape-coordinate plane.

242

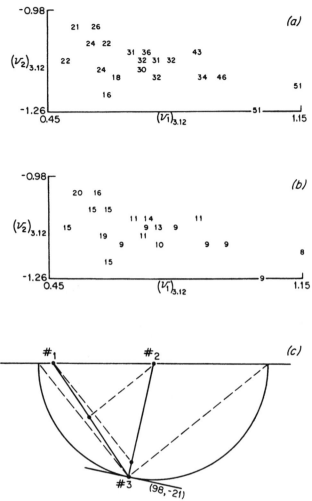

Figure 6.5.9. Shape coordinates for 20 mean forms of *Globorotalia truncatulinoides*. The movable point is landmark #3, the tip of the axis in Figure 3.4.11. (*a*) Number plotted at shape-coordinate pair is latitude in degrees S. (*b*) Number plotted at shape-coordinate pair is mean area, in 0.001 mm^2. (*c*) Circle construction for the interpretation of the principal axis of this scatter as a shape variable.

6.5.2.2. Size allometry. —

The regression of Centroid Size on the pair of shape coordinates in the figure is substantial. We have

$$\sqrt{p^2} \sim 136 - 54\nu_1 + 16\nu_2,$$
$$\quad\quad\quad (13) \quad\quad (37)$$

with $R^2 = .65$, $p \sim .0001$. The gradient of this shape predictor is in the direction $(-54, 16)$, satisfactorily aligned with the direction $(98, -21)$ of the principal within-group component of scatter. It would appear that this dimension of within-group variation might be considered to be "caused" by size allometry alone. (The covariances of the ν's separately with size, -1.66 and 0.37, are proportional to these regression coefficients, corroborating the factor model.) The scatter of the residuals from the regression of

243

6.5. Examples: triangles

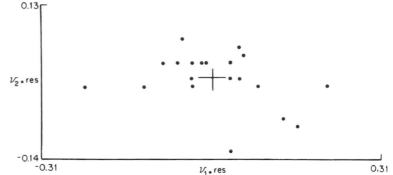

Figure 6.5.10. Scatter of shape-coordinate residuals from size allometry, 20 mean forms.

the shape coordinates separately upon size (Figure 6.5.10) appears not quite consistent with this conclusion: There is four times as much residual variance in the direction of ν_1 as in the direction of ν_2. Inspection of Figure 3.4.11 indicates the reason for this. We saw in Section 6.5.1.6 how excess of digitizing error in one direction resulted in noncircularity of shape scatters. The situation here is similar, though the directionality of error is an artifact of my landmark-location algorithm as it interacted with Lohmann's form of averaging. The eigenshape computation is conflating two convexities into one "landmark," and the precise location of the inferred maximum of smoothed curvature incorporates noise in the relative separation of those two subordinate landmarks. This noise happens to be horizontal to this baseline. The additional variance is not sufficient to cast much suspicion on the single-factor model of dependence, however, as the multiple-regression coefficients are proportional to the simple-regression coefficients.

Certain departures from the null model will be labeled as allometry by this test procedure. For instance, if in a configuration of three landmarks two were rigidly constrained to a constant separation (violating the independence assumption), allometry would be detected in the second shape coordinate of the third landmark to that baseline, just as was detected here. But under such a model we would not expect the presence of a clear axis in the shape-coordinate scatter aligned with the computed gradient of allometry. Under the condition $\epsilon_{1x} = \epsilon_{2x}$ in equations (5.3.1), the scatter of shape coordinates would still be nearly circular for many mean triangular forms, with shape-coordinate variances under the null model now expected to be $2 + 2s^2$ and $1 + r^2 + (1 - r)^2$, and their covariance $s(1 - 2r)$. Alternatively, the shape residuals after size is partialed out (Figure 6.5.10) would be distributed along a narrow curve if only one point were free to change its relative position with respect to two others. That is not the case here: Landmark-location error alone is not capable of explaining this scatter. The size allometry is certainly real.

244

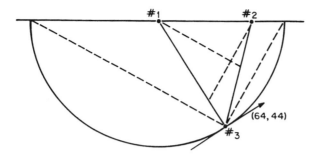

Figure 6.5.11. Shape variable best predicting latitude.

6.5.2.3. *Latitude.* —

The dependence of the shapes of these forms upon latitude is not so simple. The prediction gradient for latitude is

$$\text{latitude} \sim 35° + \underset{(6)}{64°\nu_1} + \underset{(19)}{44°\nu_2},$$

with $R^2 = .88$, $p < .0001$. Latitude is more systematically associated with these shapes than is size. But the shape variable that best predicts latitude is not at all aligned with the principal component of the scatter in Figure 6.5.9. The vector $(64, 44)$ makes an angle of more than 45° with the direction $(98, -21)$ of that component. It corresponds instead to the ratio of distances constructed in Figure 6.5.11. By Table 6.3.1, this aspect of shape is effectively measured by the angle at landmark #1. This variable is unrelated to the best measure of the principal axis of this scatter, the aspect ratio to baseline #3#1 or, equivalently, the angle at landmark #2.

The simple regression coefficients of the shape coordinates separately upon latitude, 0.153 and -0.020, are *not* proportional to these multiple-regression coefficients. (For instance, 44° is significantly different from zero and even more significantly different from $-66°$, the simple regression coefficient for latitude on ν_2 separately.) It follows that the factor model fails; shape is not the result of dependence upon a single effect of latitude by circular normal perturbations. The strong upward cant of the predictor of latitude in this shape-coordinate scatter can be detected in retrospect in Figure 6.5.9. Its origin is in the position of the shapes for latitudes 16° and 18° at one extreme of the hull under these points, balanced against points at latitudes 36° and 43° on the opposite side. The deviation between these apparently reliable forms is greater than can be accounted for as perturbation around a factor prediction.

6.5.3. Comparison of two craniofacial syndromes

The same design we applied to longitudinal data can be used for any other matched design. In particular, for statistical purposes **we**

245

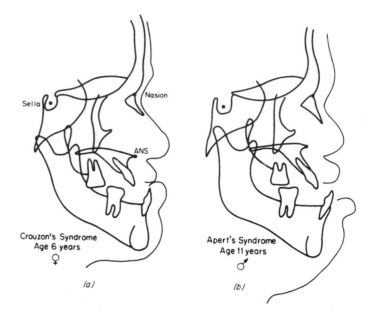

Figure 6.5.12. Typical forms of (*a*) Crouzon syndrome and (*b*) Apert syndrome as seen in the lateral cephalogram. After Bookstein (1984*b*:Figure 11).

may construe deformity as deformation. Any instance of a craniofacial syndrome, for instance, may be measured not as a form but as a deformation of the "normal," specifically, of the age- and sex-matched University School Study normative mean. The ratio of distances along the principal axes then represents the shape measure that is "most abnormal" in the deformity. When the null model applies to variation around the group mean landmark locations, this shape measure is the optimal Fisherian discriminator as well.

For example (Bookstein, 1984*b*), consider two variants of craniofacial synostosis: Apert syndrome and Crouzon syndrome (Figure 6.5.12). A synostosis is a premature closure of bony sutures; these two syndromes involve the intracranial bony sutures about the maxilla (upper jaw) and frontal bone (forehead). Apert syndrome, or acrocephalosyndactyly, shows synostosis of the cranial base and deformities of the extremities as well. Facially, these syndromes typically include a high, bulging forehead and a short maxilla positioned farther back than normal. The most obvious aspect of these deformities is the "caved-in" appearance of the midface. This section presents an analysis of the lateral facial aspect of the syndromes as represented by the triangle Sella–Nasion–Anterior nasal spine (ANS) (see Section 3.4.2). For the form of the mandible in these syndromes, see Section 3.5.

For the landmark ANS to a Sella–Nasion baseline, Figure 6.5.13*a* scatters the shape coordinates of each case with respect to the age- and sex-matched normal mean forms. In effect, each point is the deformity of one case, construed as a deformation from the form it "should have had." (Sampling variation of the

246

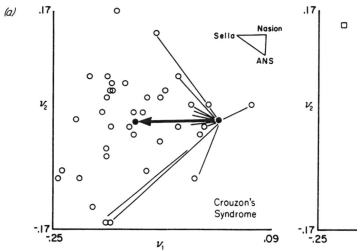

(a)

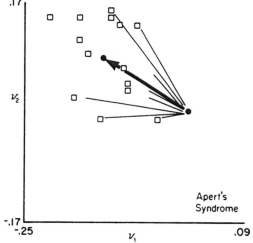

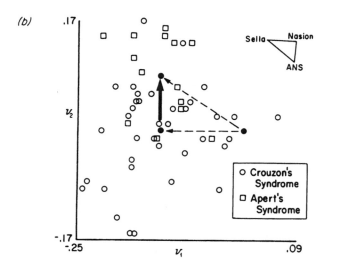

(b)

○ Crouzon's
Syndrome
□ Apert's
Syndrome

Figure 6.5.13. Comparison of Crouzon and Apert syndromes. (*a*) Translated pin plots (cf. Figure 6.5.3) for ANS to the Sella–Nasion baseline in Crouzon syndrome ($N = 37$) and Apert syndrome ($N = 14$) as deformations of the matched University School Study normal means [which are all to be taken at (0, 0), the right endpoint of the heavy vectors]. Data from the Institute for Reconstructive Plastic Surgery, New York University. (*b*) Vector for the difference between Apert and Crouzon syndromes: difference of the mean vectors for the syndromes separately. (*c*) Operational proportions, with sampling standard errors, representing the mean vectors in (*a*) and (*b*) and their difference. In the syndromes separately, all dimensions are reduced from normal, but some are reduced much more than others. The deformation that represents Apert syndrome for this triangle is not an intensification of that which represents Crouzon. After Bookstein (1984*b*:Figure 12).

(c)

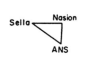

Crouzon's
Syndrome
$N = 37$

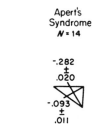

$-.230$
$\pm$
$.010$

$-.079$
$\pm$
$.013$

Apert's
Syndrome
$N = 14$

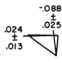

$-.282$
$\pm$
$.020$

$-.093$
$\pm$
$.011$

Apert's
vs.
Crouzon's

$-.088$
$\pm$
$.025$

$.024$
$\pm$
$.013$

247

normal mean forms is ignored in this analysis.) These vector means, which clearly show statistically significant mean shape differences, may be represented by the proportions indicated in Figure 6.5.13c. In neither syndrome are the principal axes aligned with familiar anatomical orientations, horizontal or vertical; nor are they aligned with each other. In terms of this triangle of landmarks, the difference between the syndromes is an additional deformation of normal, expressed in the difference between those mean deformity vectors (Figure 6.5.13b). This vector, itself highly statistically significant, corresponds to the principal axes and strains shown at the right in Figure 6.5.13c: additional shortfall of the distance from Nasion to ANS without further shortfall of normal along the cranial base. The vectors representing the two deformities are not parallel. The typical Crouzon form is thus not "in between" the normal and the typical Apert, and the difference between the effects of the two syndromes is best measured by a proportion different from those that characterize the deformities separately. We shall return to consider more of the landmarks of these Apert patients in Section 7.5.5.

6.5.4. Normal mandibular growth in three dimensions

The University of Michigan University School Study data base (Section 3.4.2) includes pairs of films at 90° for about 100 subjects at an average of four ages each. The data base includes 20 such film pairs for 8-year-old males and another 20 at 12 years of age; of these, 12 pairs correspond to serial studies. This example describes the mean changes of a mandibular landmark configuration (a pentahedron: Menton, left and right Condylions, left and right Gonions) for this small sample of boys. Section 5.4.4 has already presented the statistics of these landmarks; we now have the techniques to interpret those statistics. The analysis to follow, which appeared in Grayson et al. (1988), incorporates a sufficient number of triangles to exhaust the findings of any other biometric analysis dealing with the same five points.

The three-dimensional findings are summarized in Figure 6.5.14. These represent three-dimensional descriptions of mandibular size and shape change free of perspective distortions. For instance, the summary of change in the triangle Menton–Condylion–Condylion indicates that the bicondylar breadth (distance between the condyles) has increased at an average rate of 1.53% per year, the smallest specific rate of growth of any distance definable using these three landmarks, whereas the true (three-dimensional) distance from Menton to the intercondylar line has increased by an average of 2.48% per year over this interval, the largest of any distance. The standard deviation of the rate of increase of this latter distance is 0.40%; that for bicondylar breadth is twice as great, owing to the greater uncertainty of location of the condyles in this direction.

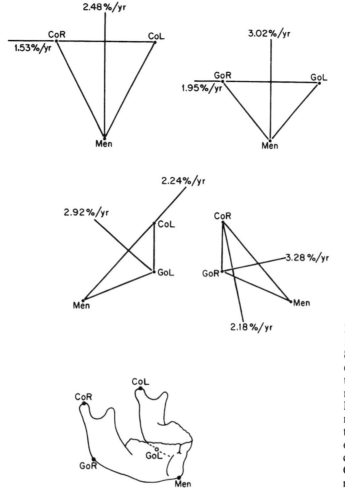

Figure 6.5.14. Mean growth for 12 boys observed between ages 8 and 12, represented by the changes in four triangles relating five points (Gonions left and right, Condylions left and right, Menton). All triangles have been rotated to lie flat in the plane of the paper before averaging. The difference of the mean growth changes for the two triangles Condylion–Gonion–Menton is not significant.

In the two-dimensional frontal view (Figure 6.5.15a) this same triangle shows a rate of increase of (projected) distance of Menton from the line between the condyles of 3.07% per year. This number is too large, indicating a decrease in foreshortening of this triangle at the same time that growth is occurring. By contrast, in the basilar view (the view upward "from the floor," not typically realized on actual x-ray film), the same distance shows a rate of increase of only 1.60% per year, considerably less than that seen in the three-dimensional analysis (and statistically indistinguishable from the growth rate of 1.53% in the distances between the condyles – there is no mean shape change for this triangle in this view).

In the triangle Menton–Gonion–Gonion (Figure 6.5.14) the bigonial breadth (distance between the gonions) grows most slowly, less than 2% per year, whereas the distance of Menton from that line grows at a rate of more than 3% per year. This rate of change

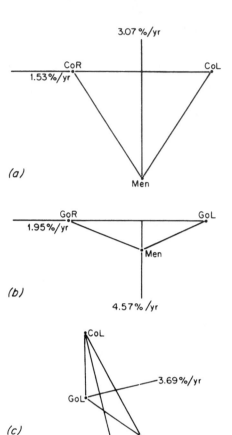

Figure 6.5.15. Conventional projections of the same data as in Figure 6.5.14, showing a combination of growth and changes in foreshortening. (*a*) Frontal view of the triangle on Menton and the condyles, showing too large a rate of growth of Menton away from the condylar axis. (*b*) Frontal view of the triangle on Menton and the gonions. (*c*) Lateral view of mandible.

is exaggerated in the frontal view (Figure 6.5.15*b*) by a decrease of foreshortening as the plane of the triangle in question rotates downward. The change in this projected distance appears to be at a rate of more than 4.5% per year; in the basilar view, changing according to the opposite foreshortening, the rate of growth appears to be only 2.8% per year.

As the bigonial breadth grows relatively faster than the bicondylar, the observed changes of distances in the lateral view of the mandible are likewise altered by foreshortening. The rate of increase of mandibular "width," as measured along the bisector of the gonial angle, is nearly the largest of any distance involving these three landmarks. Analysis of the lateral cephalogram overstates both this rate and the rate of growth in the perpendicular direction. Over the course of normal growth, the whole lateral view of the mandible "turns to face the camera." Whereas the lateral view increases in apparent area by about 6.1% per year (Figure 6.5.15*c*), the triangle of landmarks in space increases in area by only about 5.4% per year (Figure 6.5.14).

Using the shape coordinates for this pentahedron set out in Section 5.4.4, these features are reliable separately as follows: The

250

changes of the ordinate of Menton to the baselines Gonion–Gonion and Condylion–Condylion are significant by Student's t at $p \sim .002$ and $.001$, respectively; the shape change of the lateral triangle separately is not significant ($p \sim .20$) as a T^2 on two degrees of freedom.

6.6. A COMMENT ON "FINITE ELEMENTS"

There is another technique available for the description of biological shape change, the technique of *descriptive finite elements* (e.g., Skalak et al., 1982; Moss et al., 1985, 1987; Cheverud and Richtsmeier, 1986; Diewart and Lozanoff, 1988; Richtsmeier, 1988). In this approach, an arbitrary model of the homology map (Section 3.1), smooth except at landmarks or on curves connecting landmarks, is exactly fitted as an error-free interpolant to a pair of landmark configurations, and certain aspects of its derivative are reported graphically. My own biorthogonal grids (Bookstein, 1978) seem to have been the earliest technique of this sort. That interpolant is smooth throughout the interior of a curvilinear polygon having the landmarks for vertices: That is, there is just the one "finite element." Analyses of this class must be distinguished from *constitutive* finite-element modeling, in which stress–strain relations are specified in advance (based on earlier measurements), and that map is computed that minimizes the real physical energy of the system under assigned boundary conditions. In constitutive finite-element analysis, deformations are generated or maintained by real forces; not so in the descriptive applications. Finite-element pictures in this book include Figures 6.1.1, 6.1.2d, 7.2.8, and 7.4.2, as well as Figure 6.6.1 in this section.

The finite-element techniques treat the derivatives of the mapping, the little squares-to-parallelograms in figures like Figure 3.4.2, as if they specified actual transformations of patches of tissue. The same computations as those of Section 6.1 or 6.2 are applied to pull out principal strains and principal directions, in two dimensions or three, which are then diagrammed in various suggestive ways. Biorthogonal grids are integral strain trajectories of these little crosses all across a form (Bookstein et al., 1985). Other approaches diagram a sparse assortment of these strain tensors at some points of the picture, or extract even less informative, such as their averages "at" landmarks or their strain ratios alone without information about principal directions.

The analyses of this chapter are finite-element analyses for the simplest finite element, a single triangle, and the statistics I have demonstrated are the unique multivariate statistics appropriate to analysis of such finite elements regardless of the computational environment, such as an engineering computing package, in which they are produced. For configurations of landmarks more complex than triangles, what is called "finite-element analysis" in the morphometric literature is essentially restricted to interpolation and differentiation only and thus is quite divergent in spirit from the statistical data analyses of this book. The typical "applications" of finite-element analysis in morphometrics treat principal axes of interpolants as if their application to structures more complex than triangles is unambiguous. But, as I shall argue in detail in this section, it is only the statistics of the finite-element analysis that are unambiguous, not the analyses themselves. Diagrams that are restricted to samples of a few principal axes, without the statistics of the landmark configurations, can be arbitrarily misleading both about the shape changes or shape differences reported and about the statistics of those comparisons.

For modest amounts of shape variability, there is nothing intrinsically wrong with these representations from the statistical point of view. The multivariate statistics of an adequately long list of tensor descriptors are equivalent to those of any other candidate basis for the space of shape coordinates of the landmarks at hand (Bookstein, 1987a). It is not sufficient, however, to use only the principal strains or the so-called *tensor invariants*, which are the coefficients of the characteristic equation of which the principal strains are the solutions. This supplies two numbers only (in two dimensions; three, in three dimensions), whereas three (in three dimensions, six) are necessary: The missing parameters encode the directions of the principal axes upon the form. When the additional parameters are entered into the multivariate analysis, the resulting scheme has all the information of our Centroid Size and shape-coordinate pair. But it is considerably less convenient to carry out statistics on a list of invariants *and* a list of angles than on a vector of shape coordinates together with a single size variable. Now circular normal noise in the data no longer leads to patterned covariance matrices for the shape descriptors, and so forth.

Moreover, most published examples of biometrics based on descriptive finite elements do not supply the correct number of descriptors for statistical purposes. (We need $2K - 3$ for K landmarks in two dimensions, $3K - 6$ in three dimensions; the integers subtracted total the degrees of freedom for translation and rotation.) Presentations will typically instead draw out a few strain crosses in certain regions of a sketch of a typical form: perhaps "in the middle" of a large region without landmarks (Diewart and Lozanoff, 1988), perhaps "at" a landmark (Richtsmeier, 1988), perhaps "in" a triangle arbitrarily hewn out of the picture as one in a mosaic of little neighborhoods (Moss et al., 1985, 1987). Naturally these displays express the arbitrary properties of the chosen interpolation to a greater or lesser extent, and always nonlinearly. Different interpolation functions (e.g., my thin-plate splines, versus the "hexahedra" of Lewis, Lew, and Zimmerman, 1980) will result in different crosses *for exactly the same data*. This criticism applies just as much to my biorthogonal grids as to any of

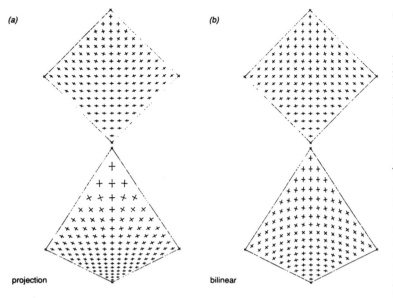

(a)   (b)

projection   bilinear

Figure 6.6.1. Two interpolations for the square-to-kite transformation as a single finite element, presented via the interpolated maps along with the symmetric tensor field of affine derivatives, analogous to Figure 6.2.1 (Bookstein, 1985*b*). (*a*) Ordinary projection. (*b*) Bilinear transformation (compare Figure 7.4.2). Nothing about the statistics of these four landmark locations can differentiate between these two models (or among an infinite number of others); additional data are necessary. The statistic of Section 7.2, however, will reject *all* of these alternatives in favor of a uniform grid if shape variability is sufficiently high.

the other techniques of this family. A not unreasonable example is shown in Figure 6.6.1.

The issue is not one of "sampling variability" over cases. The standard error of a principal axis for the mean transformation of a triangle of landmarks has already been shown in Figure 6.5.5, and a similar calculation based on digitizing error can apply to changes of landmark locations over growth for a single specimen. But such standard errors apply to the uniform transformation fitted to the landmarks, not to specific interior points of tissue. In effect, by the transect theorem, the "sampling variation" appropriate to the question is over triangles (Bookstein, 1987*a*), and the only methods known to me that correctly handle variability of this sort are those of this book. Pictures of tensors are always conditional statements: A certain ratio of lengths between constructed landmarks shows the extremes of change, but it corresponds to the drawing only *if* straight lines stay straight and parallels parallel. As Figure 6.6.1 shows, for more than three landmarks the additional uncertainty of choice of model is *not* in the form of a standard error converging to zero as $1/\sqrt{n}$ as data accumulate. No thin-plate spline in this book, for instance, has a "reliability"; as drawings they are purely visual aids. Resolution of disagreements like that in Figure 6.6.1 is *impossible* without additional data at smaller scale. Properly speaking, the locus of singularity in the figure (the place where the cross of principal axes of the derivative is indeterminate in direction) does not have a standard error. That special point, at which the map stretches distances at the same rate in all directions, could be anywhere inside the square. The disagreements among these and other maps can be substantial. At one locus along each edge, for instance, the imputed principal axes differ by the maximum extent possible, 45°; likewise they differ by nearly 45° along the horizontal segment through the center of the square for some distance to either side. These disagreements can be "resolved" only when additional data are tested that will *disconfirm* one model or the other, or both, by the methods of Chapter 7. Of all aspects of morphometrics, this theme bears the most Popperian (falsificationist) logic.

Nothing in the development of this or previous chapters is inconsistent with such methodological conscientiousness. Methods for analysis of landmark locations, by shape coordinates or other algebra, are just that: methods for analysis of landmark locations. The size variables $|\Sigma c_i Z_i|$ are distances between weighted averages of homologous points; the constructed averages need not be, and probably will not be, biologically homologous themselves, nor can straight-line distances be expected to stay straight over real biological changes. Indeed, for more than three landmarks, interior points can be expressed as constructed landmarks in more than one way, and whenever a transformation is nonlinear, these alternative barycentric coordinates will "correspond" to different points in every other form (Figure 6.6.2). The shape-coordinate method refers to landmark locations only; everything drawn "inside," including the thin-plate spline mappings of the next chapter, is a mere diagrammatic convenience. Thus the shape coordinates are not associated with an estimate of the homology map (i.e., the interpolation); instead, they support statistical fits of simple maps to the available data.

Because it is difficult to indicate the standard error of uniform principal axes on such diagrams (cf. Goodall, 1983), and because it is impossible to know the systematic error in between landmarks for the uniform or any other model, most current versions of descriptive finite-element modeling are inappropriate for the understanding of landmark data. They are suited instead for the analysis of fiducial or reference points at rather close spacing, like the ink spots on Avery's tobacco leaves (Section 2.4.3). Where patterns are announced for tensor representations of the difference between a pair of mean forms, it is uncommon to see either acknowledgment that the reported patterns depend on the choice of interpolant or tests of the ordinary statistical significance of the pattern in the face of sampling variability in the landmark locations (which are, after all, the only data available). In Section 7.2 I shall comment on an appropriate statistical test for the meaningfulness of any single symmetric tensor (cross) as it is claimed to apply inside any region bounded by more than three landmarks. The criteria by which those visualizations may be judged meaningful, rather than misleading, are quite separate from the statistics of landmark location that the elements, even when parameters are sufficient in number, rather inconveniently support (Bookstein, 1987a).

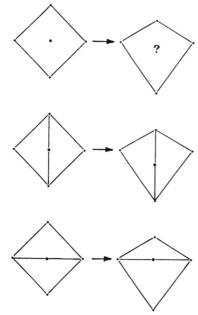

Figure 6.6.2. Incompatibility of the finite-element and the shape-coordinate approaches. To one interior point on the left correspond two constructed landmarks and thus two corresponding constructed points on the right.

In my present view, *descriptive finite-element analysis should never be used for actual configurations of more than three landmarks*. The role of finite-element models in morphometrics should be restricted solely to the display of smooth models for which there exists a biological justification and the residuals from which are found nonsignificant by appropriate statistical test. This implies, in particular, that there must *be* a residual or other source of variance (Bookstein, 1990*g*) for the denominator of the test; "models" cannot be interpolants, but must be overdetermined. Even then, the dependence of the derivatives drawn upon algebraic details of the choice of smooth model must be explicitly noted. In practice, in the absence of *constitutive* models of how tissues deform under particular biological forces, this restricts the biometric use of finite-element diagrams to uniform components (Section 7.2). Elsewhere in biometrics, except as a graphical summary of analyses erected and verified by other means, their technology detracts greatly from the simplicity of the shape-coordinate and shape-space methods, while adding no statistical power at any stage and greatly tempting the analyst into the inadvertent discarding of crucial degrees of freedom. For an application in a wholly different area to which these objections do not apply, see Sampson et al. (1991).

7

Features of shape comparison

For a data base consisting of Cartesian coordinates of homologous landmarks upon forms not too dissimilar, there is at root only one statistical analysis of shape. The analysis resides in a space of $2K - 4$ dimensions, where K is the number of landmark points involved. For triangles, this space is two-dimensional, like the space in which the data were gathered. For any larger number of landmarks, the space of shape descriptors has higher dimensionality than the physical space of the data. Then diagrams of tensor analysis are necessary to reexpress these findings in terms of vectors distributed over the space in which the data were gathered: $K - 2$ 2-vectors corresponding to the $2K - 4$ dimensions of shape.

But that vector space must not be confused with the real space inside the organism whose growth or evolution led to the images we are comparing. What should be distributed over the organism are *processes*, not vectors. We began our intellectual journey in Chapter 2 by abstracting the richness of the notion of biological homology into the stark simplicity of a mathematical point-to-point mapping. This seemed like the most direct way of casting our biological understanding of form into a language susceptible to statistical analysis. From these mapping functions we could systematically select discrete samples, the landmark points. Multivariate statistical analysis could be wrestled into a form adequate to deal with these data in a manner drained of all dependence on such nonbiological matters as choice of triangles or of a coordinate system.

We have not yet justified the severity of this abstraction. It can be defended only by appeal to findings it may expedite that answer to questions from the original context of comparative anatomical analysis. We need to reexpress all the statistical findings "inside the organism," an organism that only by accident finds itself sharing space with the mathematical manifold over

256

which the landmarks, in reality bound together biologically, have been algebraically scattered.

This chapter attempts to fulfull the old obligation, which has been the ultimate concern of biometricians ever since Galton, to measure what is *meaningful*, what serves the purposes of scientific explanation. We need to leave the language of statistics behind and revert to descriptions using biological terms wherever possible. When the language must be geometric instead, we ought to speak of homology rather than of vector spaces. To that end, this chapter considers the principal modes of extracting features of maps by the more delicate consideration of changes in all interlandmark relationships taken together. It is the potential biological meaning of these features that justifies the whole enterprise of morphometrics. The machinery of the intervening chapters represent a necessary degree of reductionism in the course of achieving this goal.

Several of the interpretive metrical concepts familiar to the practicing quantitative biologist – growth gradients, rearrangements of rigid parts, localized changes – are shown here to be specific embodiments of algebraic structures built upon the shape coordinates. Often the biologist wishes to construct quantitative features such as these in the context of the sorts of statistical inference already demonstrated for triangles in Chapter 6. The subject of Sections 7.2 through 7.4 is the interplay between features of transformation and these conventional statistical tests of hypotheses involving covariance. Biologically, these refer to contrasts embodying the descriptive purpose for which particular data sets were gathered: group comparisons, effects of exogenous covariation, and the like. Following these sections, I introduce a new method, analogous to principal-component analysis, for describing aspects of shape variability that have greatest apparent geometric import irrespective of contrasts designed into the data collection. These components, representing the shape features of greatest variability of relative bending, are the analogues for landmark data of the sensible "characters" at which the systematist's search is directed, or ought to be.

For all but the most drastic changes of biological form, each of the methods explained in this chapter is practically independent of the choice of triangles underlying it. Triangles, like rulers, should be invisible to the consumer of morphometric analyses. They are not intended to be real, and one ought not to report findings in their terms; they carry the geometry, but not the biology.

In this way I hope to have arrived at **a geometry for biology**, a felicitous phrase originally coined by the late Harry Blum in a context not too distant (Blum, 1974). The purpose of these morphometric tools is not to impose the thoughtless and boring statistical metaphor of multivariate measurement vectors upon comparative anatomy. It is instead to find areas of biology for which varieties of classic analytic geometry can serve as *fruitful* mathematical models, then alter conventional multivariate methods, as aggressively as necessary, until they suit the relation of these parameters to the biological subject matter. Morphometric variables bear two structures: One, shared with more familiar types of data, is their covariance matrix. The other, the irreducible spatial ordering of landmarks, is unique to this context and must likewise be represented in the analysis. I begin this chapter by criticizing one recent development in morphometrics that, in my view, will *not* prove fruitful: the technique of Procrustes superposition. Although its multivariate statistics is technically correct, it ignores the spatial structure of morphometric explanations. The discussion emphasizes the power of the shape-coordinate formalism to support comparison of diverse algorithms. With Procrustes fits laid to rest, I proceed through a variety of classic morphometric constructs in informal order of complexity: first, homogeneous transformations (Section 7.2), then the peculiarly simple "purely inhomogeneous transformations," embodiment of rigid motions in a coordinate-free way (Section 7.3). Section 7.4 is concerned with models such as growth gradients that are not geometrically uniform but that nevertheless apply one set of parameters globally, to all regions of a configuration of landmarks. From the global we turn to the opposite language, the language of localization. Of all our morphometric strategies, this is the one closest to the original biological thrust of determining "where the phenomenon lies." Methods for localized description are offered for the two main biometric strategies: that corresponding to study of covariance (Section 7.5) and that corresponding to the study of within-group variance (Section 7.6).

Throughout this chapter are various examples that exploit the full reach of these morphometric tools. The theme is extraction, as simply and elegantly as possible, of *all* the comparative information purchased so indirectly image by image. The discrete atoms of landmark data support investigations into most of the large questions of quantitative biology. The morphometric tools of this chapter are the best I know for answering those questions in biologically meaningful ways.

7.1. PROCRUSTES SUPERPOSITION

Recently there has been some interest in **Procrustes superposition**, the computation of best-fitting superpositions of configurations of landmarks according to various geometrical criteria. All these techniques try to place one configuration of landmarks directly on top of another so that some measure of net discrepancy between homologues is minimized. For the explanation here, I shall take this criterion to be the summed-squared distance (cf. Section 5.6). There are also "resistant" methods that substitute medians for sums of squares or underweight landmarks that appear to have large residuals. The least-squares technique was introduced by Schönemann (1970) and Gower (1970, 1975) in the context of comparing diverse multivariate analyses of the same psychometric data. For recent reviews emphasizing the extension to landmark data, and placing the "resistant" methods in the proper context, see Rohlf (1990*b*) or Rohlf and Slice (1990). Goodall (1991), emphasizing the ties of these methods with the techniques of Section 5.6, clarifies many aspects of notation (while not emphasizing the superposition per se as much as Goodall and Bose, 1987). The following discussion is limited to two-dimensional data, for which the method and the critique are each more elegant. In particular, I shall exploit the great convenience of complex notation, as in equation (7.1.1), even though it is available only in two dimensions, to ease the algebra of the critique.

The Procrustes superposition is the one underlying the statistic $\cos^2\rho$ introduced in Section 5.6 for the "Procrustes distance" ρ between two shapes:

$$\cos^2\rho = \frac{\Sigma w_i z_i^C \Sigma w_i^C z_i}{\Sigma w_i w_i^C \Sigma z_i z_i^C} \tag{7.1.1}$$

This is the "net shape distance" between two landmark configurations. (Recall that it equals the mean squared ordinary Euclidean distance between corresponding landmarks when each form is scaled to Centroid Size 1 and then one is rotated and translated to a position of "best fit" to the other that maximizes precisely this cosine.) In this section I explain Procrustes superposition in terms of the shape coordinates introduced in Chapter 5. The discussion will show that these superpositions lend no particular clarity to the interpretation of deviations from the model of no shape change, a model, furthermore, that itself is of little practical value. The method can also be used to find mean shapes (Goodall, 1991), but we already have nearly equivalent ways of doing that by exploiting the shape coordinates (Section 5.4). Extensions of the Procrustes method to higher-order features, though they can exploit some of the same software, are not easily based on this distance function interpreted in the geometry of the original data space (Rohlf and Slice, 1990). They should be thought of merely as alternative algorithms for displaying the features described later in this chapter, such as the application to uniform transformations (Section 7.2.3).

This section begins with a warning: In the presence of any of the higher-order features of shape at which this chapter is aimed, the Procrustes superposition becomes systematically misleading. I demonstrate this by way of a common example, a misspecified Procrustes fit to a uniform transformation (Section 7.1.1). Following this are two subsections of more technical supporting material:

an explanation of the superposition in terms of shape coordinates, and then a demonstration of exactly how this technique violates the algebraic version of homology underlying the utility of the shape coordinates for feature analyses like that in Section 7.1.1. Yet the quantity ρ can be used effectively as a shape distance in at least one sort of study to which the underlying hypothesis of "no shape difference" is applicable: the study of *asymmetry*. The last subsection applies ρ in a variant of ANOVA for some data from honeybees. We shall return to the problem of "shape distance" late in this chapter, where we show that the Procrustes formula confounds multiple dimensions of shape difference that if kept separate will lead to appropriate feature analyses after all. There will be no successful version of superposition, however.

7.1.1. Procrustes superposition as intentional misspecification

In practice (cf. Goodall, 1991; Rohlf and Slice, 1990), Procrustes superposition of landmark data is followed by a biological interpretation of one specific pattern in the residuals: deviation between a pair of samples with respect to the residuals at one particular landmark or a few. (This is analogous to reporting the curvilinearity of a regression by examination of the residuals from a linear fit.) Comparing Procrustes residuals is an inefficient way of testing for such a difference, as the statistics of that moving point have been confounded by irrelevant variation at all the other landmarks. These, though perhaps not shifted in mean, nevertheless show small fluctuating perturbations that, by the Procrustes algorithm, are necessarily imputed in fractional amounts to all the other vertices in the course of the centroid correction. Even in this simplest sort of non-null finding, the Procrustes fit is a misspecification of the phenomenon ultimately reported. To continue our analogy, even if one suspects curvilinearity of regression by considering residuals from the linear fit, one examines and tests it by inspection of coefficients from the curvilinear fit instead.

If the extended map has true **features of shape change** such as will be introduced in the subsequent sections, then the computation of the Procrustes fit (along with its interpretation, of course) is badly confounded by landmark positioning (Rohlf and Slice, 1990). As Section 7.1.3 will show, the true relation between homologous distances out of the centroid, in this case different for different angles, is being modeled by a well-defined proportionality, which it is not; and the true relation between angles out of the centroid, which fluctuates, is modeled instead as a constant rotation. The accidental disportment of landmark locations about the form has the effect of differentially weighting different regimes of this nonlinearity, resulting in diverse regression slopes and rotations (i.e., diverse regression coefficients β) for exactly the same mapping. For instance (Figure 7.1.1), in the transformation of the square to the rectangle, which is perfectly affine and thus may be completely described by three parameters (see Sections 6.1 and 6.2), sets of landmarks emphasizing different orientations of edges lead to clearly different estimates of the "scale" component of the transformation, and quite a bit of arbitrariness in the assignment of residuals except at the centroid. For a uniform shear, one might in this way determine scale change to be any value between the two principal strains. All such values are meaningless, of course, in view of the misspecification.

In a related problem, the assumption of equally weighted, uncorrelated variations of the landmark locations in the course of the minimization is reasonable only for equilateral triangles. In any other mean configuration, the appropriate treatment must be by generalized least squares (Goodall, 1991; see also Section 7.2.3), as neighboring landmarks share displacements by processes in all intervening patches of tissue – another aspect of the pervasive misspecification. By mischievous oversampling of landmarks in certain regions, we can force the Procrustes superposition to use as "fixed point" any homologous pair of locations we choose. Finally, in the presence of nonuniformity of transformation, change by different deformations in different parts of the form (Sections 7.3 and 7.4), there are induced large local *autocorrelations* in the Procrustes residuals, which declare the misspecification yet again, in even more obscure language.

The Procrustes residual does not enter into the general theory of measuring shape change. It represents $2K - 4$ dimensions of shape change by $2K$ coordinates of "residual vectors" incorporating many varieties of visual and analytic confounding; in most interesting cases the plain visual features of shape change cannot be identified in their patterns. For instance, I am aware of no biological growth processes that do not involve change of shape; yet in the presence of growth allometry, every Procrustes fit to a pair of stages differing in age is missing a term for shape change, and thus is automatically misspecified (i.e., its residuals and their sum of squares are both wrong). Likewise, in the presence of growth gradients, any Procrustes fit, affine or not, is automatically misspecified in exactly the same way. Methods introduced later in this chapter show how to test those residuals for significance at the same time one computes a suitable fit; but these tests are not part of the standard Procrustes methods.

If indeed only one landmark is moving on a background of others that are fixed, the method of shape-coordinate analysis is much clearer than the Procrustes for both discovery and display *unless* one knows in advance that such will be the finding (i.e., the "cooked" examples of Siegel and Benson, 1982, or Rohlf and Slice, 1990). In Figure 7.1.2, which is rather more typical, a uniform change is hopelessly obscured by the optimal Procrustes superposition. These superpositions, then, are not at all useful except in situations when one knows the "correct answer" in

7.1.1. Misspecification

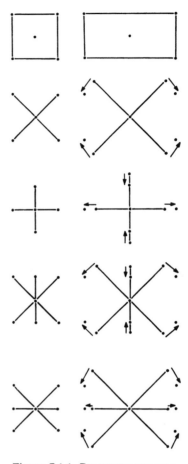

Figure 7.1.1. Procrustes superposition of a single affine transformation according to various landmark samples. All these maps represent the same shape change, but the Procrustes fit fluctuates considerably according to the landmark pattern. Scale changes for the Procrustes fits as drawn: 1.581, 1.500, 1.465, 1.665.

7.1. Procrustes superposition

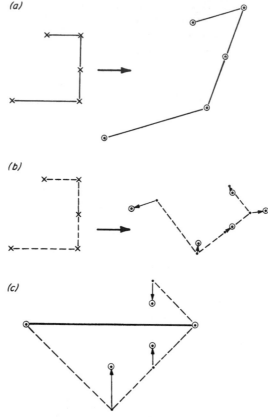

Figure 7.1.2. Ordinary Procrustes analysis of an affine transformation. (*a*) A pair of forms with five homologous landmarks. (*b*) The optimal Procrustes fit; the residual vectors are meaningless. (*c*) An affine fit with residuals zero (see Section 7.2), which is, however, not suggested by the preceding frame in any way.

advance. Trick data sets aside, the proper domain of Procrustes analysis is instead the mundane realm of *confirmation*: checking that data that should be nearly replications are sufficiently similar, and verifying that alternative multivariate scatters are related by a multidimensional rotation (Schönemann's and Gower's original application). Its extensions also supply algorithms alternative to those in the next section for extracting the linear component of shape change.

7.1.2. A complex univariate regression

This and the next subsection will explain what was just demonstrated: the failure of Procrustes analysis to accord with shape features. The problem is common to all versions of the algorithm; I shall use the least-squares algorithm here. As was explained in Section 5.6, Procrustes distance is a sort of complex correlation between shapes. To convert it into a superposition, one needs "predicted values" and "residuals" for locations of landmarks; that is, we must reexpress the same mathematics in the language of *regression*.

262

We shall reuse the setup of Section 5.3: a configuration of landmark mean locations $W_1, \ldots, W_K$ and an observed configuration $Z_1, \ldots, Z_K$ differing from the W's by perturbations $dZ_1, \ldots, dZ_K$ at each landmark. The W's, Z's, and dZ's will all be treated as numbers in the complex plane. In effect, I have assumed scale change and relative rotation to be both small. In this context, differences among alternate Procrustes algorithms (fitting the W's to the Z's, fitting the Z's to the W's, fitting both configurations to a common mean) are of no importance.

Procrustes analysis searches for an optimum member of the family of Euclidean similarity mappings, which, in complex notation, are simply the linear maps $w \to \alpha + \beta w$. The task of the Procrustes superposition is to compute the coefficients α and β of the map for which the summed-squared distance between $\{\alpha + \beta W_k\}$ and $\{Z_k\}$ is minimized. By an extension of the usual procedure for real variables, we may immediately determine that $\alpha = \overline{Z} - \overline{W}$: The regression overlays the centroids of the W's and the Z's. Henceforth, then, we can assume that the W's and Z's each have mean zero in the complex plane. There remains a regression through zero, or rather through $(0,0)$, having as its slope, just as in the real case, the normalized covariance $\beta = \Sigma W_k Z_k^C / \Sigma W_k W_k^C = 1 + \Sigma W_k \, dZ_k^C / \Sigma W_k W_k^C$. Here, once again, ^{C} is the operation of complex conjugation, replacement of $a + bi$ by its reflection $a - bi$ in the real axis (x-axis). The denominator of the formula for the regression slope is the **Centroid Size** of the standard form just as it appeared in Chapters 4 and 5. As usual in least-squares work, the scaling factor for "best fit" is asymmetric: The product of the rescaling of the W's to fit the Z's by the rescaling of the Z's to fit the W's is a term less than 1. This product is in fact the expression (7.1.1), which is the squared cosine of the Procrustes distance ρ.

The condition that centroids map to centroids is not innocuous. Buried in the algebra of these models, it seems to be asserting something about the data but is in fact untestable in that form – it is in fact stating a property of the *model* instead, a property that the data cannot falsify. The affine maps (see Section 7.2) satisfy the condition of mapping centroids to centroids as well, and they are the most general maps to satisfy this property for all sets of landmarks. For "small" regions, the **harmonic** maps of Bookstein (1978) satisfy this condition, as do the **conformal** maps that constitute a special case. The **thin-plate spline** mappings of Chapter 2 do *not* satisfy this condition in general; I believe the condition to be without biological meaning. In any case, it is enforced for Procrustes analysis by the algebra of least-squares regressions, not by any considerations based in the data. A landmark located at the centroid of its configuration in one specimen, and not located at that centroid in another specimen, will necessarily be assigned a substantial residual in the Procrustes superpo-

7.1. Procrustes superposition

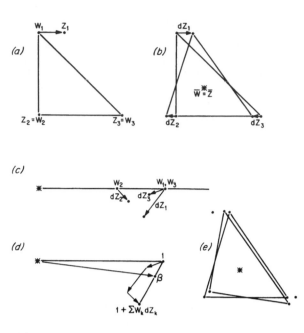

Figure 7.1.3. Procrustes analysis in terms of shape coordinates. (*a*) A change of one shape coordinate. (*b*) After the centroid is restored, displacement is distributed proportionately among the vertices in the ratio $2: -1: -1$. (*c*) Equivalent regression after rotation of all median lines to coincidence. (*d*) The regression coefficient is the weighted average of rotated and rescaled versions of the single perturbation vector; it is a linear function of that vector, as is every regression residual. (*e*) The superposition.

sition. It is not the centroids of arbitrary subsets of the landmarks that match, but only the centroid of the landmarks taken as one complete list. Centroids of arbitrary subsets *cannot* match, in general, as they have more than one formula; recall the discussion in connection with Figure 6.6.2.

We begin the reexpression of this technique in terms of the algebra of the shape coordinates by applying it to a pair of triangles taken in the two-point registration (Figure 7.1.3*a*). Let one configuration be perturbed by a vector v at the third vertex, the one free to move in the construction. Superposition at the centroids results in a distribution of the perturbation among all three vertices, rather than just one, in the ratio $2: - 1: - 1$. That is, we have $dZ_1 = 2v/3$, $dZ_2 = dZ_3 = -v/3$.

Notice, in the formula for β, that (after adjustment of centroids) the factor dZ_k enters conjugated. If we rotate both this quantity and its weight (unperturbed position) W_k by the same angle (i.e., multiply both by a unit complex number), the factor and its conjugate multiply to 1, and the contribution to β will not have changed. We take advantage of this opportunity by closing up our original triangle like a Japanese fan, rotating all W's around the centroid of the W-triangle until they are collinear along the x-axis (Figure 7.1.3*c*). (A similar maneuver allowed us to normalize the shape of any triangle as the degenerate form of Figure 5.6.2, from which we could directly transcribe the exact Mardia–Dryden distribution of the shape coordinates under the null model.) The perturbation v has rotated along with the ribs of the form; it has now reappeared in the form of a complex multiple at each of the three new "vertex" locations. Each perturbation is of the form $v_k = vf_k \exp[-i \arg(W_k - \overline{W})]$, where arg is the com-

264

plex argument (angle) function and f_k is $\frac{2}{3}$ or $-\frac{1}{3}$ as appropriate. In this form the expression for β is clearly linear in the vector v, as are all the observed dZ_k. Hence so is every residual $dZ_k - \beta W_k$, $k = 1, 2, 3$. The weights W_k in the formula for β are now real; the argument of β is the negative of the length-weighted average of torques exerted by the multiples of v at every landmark, and the amplitude of β differs from the ratio of centroid sizes by a factor that is the absolute value of $\Sigma Z_k W_k^C / (\Sigma Z_k Z_k^C \Sigma W_k W_k^C)^{1/2}$, the value $\cos \rho$ underlying equation (7.1.1).

A parallel construction applies to Procrustes analysis of the perturbation of one single point in a configuration of K landmarks W_k, $k = 1, 2, \ldots, K$. In the first step, the restoring of centroids, any perturbation v at one landmark is replaced by a displacement of $[(K - 1)/K]v$ there and displacements $-v/K$ at each of the other $K - 1$ landmarks. The regression may then proceed by rotation of all unperturbed landmarks around the centroid to a position of collinearity. The regression coefficient β is again linear in the original displacement v, and thus residuals at each landmark are likewise linear in v. In a sample of multiple forms scaled to the same "standard," if displacement involves only a single landmark, then all residuals are multiples of a single scatter by diverse rotations and rescalings. In particular, as shape change for a triangle can be considered to have occurred "at" any landmark one pleases, **all three residuals from the Procrustes fit for a triangle of landmarks have exactly the same scatter, the same information.** It is displayed with remarkable redundancy, however, six degrees of freedom replacing the original two. (A numerical verification of the observation proceeds best by application of – a Procrustes fit! Indeed, this was its original application, to the measurement of concordance of diverse multivariate analyses. I thank Colin Goodall for this point.) The general Procrustes fit may be thought of as the superposition of the redistributed effects of K of these perturbations, one from each landmark.

7.1.3. Its relation to two different registrations

For ease of exposition, let us index the landmarks by their angles out of the centroid. We can then connect adjacent entries on this list by line segments to form a polygon. We shall refer to functions that take values on this polygon. Consider the points $(1 - \alpha)Z_k + \alpha Z_{k+1}$ on segments between consecutive vertices of the hull. (The arithmetic of subscripts is modulo K.) We can consider these points as functions of a single angular variable θ in $(0, 2\pi)$: $P_Z(\theta)$ is the point given by the preceding equation when k is the integer part of $K\theta/2\pi$ and α is the fractional part of the same quantity. Write $(d_Z(\theta), t_Z(\theta))$ for the polar coordinates of $P_Z(\theta)$ out of the centroid of the landmarks to any convenient azimuth, and similarly polar coordinates $(d_W(\theta), t_W(\theta))$ for $P_W(\theta)$, the homologous polygon on the W's. The points $P_Z(\theta)$ and $P_W(\theta)$ are homologous

265

7.1. Procrustes superposition

(in the sense of Section 4.1), and likewise the centroids are homologous; hence distances from the centroid to points $P_Z(\theta)$ and $P_W(\theta)$ are homologous as size variables and supply legitimate baselines for construction of shape coordinates.

Because the relative repositioning of the images was a least-squares fit, there is variation of sign in the differences $d_Z(\theta) - d_W(\theta)$ of "observed" and "fitted" values of the radial coordinate. (Otherwise, we could execute an obvious rescaling to reduce the sum of squares about the fit.) As a function of θ, the ratio of lengths d_Z/d_W varies from side to side of the value 1.0. It must therefore cross that value at at least two distinct values θ_{1r} and θ_{2r}. (The subscript r means "radius.") At these two values of θ, lengths of segments out of the centroid to homologous points of the convex hulls are the same in the two forms. The endpoints of these segments are homologous, by the criterion of Section 5.1, and their scaled lengths are the same. **But nothing suggests that these line segments overlie each other.** One of the endpoints, the centroid, is fixed in location; the other rotates according to the global criterion of best fit. It is by exactly this discrepancy of orientation that the residual vectors $Z_k - (\alpha + \beta W_k)$, landmark by landmark, fail to represent tensors of deformation. They have been rotated out of a proper registration.

Similarly, because the relative rotation of the images was least-squares (in effect, setting the weighted mean of angles between W_k and Z_k to zero), there is variation of sign in the differences of azimuth $t_Z(\theta) - t_W(\theta)$ around the landmark polygon. (Otherwise, we could execute the obvious rotation to reduce the error sum of squares.) Just as it was for the radius function d, the function $t_Z - t_W$ embodying angular discrepancy after the Procrustes fit will have at least two zero-crossings as we pass around the landmark configuration. At these azimuths θ_{1a} and θ_{2a} (a is for "angle"), segments out of the centroids to corresponding points of the convex hulls have the same relative orientations, **but not the same lengths.** Hence, again, the residual vectors likely fail to be interpretable. Some baseline size information has been inadvertently left in the superposition.

We see in this manner that superposition at the Procrustes optimum splits the difference among a number of superpositions that if executed correctly would separately satisfy the requirements of the shape-coordinate statistics. In many cases (cf. Figure 7.1.4) the two sets of crossings separate one another as they leapfrog their way around the landmark polygon. To the extent that the transformation bears a large affine component, the "registrations" associated with polygonal parameters θ_r for which relative segmental scale is correct will be considerably rotated from correct orientation, and the "registrations" associated with polygonal parameters θ_a for which orientation is correct will be considerably discrepant in scale. As a result, even the simplest of the nontrivial shape changes, those that are uniform shears (see

266

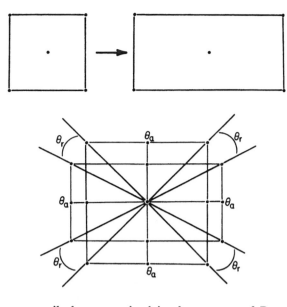

Figure 7.1.4. Interlacing of zero-crossings of radius-comparison and azimuth-comparison functions for a Procrustes superposition: θ_r, homologues with correct relative segmental scale out of the centroid (usually, angles disagree); θ_a, homologues with correct relative orientation of segments out of the centroid (usually, lengths disagree).

Section 7.2), cannot easily be recognized in the pattern of Procrustes residuals. Procrustes superpositions are ill-suited for diagnosing most effects on biological shape as they are observed in practice.

Under certain circumstances, some θ_r will coincide with some θ_a, whereupon the computed least-squares map becomes an acceptable baseline superposition. For instance, consider two triangles having one angle very small and the side opposite that angle very short. The Procrustes optimum will match the vertices of small angle and the midpoint of the sides opposite (so that the residuals at the sharp vertex will be almost exactly zero), and this is an acceptable superposition according to the tensor methods. I know of no nontrivial case of this agreement for configurations of four or more landmarks or for triangles of area substantially different from zero.

7.1.4. Application: asymmetry

Although the Procrustes superposition is rarely of any morphometric use, the measure ρ of Procrustes distance may be quite interesting. In the following example, taken from Smith, Crespi, and Bookstein (1990), it supports an equivalent to the analysis of variance for direct quantification and partition of effects upon asymmetry into the **directional and fluctuating components** introduced by Van Valen in 1962.

In 1988, Deborah Smith (Division of Biological Sciences, University of Michigan) sampled honeybees: nine hives each of *Apis mellifera mellifera*, *A. m. carnica*, and the hybrid "Nigra" strain from various locations in Europe. Wings were removed from 10 workers and up to 5 drones per hive, and the 19 forewing

7.1. Procrustes superposition

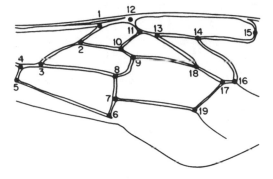

Figure 7.1.5. Nineteen landmarks for 380 wing pairs in three strains of *Apis mellifera*. Differences between strains, which are not our concern here, are concentrated in the relative position of landmark #14.

landmarks of Figure 7.1.5 were digitized. The larger design of the study correlates allozyme data to morphological asymmetry and also to venation abnormalities; here I report only the asymmetry data.

As can be seen in Figure 7.1.6, the variance of this landmark configuration is very low; its development is highly canalized. (A comparable figure for mosquito wings may be found in Rohlf and Slice, 1990.) We may nevertheless inquire about left-to-right differences, as they might relate to hybridization or other indications of developmental stress. Our measure of asymmetry will be an approximation of Procrustes distance ρ: the quantity $A = (1 - \cos^2\rho)^{1/2}$, where the inner quantity is Procrustes shape distance, equation (7.1.1), between the 19 left landmarks and the mirror image of the 19 right landmarks wing by wing. This value is exactly analogous to the usual standard error $(1 - r^2)^{1/2}$ for the regression of one scalar variable upon another. In this translation, all variances and covariances are taken across landmarks *within specimen*. The "sample" is one single set of landmark locations in the left wing compared with the corresponding (reflected) locations on the right; the "sample size" is, for the moment, 19.

In plain words and pictures, the value A is the expected (root-mean-squared) deviation between corresponding landmark points, left versus right for that particular pair of wings, after they are superimposed "optimally" at unit size. Here "optimally" means "so as to obtain the minimum value for A." In Figure 7.1.7, the quantity A is the root mean square of the radii of the circles, and so A^2 is proportional to their mean (or total) area. The quantities

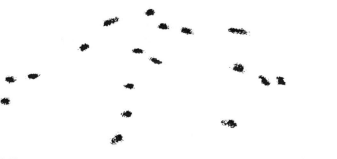

Figure 7.1.6. Procrustes superposition of 380 right wings of *A. mellifera* upon the mean landmark configuration.

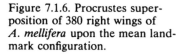

268

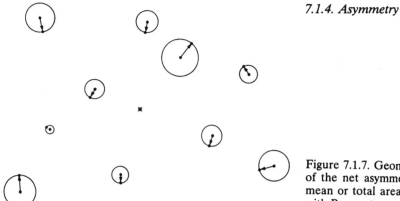

Figure 7.1.7. Geometric meaning of the net asymmetry score A: mean or total area of the circles with Procrustes residuals as radii.

A and A^2 are unit-free, analogous to "fractions of variance explained."

We averaged our asymmetry measure over the 380 bees of our sample in the form of its mean square, the quantity

$$\overline{A_i^2} = \sum_{i=1}^{380} A_i^2/380,$$

where $1 - A_i^2$ is the measure given by formula (7.1.1) for the ith bee. This value is 0.000659 for our data, representing a "typical" residual deviation of left from right landmark, after the regression fit, of 0.0257. Of the mean square 0.000659, 0.000293 is *directed asymmetry*, the measure $\overline{A}^2$ of asymmetry between the sample mean configurations of left and right wings. The remainder of $\overline{A_i^2}$, 56% of the total, is *fluctuating asymmetry* (Van Valen, 1962). Whereas the amount of directional asymmetry is larger for males ($\overline{A} = 0.0237$) than for females ($\overline{A} = 0.0148$), the root mean squares of fluctuating asymmetry are virtually the same in the two sexes (0.0167 versus 0.0178). As it happens, there is no significant difference in mean total asymmetry among females of the three strains. The difference in total asymmetry among males was primarily directional, with *carnica* lower than *mellifera* and the hybrids. Further findings are set forth in Smith et al. (1990).

This measure A of asymmetry is not among those reviewed in Palmer and Strobeck's survey (1986) of the literature of asymmetry measurement. The formulas they review all refer to *character values* measured separately on left and right sides. The closest approach to our formula (7.1.1) in Palmer and Strobeck's table is their formula (9), the measure $(1 - r^2)^{1/2}$. The r they mean is the correlation between left- and right-sided measures *across a sample*. When landmark locations are available in place of "characters," the richness of their algebra supports an analogous quantity, our index A, for computation *case by case*: a very important difference.

The measure A, by comparing the two observations of the "same" landmark configuration in one direct measurement, neatly avoids the typical problems of multivariate morphometrics, as reviewed by Palmer and Strobeck (1986), Reyment et al. (1984), and others. Coverage of the form is as even as the pattern of landmarks itself. The problems of character sampling, and the character correlations endemic to computed distances and ratios, are completely circumvented. There is no problem of standardizing "character size" prior to aggregation (cf. Bookstein et al., 1985: scct. 2.3), because there is only one "character," the shape of one configuration of 19 landmarks. Only a single "size" applies to the analysis, the familiar Centroid Size of Chapter 4. The value A has a plain geometric meaning (Figure 7.1.7), with no uncertainty as to its units. Finally, because the algebra underlying the measure A is limited to sums of squares and cross-products, the comparison of directed asymmetry and fluctuating asymmetry is itself just another partition of sums of squares, as we demonstrated earlier.

7.2. THE UNIFORM COMPONENT OF SHAPE DIFFERENCE

We have seen in Chapter 6 that any single comparison of a pair of landmark triangles can be reported as a single **symmetric tensor** or deformation ellipse, and we have proved in Chapters 5 and 6 that any study of group difference or group change in a triangle of landmarks may be reported as a change of shape coordinates to any baseline, tested in shape-coordinate space for statistical significance, and interpreted as a symmetric tensor (or equivalent ratio or angle) relating the group means or describing the mean change.

Most landmark data sets include more than three points. There are then many triangles that might be used for construction of shape coordinates, and it is not obvious under what circumstances they would result in the same explanations. Any rigid set of triangles, together with a choice of baseline for each triangle, can make up a *basis* for shape space in the vicinity of a mean form – a set of coordinates permitting reconstruction of any conventional shape variable (see Section 5.2). The *statistical* aspects of alternate bases are unambiguous: A significance test applied to one basis for shape space gives approximately the same p-level as that to any other basis. This means that the tests for existence of group differences, mean growth, allometry, ecophenotypy, and so forth, are nearly unambiguous over all rigid triangulations of a configuration of landmarks. Then the multivariate analyses of all the sets of shape coordinates in Figure 7.2.1 are equivalent (except for the nonlinearities ignored in the shape-coordinate formalism).

Yet this invariance of statistical output does not tell us how to report what it is that we find. The vector space of shape coordi-

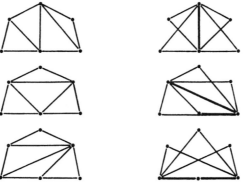

Figure 7.2.1. Alternate sets of shape coordinates: alternate bases representing shape space for purposes of statistical hypothesis testing. Left: Ordinary triangulated trusses. Right: Alternate two-point registrations. Note the flat triangle of zero area in the third triangulation on the right. Significance levels are nearly unchanging across these and all analogous bases for shape space.

nates is unambiguous; but, on the whole, it is incomprehensible to the practicing biologist. We do better to report effects that are either **global** (uniform throughout a form, or graded smoothly from edge to edge) or very **local** (limited to a particular neighborhood of landmarks or to a particular organ or tissue). By the statistical invariance just reviewed, these reports must consist of reexpression of shape difference or shape covariance using one or another basis set (choice of triangles and baselines) determined in advance to be of particular utility for certain sorts of descriptions. We are, in other words, engaging in the analogue of *factor rotation* to *simplify* reports of shape changes the existence of which is already unambiguously demonstrated. But the analogy to rotation is limited in one crucial aspect: The biometrically relevant features of shape change can be specified in terms of the configuration of mean landmarks well before any changes or other covariances of shape are observed. These features of shape change are particular *predetermined subspaces* of the full space of shape coordinates, and our "descriptions" will all be applications of the single mathematical operation of **projection.**

In this section we introduce the simplest of these predetermined subspaces, that representing the **uniform** (or *linear*, or *affine*) model for shape change. We describe its appearance in terms of any system of shape coordinates and demonstrate a method for fitting it to data that is just as invariant as the T^2 under changes of the shape basis underlying those coordinates. Most of the components of shape change to be discussed subsequently will pertain to the residuals from this fundamental fit: For instance, the thin-plate spline fit (Section 2.2) describes primarily residuals from such a linear term.

7.2.1. The appearance of uniform shape changes

Figure 7.2.2 shows an arbitrary uniform shape change. Temporarily fixing the baseline to be the segment from landmark A to landmark B (Figure 7.2.2b), we may consider its effect on shape coordinates that represent many initial triangular forms ABX. A

271

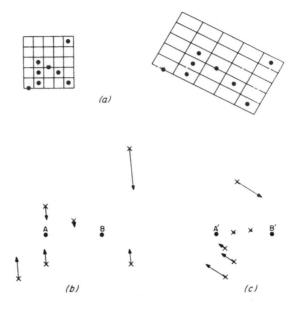

Figure 7.2.2. Uniform shape change (*a*) and its representation in terms of shape coordinates to two arbitrary baselines (*b, c*).

regularity leaps to the eye: All changes of shape coordinates are parallel, and the length of each is proportional to the distance of the starting (or ending) position from the baseline. Notice that the vectors of displacement for landmarks below the baseline are reversed in direction. The distance from baseline that serves as our factor of proportionality must be taken as **signed**. In symbols, there is a vector α with $(\Delta v_1, \Delta v_2) = v_2 \alpha$ for all shape-coordinate pairs (v_1, v_2).

Series of vectors that are parallel and proportional in this way count as **one single feature** for the reporting of a shape comparison. The proof of this assertion is a straightforward deduction

Figure 7.2.3. Proof that uniform shape changes yield shape displacements proportional to signed distances from the baseline. (*a*) Because affine transformations leave parallel lines parallel, the effect of affine transformation on the shape of congruent triangles like these is the same regardless of position. (*b*) Affine transformations transform similar triangles similarly. It follows that even though affine transformations per se make no reference to any sort of "baseline," once a baseline is (however arbitrarily) imposed, the effect of the transformation on any shape-coordinate pair, interpreted as a displacement, is proportional to its distance from that baseline.

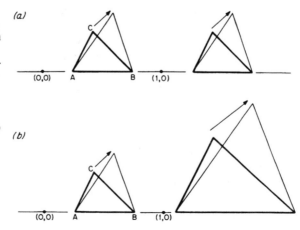

from the theorem that affine transformations leave parallel lines parallel. The graphical demonstration in Figure 7.2.3 should suffice.

> **A uniform transformation shifts all shape-coordinate pairs by multiples of a single vector. The multiple is proportional to signed distance from the baseline.**

7.2.2. Baseline-invariant fitting

Uniformity of transformation is not a matter of baselines. The finding of parallelism must be the same if we switch to any other baseline (Figure 7.2.2c). The vectors are now of different lengths than in the preceding frame, and different landmarks are assigned retrograde displacements below the baseline. The projection operation that will realize least-squares fits to representations of this sort ought to be likewise invariant against changes of baseline.

Description of the subspace onto which we are projecting is fairly immediate. The changes at all landmark locations for the uniform change are all multiples of one single vector (α_1, α_2) by factors that represent the means $\bar{\nu}_{2i}$ of the second shape coordinate landmark by landmark. [The vector (α_1, α_2) may be taken to be the effect of the transformation upon a landmark located just as far from the baseline as the length of the baseline.] Let us number landmarks so that the baseline runs from landmark 1 to landmark 2, thus using for shape coordinates the pairs (ν_{1k}, ν_{2k}) $= (Z_k - Z_1)/(Z_2 - Z_1)$, $k = 3, \ldots, K$. We can write changes in this set of coordinates as the column vector $\Delta \mathbf{V}^T =$ $(\Delta\nu_{13}, \Delta\nu_{23}, \ldots, \Delta\nu_{1K}, \Delta\nu_{2K})$. Then the appearance of a uniform transformation in shape space is that of a vector of $2K - 4$ changes:

$$\Delta \mathbf{V} = \alpha_1 \big(\bar{\nu}_{23}, 0, \bar{\nu}_{24}, 0, \ldots, \bar{\nu}_{2K}, 0\big)^T + \alpha_2 \big(0, \bar{\nu}_{23}, 0, \bar{\nu}_{24}, \ldots, 0, \bar{\nu}_{2K}\big)^T$$
$$= \alpha_1 \mathbf{V}_1 + \alpha_2 \mathbf{V}_2,$$

where $\mathbf{V}_1$ and $\mathbf{V}_2$ (written as column vectors) are the patterns of interlaced $\bar{\nu}_2$'s and zeros expressing the dependence of each component upon distance from the baseline. When the equation is written out in this basis-specific form, it is not obvious that the subspace in question is invariant against change of basis; the proof is by noting the irrelevance of choice of baseline to the fact of being a uniform transformation, as we argued earlier.

Although the general linear function in two dimensions is of the form $ax + by + c$, the linear component of any change in shape space is of the form $a\bar{\nu}_2$, that is, ay only. The other two terms are

273

missing because the method of shape coordinates requires that locations $(0,0)$ and $(1,0)$ be fixed; for linear transformations, it follows that both the coefficient of x and the constant term must be zero. We shall observe the unique contributions of points along the baseline to various nonlinear components of transformation in Section 7.3.

We seek a method of projecting the observed data down onto this (invariant) subspace that is likewise invariant against change of basis. The simplest means of achieving *this* invariance is by the method of generalized least squares. We project in a direction orthogonal to the (invariant) subspace in terms of an orthonormalized basis for the shape coordinates of $\Delta \mathbf{V}$. This orthonormalized basis will not change geometrically under change of basis for shape coordinates, and so the fitted uniform term will be the same regardless of the baseline in which the shape coordinates are expressed.

Set forth in this way, the statistical modeling reduces to a multiple multiple-regression equation. If S is the sample variance-covariance matrix of the $\mathbf{V}$'s, and $\mathbf{W}$ is the $2 \times (2K - 4)$ matrix of the vectors $\mathbf{V}_1$ and $\mathbf{V}_2$, then the generalized least-squares estimate of the parameter vector $\alpha = (\alpha_1, \alpha_2)$ is

$$\hat{\alpha} = (\mathbf{W}^T S^{-1} \mathbf{W})^{-1} \mathbf{W}^T S^{-1} \Delta \mathbf{V}. \tag{7.2.1}$$

The squared length of the projection $(\mathbf{W}\hat{\alpha})^T S^{-1}(\mathbf{W}\hat{\alpha})$ is the explained variance of this regression in the S^{-1}-metric. The predicted "values" are $\widehat{\Delta \mathbf{V}} = \hat{\alpha} \mathbf{W}$.

For the estimation of the linear part of a difference between two groups, the matrix S will be the usual pooled estimate of within-group covariance. For the estimation of the linear part of a mean change, we can convert the computation into a matched form by replacing S with the covariance matrix of the change scores themselves; the term $\Delta \mathbf{V}$ is unchanged, as are the vectors $\mathbf{V}_i$.

7.2.2.1. Examples without data. —

When one can presume that the null model of circular landmark noise applies around the mean change, then the matrix S in the preceding exposition may be replaced by the matrix $\bar{S}$ of expected covariances of the shape coordinates about their means set out in equations (5.3.2). [See also Mardia and Dryden, 1989a; this is their matrix $A(\Theta)$.] Consider, for instance, the starting square set on a baseline as in Figure 7.2.4a, with $(r_3, s_3) = (0.5, 0.5)$, $(r_4, s_4) = (0.5, -0.5)$. Then the terms $\mathrm{cov}(\nu_{i3}, \nu_{j4})$ of the off-diagonal block are all zero, $i, j = 1, 2$. (This is one instance of the involution introduced in Section 5.3.2.) It follows that $\bar{S}$ and $\bar{S}^{-1}$ are both multiples of the identity matrix, so that our computation

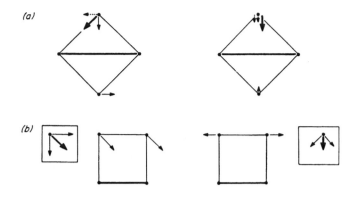

Figure 7.2.4. Examples of the uniform component α (heavy lines) for changes of a square (lighter solid lines) under the assumption of i.i.d. noise landmark by landmark about the mean change. (a) Diamond position. The component is the change vector at the top minus that at the bottom; dotted lines, 180° reflection of displacement of lower shape-coordinate pair before combining with displacement of upper pair. (b) Righted position. The component (insets) is $1/\sqrt{2}$ times the mean of observed changes at $(0, 1)$ and $(1, 1)$ rotated 45° counterclockwise and clockwise, respectively.

reduces to ordinary least squares; furthermore, equation (7.2.1) reduces to $\hat{\alpha} = \Delta Z_3 - \Delta Z_4$, the simple vector difference of the observed mean changes of shape coordinates at top and bottom of the diamond. If these vectors are equal and opposite, the change is purely uniform – there is a residual of $(0, 0)$ from the regression at both moving landmarks. If the vectors are equal but *not* opposite (Figure 7.2.5a), then the uniform component is $(0, 0)$, and the entire observed change is "residual."

As another example (Figure 7.2.4b), we consider the same square to a different baseline. The starting shape-coordinate means are now $(r_3, s_3) = (0, 1)$, $(r_4, s_4) = (1, 1)$. From equations (5.3.2) we derive

$$\tilde{S} = \begin{bmatrix} 4 & 0 & 2 & 2 \\ 0 & 4 & -2 & 2 \\ 2 & -2 & 4 & 0 \\ 2 & 2 & 0 & 4 \end{bmatrix}, \quad \tilde{S}^{-1} = \frac{1}{4} \begin{bmatrix} 2 & 0 & -1 & -1 \\ 0 & 2 & 1 & -1 \\ -1 & 1 & 2 & 0 \\ -1 & -1 & 0 & 2 \end{bmatrix}.$$

From

$$\mathbf{W} = \begin{bmatrix} 1 & 0 & 1 & 0 \\ 0 & 1 & 0 & 1 \end{bmatrix}$$

there follow $\mathbf{W}^T \tilde{S}^{-1} \mathbf{W} = \frac{1}{2}\mathbf{I}$ and

$$\hat{\alpha} = 2\mathbf{W}^T \tilde{S}^{-1} \Delta \mathbf{V} = \frac{1}{2} \begin{bmatrix} 1 & 1 & 1 & -1 \\ -1 & 1 & 1 & 1 \end{bmatrix} \begin{bmatrix} \Delta \nu_{13} \\ \Delta \nu_{23} \\ \Delta \nu_{14} \\ \Delta \nu_{24} \end{bmatrix}$$

$$= \frac{1}{2} \begin{bmatrix} \text{sum } \Delta \nu_1 + \text{diff } \Delta \nu_2 \\ \text{sum } \Delta \nu_2 - \text{diff } \Delta \nu_1 \end{bmatrix}.$$

7.2. Uniform component

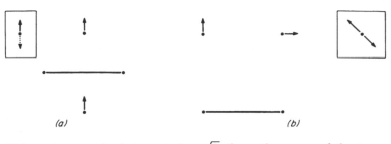

Figure 7.2.5. Examples with uniform component zero, as shown by vector cancellation (insets). (*a*) Diamond configuration; equal vectors of shape-coordinate change at opposite corners of the diamond. (*b*) Upright configuration; change at (1, 1) rotated by 90° clockwise from change at (0, 1).

This vector may be interpreted as $\sqrt{2}$ times the mean of the two vectors of mean change after a relative rotation: that at (0, 1) 45° counterclockwise, that at (1, 1) 45° clockwise. If this rotation sends the sum of the rotated vectors to zero (Figure 7.2.5*b*), then the uniform component using this $\tilde{S}$ is the zero vector.

Notice that the uniform component fitted to displacements at (0, 1) and (1, 1) that point oppositely along the *x*-axis will point *vertically*. The uniform component here is an average of horizontal length changes leaving the baseline unchanged but increasing (or decreasing) a parallel interlandmark distance; it is therefore represented by a principal strain that is horizontal at half the rate of increase of the distance between the upper pair, and to a baseline aligned with that strain it will be recognized in the purely vertical behavior imputed to the landmarks by the other principal strain.

7.2.3. Other algorithms

The two versions of the linear component just introduced – both fits by generalized least squares, one to the null-model covariances $\tilde{S}$ and one to a covariance matrix S of shape coordinates actually given by data – are only two possibilities out of a considerable adaptive radiation of techniques for this estimation that have all appeared in the last two or three years.

Mardia and Dryden (1989*a*) have introduced a maximum-likelihood approach to the estimation of the same uniform component we are discussing here. Under the model of identical circular normal deviations about mean landmark locations, using the exact (Mardia–Dryden) joint distribution of sets of shape coordinates for multiple triangles, they maximize likelihood over a reasonably parameterized family of such distributions subject to the constraint of geometric uniformity as introduced here. Their result is thus an exact version of the present algorithm using $\tilde{S}$ instead of S. Although the substitution of exact maximum likelihood for the normal approximations of this book is relatively innocuous, using a modeled matrix $\tilde{S}$ in place of observed covariances S can make a radical difference for one's computations. In large samples, a choice between the two approaches might well hinge on prior knowledge from the domain of application. When landmarks are widely spaced over a form, and processes regulating different parts of the form correspond to different epigenetic rhythms, different patterns of environmental influences, and so forth, then it might be tenable to presume independence of variations at the landmark locations separately. (Of course any such assumption must be checked by inspection of shape scatters.) When landmarks are taken at close spacing, are located in parallel on replicate or symmetric structures, seem to show common factors, or develop in a context of biological functioning that forces a correlation of features of deviation, then it seems unwise to presume a simple model of error structure without verifying it against the actual features of the variance-covariance structure of the data.

The generalized least-squares procedure using the matrix S derived from the data in effect allows the covariance structure observed in the shape coordinates to approximate an exactly normal joint distribution; in this version we do not concern ourselves with "which normal distribution it is." If the data did originally arise by circular normal variation at landmarks separately, a considerable loss of effective degrees of freedom is thereby incurred. (For instance, the generalized least-squares procedure requires sample sizes larger than twice the count of nonbaseline landmarks; the maximum-likelihood procedure of Mardia and Dryden can operate on much smaller samples.) When the maximum-likelihood methods or the least-squares Procrustes methods are extended to include any realistic distribution of correlated "errors" (Goodall, 1991; Mardia and Dryden, 1990), the only remaining difference from the approximations here is in the linearizations. In contrast, Rohlf and Slice (1990) likewise use a "Procrustes method" for a linear part, but their intention seems to be limited to ordination and display. They offer no statistical summaries or tests and exploit no equivalent of a sample covariance structure.

7.2.3.1. A serviceable factor estimate. —

Section 7.6 of this book is devoted to explicit analyses of features of this organization beyond the uniform – the pattern of all this "covariation of local deviations." Yet, even if the estimation of the "linear part" of a shape change or a shape scatter is thus bound up with estimation of all its other features at the same time, it will be very useful to have an approximation applying quickly even without all the machinery for testing. One technique for generating such sample scatters of the uniform part is demonstrated in Rohlf and Slice (1990). Here I present an alternative that can be produced in any conventional statistical package without any matrix computations.

Notice that the picture of a uniform change to an arbitrary baseline (Figure 7.2.2) is, formally, the same as the usual single-factor model (Figure 7.2.6a; compare the discussion in Section

7.2. Uniform component

Figure 7.2.6. The linear term as a factor. (*a*) Data (shape change of a pentagon). (*b*) The model: Each displacement is a known multiple $\bar{y}_i$ of a single vector-valued factor score α, plus circular noise. (*c*) The estimate $\tilde{a}$: weighted sum of the observed displacements. When the baseline runs through the centroid of the landmarks (not the case in this sketch), the estimate best attenuates the contribution of purely inhomogeneous transformations (Section 7.3).

4.2.2). For any change $(\Delta x_i, \Delta y_i)$ of shape-coordinate pair (x_i, y_i) from its mean or from an earlier observation, the "factor prediction" will be $(\Delta x_i, \Delta y_i) \sim y_i \mathbf{F}$, where $\mathbf{F} = (f_x, f_y)$ is a "standardized" factor score. In conventional analysis, the factor is standardized to have variance 1; in this application, it is better to standardize it to match the expected displacement at distance 1 from the baseline.

For transformations that are truly linear, up to landmark noise, the effect of the transformation at every landmark is a multiple of one single vector $\mathbf{F}$, the multiple being the mean height of the landmark above the baseline. If the uniform part of a shape change acts like a factor, we ought to be able to estimate it like one (Figure 7.2.6*b*). Assuming uncorrelated residuals (Section 2.3.2; but see the subsequent discussion), we estimate $\mathbf{F}$ by a weighted sum of its observed indications, each multiplied by the

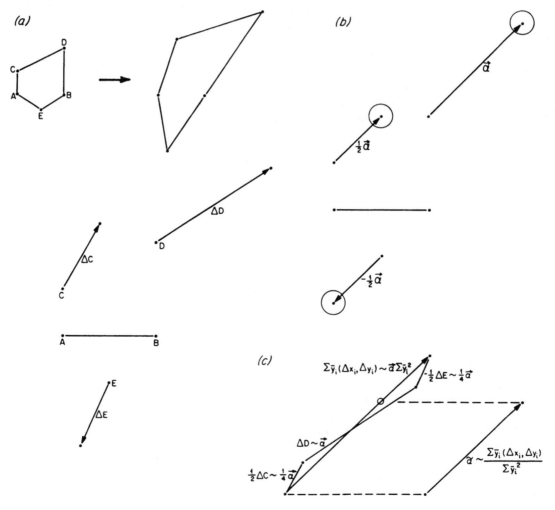

278

appropriate mean height (the relevant "loading" y_i). In this way we are estimating a single vector-valued factor score by the weighted sum $\Sigma y_i(y_i\mathbf{F})/\Sigma y_i^2$ of its (vector-valued) simple indicators, the sums to be taken over all the indications of the factor – all the movable landmarks. The denominator arranges for the normalization to baseline distance 1, as we desired. The normalized score $\mathbf{F}$ applying to a "standard" landmark exactly one baseline length's distance from the baseline will be independent of change of baseline when interpreted as a tensor in the usual way (Chapter 6). The formula for our estimate of this "uniform factor" is thus

$$\mathbf{F} = \left(f_x, f_y\right) = \Sigma_i \bar{y}_i(\Delta x_i, \Delta y_i)/\Sigma_i \bar{y}_i^2. \qquad (7.2.2)$$

This factor takes on a value for each specimen in a sample; the resulting scatter may have one or two sample principal components (Tabachnick and Bookstein, 1990*b*) that maximize the ratio of variance to anisotropy (distance in the shape-coordinate plane, Section 6.3). We shall not need this further decomposition here (although it is approximated to ease the explanation in Figure 7.6.5*c*).

This estimate of $\mathbf{F}$ seems too simple and arbitrary to be credible. Indeed, it is subject to two immediate and obvious objections. The estimate of the single factor score $\mathbf{F}$ by the weighted sum of its indications assumes, as explained in Section 4.2.2, that the errors about this factor prediction are independent. In the current application, there are two different ways in which that independence might fail: by correlation of actual landmark displacements and by the joint dependence of all the shape coordinates on the single pair of baseline landmarks to which they have been referred. Perhaps surprisingly, we can bring both of these sorts of errors under reasonable control by carefully choosing the baseline.

1. *Correlation of landmark displacements beyond the uniform term.* The next section will show how to describe the simplest patterns by which data can deviate from uniformity: the *purely inhomogeneous transformations.* It will be seen there that these transformations can be characterized, to a first approximation, as those that displace shape coordinates by the same directed distance on either side of the diagonal. In the formula (7.2.2), therefore, *they will approximately cancel out*, as long as the baseline is chosen to run approximately through the centroid of the data. The resulting "factor estimate" may still be confounded by higher-order (more localized) components of shape variation, but in most applications these represent far less variance.

2. *Correlation of baseline errors.* Let us suppose, now, that the two baseline landmarks participate in no nonlinearities, but instead deviate from the presumed linear model only by their own developmental or measurement errors $(\varepsilon_{1x}, \varepsilon_{1y})$ and $(\varepsilon_{2x}, \varepsilon_{2y})$. The net contribution of these errors to the factor estimate $\mathbf{F}$ of (7.2.2) will be the sum of all the terms from all the equations like

(5.3.1) for all the landmarks that are not on the baseline: the expression

$$\{\varepsilon_{1x}[\Sigma(r-1)s] - \varepsilon_{1y}(\Sigma s^2) - \varepsilon_{2x}(\Sigma rs) + \varepsilon_{2y}(\Sigma s^2),$$

$$\varepsilon_{1x}(\Sigma s^2) + \varepsilon_{2x}[\Sigma(r-1)s] - \varepsilon_{2x}(\Sigma s^2) - \varepsilon_{2y}(\Sigma rs)\},$$

where all sums are taken over the mean positions (r, s) of the "movable" landmarks. This expression is then divided by Σs^2 to provide the normalized factor estimate.

The normalized estimate **F** picks up a perturbation $(\varepsilon_{2y} - \varepsilon_{1y}, \varepsilon_{1x} - \varepsilon_{2x})$ regardless of the other components of error. That is, the factor estimate based on the shape coordinates is *attenuated* by twice the error variance of the baseline landmarks separately. On the null model, this attenuation is the same regardless of baseline chosen.

The remaining terms, having coefficients $\Sigma(r-1)s$ and Σrs, may be sent to zero by careful choice of baseline. If the baseline passes through the centroid of all the landmarks (a condition already desirable for annihilating the largest-scale nonlinearities), the term Σs will be equal to zero. If the baseline is also chosen along a principal axis of the mean landmark configuration, we shall have $\Sigma rs = 0$ (noncorrelation of the mean shape coordinates around the baseline). These two conditions, together, imply $\Sigma(r-1)s = 0$, so that all the terms except in Σs^2 will vanish. One might run a baseline exactly along this principal axis, by suitable weighting of landmarks toward either end (cf. Section 4.1.3), or simply choose the best of the available interlandmark segments, as we have done in the example following.

We can estimate the remaining errors around these factor scores in the usual psychometric way. If $x_i = a_i \mathbf{F} + \varepsilon_i$ for independent ε's, then the error variance of the most simply weighted estimate of **F**, $\Sigma a_i x_i / \Sigma a_i^2$, is $\Sigma a_i^2 \text{var}(\varepsilon_i)/(\Sigma a_i^2)^2$. Assuming $\text{var}(\varepsilon_i)$ a constant, σ^2, this is $\sigma^2/\Sigma a_i^2$. But in the current application each loading a_i is y_i, the mean shape ordinate of the ith landmark. Hence, as a first approximation,

$$\text{s.e.}(\mathbf{F}) = \sigma/(\Sigma y_i^2)^{1/2}, \tag{7.2.3}$$

where σ^2 is the mean variance of prediction error of the landmarks by the uniform factor **F**, averaged over both coordinates of all the movable landmarks. In this form, σ^2 includes the effects of all systematic nonlinearities and also all the terms like Σrs in the baseline landmark errors, regardless of baseline choice.

7.2.3.2. Example: rat calvarial growth. —

To demonstrate this simple factor estimation I have chosen some data about rat calvarial growth to be evaluated statistically in Section 7.2.5. Data for eight landmarks have been introduced in

280

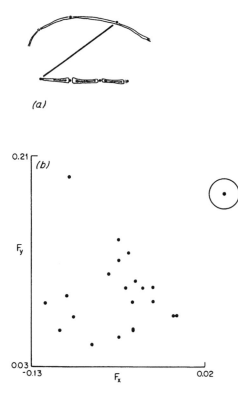

(a)

Figure 7.2.7. A linear component for rat calvarial growth from age 7 to age 14 days; Opisthion omitted. (*a*) Baseline chosen in accordance with the recommendations in the text, and population mean estimate of the component. (*b*) Sample scatter together with circle of uncertainty, radius 0.0131, derived from prediction variances. (Note the outlier; this point seems correct.)

Section 3.4.1. Figure 7.2.7 shows the mean positions of seven of the landmarks, those that proved in retrospect to participate in a systematically linear component of this change. The baseline most in keeping with the recommendations of the text – through the centroid, aligned with a principal moment of the mean configuration – runs from Basion to Bregma, as shown in panel *a*. The sample scatter of estimated **F**'s for growth changes in these 21 rats to this baseline, as computed from formula (7.2.2), is displayed in panel *b*, along with a circle of imputed factor-score uncertainty, radius 0.0131, computed according to equation (7.2.3). (For the regressions of changes in these 10 shape coordinates on **F**, we have $\overline{\mathrm{var}\,\varepsilon_i} \sim 0.0189^2$ and $\Sigma a_i^2 = 2.088$.) We shall explore the misspecification of this analysis in Section 7.3.3.1.

7.2.4. Two T^2-tests regarding linearity

The following material and that in Section 7.2.6 are drawn from Bookstein and Sampson (1987, 1990). Real biological data never show exactly the same change in any two triangles because of the distributed control of biological processes (i.e., developmental "noise") and because of measurement imprecision in the location of landmarks. We may nevertheless be interested in the extent to which an observed change of shape can be considered to have been generated by a process that was uniform up to sampling error. Such uniformity obviously would simplify one's report of the phenomenon greatly. To proceed along this line of inquiry, let us assume a sample of size N somewhat larger than the number of shape coordinates we are using. There are then enough degrees of freedom about to permit two separate tests of the linear fit: the deviation of the data from the homogeneous model, and the deviation of the homogeneous model from the case of no shape change.

The model of uniform shear may be tested against the alternative of a "general" mean shift – that is, changes of shape coordinates by amounts that are unrelated from landmark to landmark, not necessarily parallel and not necessarily proportional – by a version of Hotelling's T^2 due to Rao (1973:565). The fitted mean shift vector $\mathbf{U} = \mathbf{W}\hat{a}$ was obtained by fitting two parameters, imposing $q = 2K - 6$ linear restrictions on the vector of $p = 2K - 4$ shape coordinates. Then, under the null hypothesis of an exactly linear model, the scaled lack of fit

$$T_r^2 = N(\Delta \mathbf{V} - \mathbf{U})^T S^{-1}(\Delta \mathbf{V} - \mathbf{U}) \qquad (7.2.4)$$

has Hotelling's T^2-distribution on q and $N - 1$ degrees of freedom, where N is the sample size (presumed greater than q) and S is the sample covariance matrix of the shape coordinates. (The subscript r is for "residual.") The equivalent $F = \{(N - q)/[q(N - 1)]\}T_r^2$ has q and $N - q$ degrees of freedom.

Supposing that this T^2-test accepts the "null" hypothesis of no deviation from the linear fit, we should proceed to test that fit itself against zero – the additional null hypothesis $\alpha = 0$. The testing framework is the same as that in Srivastava and Carter (1983:sect. 6.2) for restricted (fitted) means. If

$$T_l^2 = N\hat{a}^T \mathbf{W}^T S^{-1} \mathbf{W}\hat{a}, \qquad (7.2.5)$$

then $F = [(N - p)/2]\{T_l^2/[(N - 1) + T_r^2]\}$ has 2 and $N - p$ degrees of freedom under a null hypothesis of linear term $\alpha = (0, 0)$. (The subscript l is for "linear.") If T_r^2 is significant, there is no point in testing T_l^2 – the model is already known to be a misspecification.

Because the estimate $\hat{\alpha}$ is a projection of the sample mean or mean change into a subspace relatively fixed in orientation, we can interpret the fraction $T_l^2/N\Delta\mathbf{V}^T S^{-1}\Delta\mathbf{V}$ as the fraction of mean landmark shift "explained" by this linear model. The R^2 to which this is analogous is over a "sample" of all the landmarks taken with one (mean) shift each, not over the sample of cases in the data set.

This test can be carried out as well using $\bar{S}$, the covariance matrix on the null model, in place of S. The variance σ^2 of the landmark noise underlying the shape coordinates must then be estimated. Mardia and Dryden (1989*a*) derive this value by maximum likelihood. One can instead approximate it by matching the trace of $\tilde{S}$ to that of the observed S, exploiting the formula var $\nu = \sigma^2 p^2 / b^4$ for shape coordinates to a baseline of length b on the null model (Section 5.3.1). (It should be possible to test for proportionality of S and $\tilde{S}$ at the same time σ^2 is estimated, by reference to the Wishart distribution. I hope someone works out such a test soon.) I resort to $\tilde{S}$ in two circumstances: when there are insufficient cases in the data to invert S reliably, and when the observed scatter of shape coordinates includes a strong single factor expressing an exogenous cause whose effects should not be foreshortened. It would be better to estimate the effect of this factor, partial it out, and consider the true residual correlations of the shape coordinates (cf. the example in Section 6.5.1.5); but if those residuals look reasonably circular and there is no mean difference in the covariate between groups, one may as well use $\tilde{S}$ directly.

For two-group comparisons, the matched T^2 of equations (7.2.4) and (7.2.5) is replaced by the usual adaptation (cf. Morrison, 1990: sect. 4.4, or Bookstein and Sampson, 1990). A program computing $\hat{\alpha}$ under either generalized least-squares procedure, S or $\tilde{S}$, and testing the partial T's based on S, as reviewed here, is distributed as part of the disk pack associated with Rohlf and Bookstein (1990).

7.2.5. Example: calvarial growth in laboratory rats

Let us return to the example of Vilmann's rats growing over the second week of postnatal life (Section 7.2.3.2). There we saw a scatter of estimated uniform factor scores that, except for one outlier, look quite homogeneous (e.g., all lie on one side of the "origin," the point of no linear shape change). But we do not know to what extent the observed shape change with growth is in fact uniform – how well it is described by this substantial uniform component.

Figure 7.2.8 shows mean growth tensors from age 7 days to age 14 days as computed for some arbitrary triangles covering the form. As these tensors appear nearly the same from region to region, it is reasonable to inquire regarding the sufficiency of the homogeneous (linear) model.

A convenient basis for the 10-dimensional space of these shape coordinates is the set of five shape-coordinate pairs taken with respect to the nearly vertical baseline Lambda–SOS. The best fit according to the generalized least-squares formula (7.2.1) in the text is $\hat{\alpha} = (0.098, 0.021)$. When the angles formed between the perpendicular to this direction and the baseline are bisected, just as in the general construction of principal axes from small changes of shape coordinates (Section 6.2.4), there results the orientation

7.2.5. Example: rats

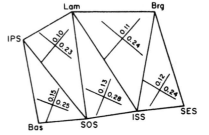

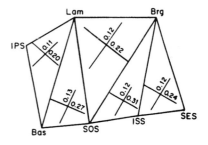

Figure 7.2.8. Growth of 21 male rats, age 7 days to 14, according to two triangulations. The growth tensors appear nearly homogeneous across the form.

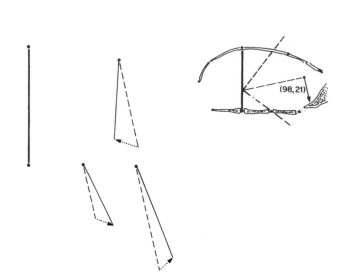

Figure 7.2.9. Fit of a uniform transformation to the observed growth in Figure 7.2.8. Shape coordinates are taken to a Lambda–SOS baseline. All vectors have been multiplied by 10 for clarity. Solid lines, observed mean shifts; dashed lines, fitted shifts; dotted vectors, residuals to be analyzed in Section 7.3.

of principal crosses in Figure 7.2.8, with anisotropy $(0.098^2 + 0.021^2)^{1/2} \sim 0.100$.

For the deviation of the fitted means (dashed vectors) from the actual means (solid vectors) in Figure 7.2.9, the F-ratio derived from Hotelling's T^2, equation (7.2.4), is 4.3 on 8 and 13 degrees of freedom, significant at the .005 level. That is, there is some signal remaining in the residuals from this fit, the dotted vectors in the figure; we shall return to the interpretation of this residual in Section 7.3. But even though this residual is significant, most of the observed shape change is encompassed by this linear fit. The sample mean has (generalized) squared length $\Delta V^T S^{-1} \Delta V = 29.4$; the homogeneous component just fitted has length $(W\hat{a})^T S^{-1}(W\hat{a}) = 26.9$, or 91.4% of the total. This percentage may be interpreted by analogy to the fraction of variance explained by the linear term in a regression to a curvilinear function without error term. The T^2 for this fit [equation (7.2.5)] is, of course, highly significant, even though the model it represents is slightly misspecified. The corresponding T^2 for Figure 7.2.7, showing individual scores on this component, is of course a great deal more significant – none of the 21 points have positive Δx – but that is because we have "arbitrarily" (i.e., by contemplation of Figure 7.2.8) reduced the apparent degrees of freedom from 8 to 2.

The near-invariance of this fit under change of basis for the shape coordinates may be demonstrated by repeating the computations to a different baseline. Figure 7.2.10 shows the same uniform component extracted from shape coordinates to the baseline Basion–Bregma, rotated from Lambda–SOS by some 54°. The computed coefficient vector $\hat{a}$ is now $(-0.060, 0.088)$, rotated some 110° in the opposite direction from the equivalent vector computed with respect to the baseline Lambda–SOS. The F-tests agree closely between the baselines. The anisotropy is $(0.060^2 + 0.088^2)^{1/2} \sim 0.106$, close enough to the estimate for the other

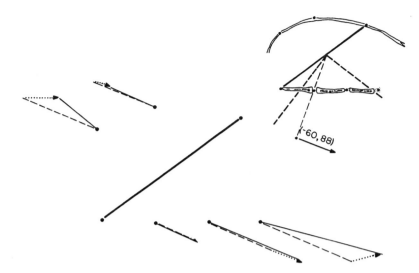

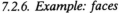

(-60, 88)

Figure 7.2.10. The same linear fit to the two-point registration Basion–Bregma.

baseline. The remaining small discrepancies involve the nonlinearities ignored in the shape-space formalism. By comparison, the factor scores estimated separately (Figure 7.2.7) averaged $(-0.056, 0.090)$ to the same baseline. The anisotropy is again 0.106. The principal axes of these two fits agree well with one another and with those in Figure 7.2.8.

The direction of the major principal strain is closely aligned with the direction of most rapid growth of the cerebrum in these rats. That this single feature dominates the shape change accords with the functional-matrix hypothesis of Moss et al. (1985), whereby processes internal to the growing skull determine changes in the form of the surrounding "functional matrix."

7.2.6. Example: the effects of prenatal alcohol on children's faces

In the Seattle Longitudinal Prospective Study of Alcohol and Pregnancy we located 23 landmarks from photographs of 36 children, as reviewed in Section 3.4.4. Twenty-eight of these children had been exposed to low doses of alcohol prenatally; the other 8 children had been considerably exposed. The two groups differed significantly in mean shape; here we shall concentrate upon interpretation of the differences in their lateral views. It appears from the mean shifts (Figure 7.2.11) that six of the landmarks, along with the endpoints #19 and #23 of the baseline, may participate in a uniform transformation. *For these six pairs of shape coordinates* the fitted linear transformation is as shown in Figure 7.2.11*b*; the residuals from this fit for the eight landmarks to which it was fitted are not significant. In view of the arrangement of all but one of these landmarks near a line, the simplest interpretation of this change is as involving *one* landmark only: relative motion of the earhole upward with respect to the line of

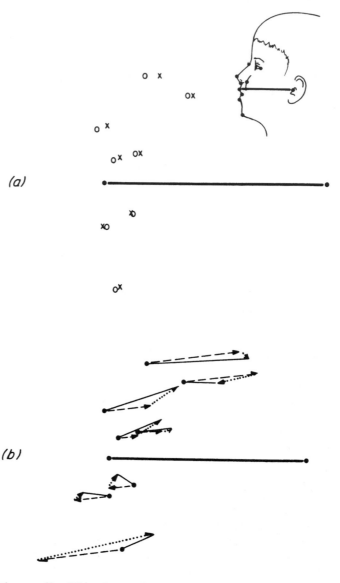

(a)

(b)

Figure 7.2.11. Mean positions of 10 landmarks from lateral photographs for two groups of children. The shape coordinates are taken to a baseline from upper lip to earhole. (a) Mean forms; O, mean shape coordinates for 28 unexposed children; X, means for 8 exposed children. (b) Analysis of difference vectors, multiplied by 8 for legibility. Solid lines: change vectors observed; dashed lines: linear fit to six of the eight vectors; dotted lines: residuals for all eight.

the profile. This change is consistent with the presumed etiology of alcohol teratogenesis in terms of damage to midline cerebral structures; alas, there is no other evidence for such a process in these data.

Landmark #15 is well off the plane of the profile landmarks with which it appears to group in the lateral projection. In reality it is some 5 cm from landmark #14, but appears adjacent. Most of its observed relocation between the groups lies in the frontal view (not presented here), where its displacement is indeed substantial. In hindsight, it might better have been omitted from the lateral analysis as too prone to artifacts of foreshortening. Landmark #22, the chin point, cannot be dismissed so easily. Its vector of alcohol effect, which "should" be antiparallel to those for points #17 and #18 (on the hypothesis of a transformation that is uniform), is more nearly parallel to them instead. If this particular deviation from the uniform model is significant, it represents a geometrically independent anomaly – a "weak chin" – unrelated to the uniform change we have previously discerned.

A convenient way to test whether or not that chin motion is indeed significant is by the T^2 [equation (7.2.4)] of a quadrilateral of points for uniformity, in which three of the points are selected from those participating in the uniform transformation we have already recognized, and the fourth is #22. (To avoid a need for Bonferroni corrections, one might use the composite of all remaining landmarks upon the uniform component, rather than selecting, as here, the one farthest from the baseline.) In this simplified setting, Rao's residual T^2 is equivalent to a direct (linearized) comparison of the two shape-coordinate changes: The question becomes one of equality between the two mean group differences of shape coordinates, each divided by its mean displacement from the baseline. For the baseline in Figure 7.2.11, this T^2 is 23.69, $p \sim 0.0002$. (To the five other possible baselines in this set of four points, its values are 24.97, 25.67, 24.07, 23.01, and 24.13. This accords with the degree of invariance we have come to expect against changes of shape basis.) We infer that the deviation of the change at the chin from the uniform model applying to the rest of the landmarks is real.

7.3. PURE INHOMOGENEITY AND TRANSFORMATIONS OF QUADRILATERALS

As the preceding section indicated, there is only one sort of "uniform part" of a shape change, though there are many ways of estimating it from real data. However estimated, this feature leaves a "residual" part of shape change or shape variation that sustains descriptors of its own; and at this point some choices are available having much greater biological import. As noted at the outset of this chapter, there are two hierarchies of these descriptors, each including the uniform part as the feature "at the bottom." In one hierarchy, the uniform is the simplest in a series of descriptors of change as a superposition of steadily more complex global bivariate polynomials ("growth gradients") fitted by conventional regression methods. In the other hierarchy, based on eigenanalysis, the same uniform part is the term of "infinitely large scale" in a finite series of features that are successively more and more "localizable" in a sense to be made clear presently.

For data consisting of just four landmark locations, the choice between these descriptor ladders need not be made; for four landmarks, the feature of nonuniformity has only two geometric degrees of freedom and can be diagrammed equally well as a weighted discrepancy of shifts of shape coordinates or as a thin-plate spline. This pair of representations of the "pure inhomogeneity" is the subject of this section. Section 7.4 proceeds one level upward along the global, growth-gradient hierarchy, showing how to fit and interpret quadratic transformations. These descriptors do not depend on the mean landmark configuration, although their sample estimates require that information. Section 7.5 begins with a more detailed consideration of the thin-plate spline introduced in Section 2.2, in order to introduce the features of the other, the localizable, hierarchy. These features, the partial warps, depend strongly on the mean landmark configuration. Finally, Section 7.6 extends this set of descriptors into a useful analogue of principal components, the relative warps, that analyze the shape variation within a single sample. The computation of these descriptors refers crucially to both the mean landmark configuration and the variation of shape around that mean. There seems to be no equivalent of this analysis for the polynomial fits of the other, the nonlocal, hierarchy.

7.3.1. The description of deviation from homogeneous change

The uniform component of shape change, we have seen (Section 7.2.4), may be computed for a sample mean in a manner almost independent of the choice of a baseline for the space of shape coordinates. In this section we turn to a comparable description of the simplest sort of deviation from the uniform transformation, the **purely inhomogeneous** transformation. The word "purely" here is meant to suggest a certain simplicity of structure. We shall indicate how to recognize these transformations in explicit shape comparisons and in the residuals from uniform models, and we shall demonstrate a canonical form for such transformations, all in a coordinate-free way. The canonical form for a purely *homogeneous* strain was introduced in Chapter 6; it inheres in a pair of principal strains at 90°, a description independent of baseline choice and unrelated to any description of the starting or finishing forms separately. The canonical form for the purely *inhomogeneous* transformation has the same formal invariances of description, but a quite different algebraic form. Any such change is interpretable in two algebraically equivalent ways: as a rigid motion of two landmark segments with respect to each other, without change of lengths or angle, or as a *couple* of parallel strains, one increasing lengths, one decreasing. Nevertheless, just as in the case of the uniform transformation, once a basis is set for the space of shape coordinates, the purely inhomogeneous change of a quadrilateral is represented, for statistical purposes, by one single vector that can be scattered, correlated with exogenous variables, and the like.

A convenient setup for the introduction of these transformations is the simulation in Figure 7.3.1, the transformation of a

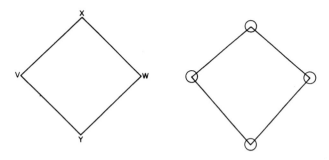

Figure 7.3.1. A purely inhomogeneous shape change: a square of landmarks changing into the form of a kite. Circles indicate localization noise at landmarks of the kite.

starting form that is square into a final form that is kite-shaped, in the presence of "noise" of unspecified source. Figure 7.3.2 shows the tensor analysis of this change of shape to three different baselines. In the following paragraphs, the analysis will be variously in terms of shifts of shape coordinates, principal crosses, and changes of scalar ratios; all arrive at the same finding. On the left in Figure 7.3.2, both mean shape coordinates move perpendicular to the baseline; hence both principal crosses are oriented parallel-and-perpendicular to the baseline. The ratio changing fastest (Section 6.2.3) in both triangles is the ratio of height to baseline. But these displacements are equal vectors on opposite sides of the baseline; for a uniform transformation, they should have been opposite vectors instead. The direction that represents the relatively fastest rate of change in length in the upper triangle, the baseline itself, is the direction of relatively least rate of change for the lower triangle, and conversely. (That is, the lower triangle is becoming taller, while the upper triangle is becoming shorter, each as measured by a vertical : horizontal aspect ratio.) We fall under the special case in Figure 7.2.5a: The uniform component is zero.

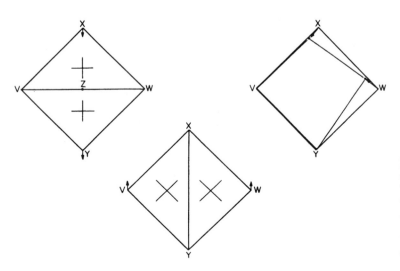

Figure 7.3.2. Three triangulations of the shape change in Figure 7.3.1. Compare Figure 7.2.5. Left to right: Principal strains parallel and perpendicular to the baseline; principal strains at ±45° to the baseline; triangulation to an outside edge.

289

The opposite internal triangulation, Figure 7.3.2 (center), results in principal crosses quite different from those at the left. The changes of the two mean shape coordinates to this baseline are parallel to it, resulting in principal axes at $\pm 45°$ to the baseline – $\pm 45°$ to their former directions. Again, the special case of Figure 7.2.5a applies. Changes that are equal and opposite for uniform transformations are instead equal, and the uniform component is zero. Again, directions that bear the larger principal strain in one of the triangles bear the smaller in the other.

A final demonstration of this opposition, Figure 7.3.2 (right), demonstrates change scores at 90° to one another, yet another case of vanishing uniform component according to Figure 7.2.5b. In all these cases the statement that there is "no net uniform component" is true, but not helpful for any descriptive biometric task. We can certainly imagine varying amounts (and, eventually, varying directions) of whatever it is we are inspecting here. These triangulations are all describing the same change. What is it?

The statistics of this change are the same for any such triangulation (any choice of baseline), because these are just different representations of the same phenomenon in shape space. If we wish to test explicitly for the change from squareness to kite-shapedness, whatever the baseline and whatever the formulas that result, the statistical discrimination of the two groups will amount to the same ordination. For instance, the contrast in question is carried by an increase in the ratio $WV : XZ$ in the top triangle of Figure 7.3.2 (left), a decrease in the ratio $WV : ZY$ in the lower, and hence an increase in the composite ratio $(WV : XZ) : (WV : ZY) = ZY : XZ$ for the combination of data from all four points. (Recall a similar combination of Procrustes-orthogonal catchers of a shape change in Section 6.4.3.) According to the triangulation in Figure 7.3.2 (center), the shape variable most sensitive to kite-shapedness is $XV : VY$ in the left triangle, $XW : WY$ in the right, combining as $(XV + XW) : (VY + WY)$. Or one might use the difference of angles VXW and VYW involving the left triangles, the ratio in which line XY is cut by line WV, and so forth. *All these contrasts have nearly the same statistical significance levels* for samples subject to variability from any source. As variables, these will all be exact linear transforms of each other, except for the nonlinearities ignored in the shape-space formalism. For instance, if the radius of the circle of landmark noise in Figure 7.3.1 and the amount of landmark shift are both 10% of the length of the diagonal, then all pairs of these measures of kite-shapedness correlate .992 (Bookstein, 1987a).

The finding of kite-shapedness is thus apparently quite robust; yet we still do not know how to report it. After all, the various triangular analyses contradict each other. The line VZW remains straight according to the triangulation in Figure 7.3.2 (left), but it is broken according to that in Figure 7.3.2 (center); conversely, X,

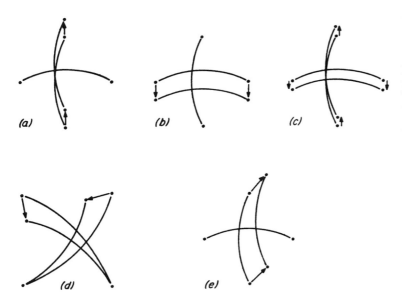

Figure 7.3.3. Report of the pure inhomogeneity as a rigid motion. The lines articulating the two "parts" are curved only so that the motion in panels *a* and *c* can be clearly viewed. (*a–d*) Four identical purely inhomogeneous shape changes. (*e*) A different purely inhomogeneous shape change: square to isosceles trapezoid (for outlines, see Figure 7.3.6*a*). This is represented as relative motion of the pair of diagonals in a different direction. Notice that it is, at the same time, a relative lengthening of one interlandmark distance and a contraction of another in the same direction (in this case, the two segments aligned northeast–southwest).

Z, and Y remain evenly spaced according to the transformation at center, but are changed disproportionately according to the triangulation at the left (cf. Figure 6.6.2). We cannot base our report on any assumed behavior of the mapping inside the form; there we simply have no data (Section 6.6). We need a description of what has happened that is wholly independent of choices of triangles and baselines: as independent of the scheme of shape coordinates used to record it as is the report by principal strains for the uniform transformations of the preceding section.

The simplest summary of this **pure inhomogeneity** is not a report of deformation at all. The change is unambiguously represented as the rigid **translation** of one pair of landmarks with respect to another without change of lengths or angle. Panels *a–d* of Figure 7.3.3 show the remaining ambiguity in the choice of baseline underlying the diagramming. The first three different "motions" represent identical shape changes. So does the somewhat different-looking configuration in panel *d*, a copy of Figure 7.3.2 (right), but with the arrows reversed. In this realization of the same transformation, the baseline was taken to straddle the different rigid components of the motion. The shape analysis of data to any of these registrations must be the same, of course. In the case of Figure 7.3.3*d*, the vanishing of the uniform component instructs us to search for the canonical form of the pure inhomogeneity. We find it here in the fact that the diagonals $(0, 0)$–$(1, 1)$ and $(1, 0)$–$(0, 1)$ have rotated by the same angles and changed scale by the same ratios, implying that to a baseline along either the other would appear to have been merely translated.

Figure 7.3.3*e* shows a *different* transformation of the same square, still having uniform component zero. The difference in

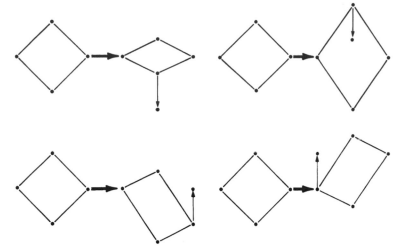

Figure 7.3.4. The inhomogeneity of the purely inhomogeneous transformation may be "assigned" to any vertex of the starting form. It is better to think of it as a single global term.

outcome (isosceles trapezoid instead of kite) is a result of the same vector structures applied in a different orientation. The distinction is the same as the distinction between the square-to-rectangle and square-to-rhombus cases in Figure 6.1.3; it owes purely to the orientation of the process upon the form. (In general, there is no reason to expect descriptions of form change to align with features of the description of form.) The equivalence of the two sorts of description of the purely inhomogeneous change – as discrepancy of shift of shape coordinates and as a couple of parallel strains, one increasing length, one decreasing – is particularly clear here.

For four landmarks, the property of being inhomogeneous and, if so, the direction of the relative motion of landmark segments entailed are **global.** It is impossible to determine any landmark in particular that is "responsible" for the transformation. Figure 7.3.4 indicates how the example of a square-to-kite nonuniformity may be considered as a "residual" at any one vertex of the square pertaining to a uniform transformation applying to any of the others. The implied uniform transformation is different in all these cases. We have seen, however, that no such component of the process exists – its value is precisely the zero vector. Thus there is nothing in the data to help us discriminate among these four equivalent interpretations of the phenomenon – all are equally misleading. The description of the rigid motion in Figure 7.3.3c happens to be that of least squared displacement; it is the average of all four of the "residual" representations. Ironically, this least-squares representation is identical with the Procrustes super-position of the pair of forms. The fact of pure inhomogeneity represented by an equal pair of shape-coordinate displacements in Figure 7.3.2 is here represented as *two* opposite pairs of equal vectors: an instance of the redundancy of the Procrustes residual as a descriptor of shape change commented on earlier.

292

We have introduced purely homogeneous transformations and purely inhomogeneous transformations separately, but it is clear that they apply together as **components** of the general change of shape of a quadrilateral of landmarks. For a starting form that is square, in the diamond orientation, the uniform component is represented by half the vector difference of the shape-coordinate displacements, and the inhomogeneous component by half their sum. In the case of a general starting form, the uniform component is fitted by the generalized least-squares machinery already introduced. The residual from that fit will show a uniform component of zero, naturally, and will suit the characterizations of inhomogeneous transformations introduced earlier in this section (opposite triangulations contradictory, etc.). In their geometrical interpretation (i.e., as inscribed upon the form), these components are both independent of the choice of baseline for the shape coordinates. Because the inhomogeneous term is a vector, in the general change of a quadrilateral there is always one direction involving no nonlinearity: the direction perpendicular to the vector describing the component. (Compare the point at infinity on the locus of the ϕ-function for conformal points in Bookstein, 1983.)

7.3.2. Picture of the pure inhomogeneity using the thin-plate spline

Recall the description of the bending of the thin-plate spline interpolant, component by component, as the deviation of the four-dimensional interpolant from flatness (Section 2.2). Applied to any quadrilateral of landmarks, it results in the same picture of the residual from uniformity regardless of what the uniform component of transformation happens to be. When we apply that formalism to changes in the form of Figure 7.3.3, we must arrive at diagrams that are multiples of the same thin plate. (The starting square is symmetrical, and changes in the x- and y-displacements at the landmarks are exactly proportional; because the spline equations are linear, the proportionality must extend to the interpolated fit at every point of the picture plane.) Then the picture of the purely inhomogeneous mapping for relative motion of the diagonals of the square in any direction is the same: It is the sheet shown in Figure 7.3.5. The plate is raised at two diagonals of the square, and lowered at the other two by equal amounts.

The thin plate here depicts change of coordinates in one particular direction only: the direction of the rigid motion. Perpendicular to that direction is a Cartesian coordinate of no change at any landmark; the corresponding splined surface is absolutely flat, the identity mapping. Thus the single thin plate in Figure

7.3. Pure inhomogeneity

Figure 7.3.5. Thin-plate spline for the purely inhomogeneous transformation. The pattern of equal and opposite landmark displacements forms an "armature" holding the plate in its bent position. This figure is the same as Figure 2.2.2, but is printed upside down.

7.3.5 describes *all* purely inhomogeneous mappings of a starting square; it merely has to be rotated and scaled to suit the data. Likewise, all nonuniform transformations of any other starting quadrilateral form share the same geometry of a different single thin plate, up to rotation, vertical scaling, and tilting.

> **The purely inhomogeneous transformation of a square always looks like the splined surface in Figure 7.3.5. It is parameterized as a vector.**

The reader may find it useful to follow the computation of this square-to-kite spline for a relative motion of the diagonals by one-eighth of their common length. Take the starting square at $(\pm 1, 0), (0, \pm 1)$. Then we have, for instance, $U(r_{12}) = U(\sqrt{2}) = 2 \log 2 = 1.3863$, and so forth, where the function U is $r^2 \log r^2$, as introduced in Section 2.2. There results the matrix

$$
P_K = \begin{bmatrix}
0.0 & 1.3863 & 5.5452 & 1.3863 \\
1.3863 & 0.0 & 1.3863 & 5.5452 \\
5.5452 & 1.3863 & 0.0 & 1.3863 \\
1.3863 & 5.5452 & 1.3863 & 0.0
\end{bmatrix}.
$$

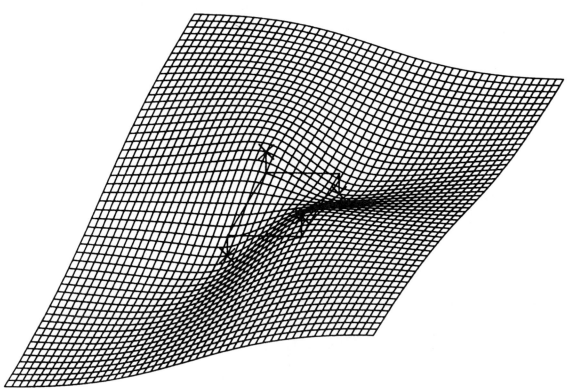

294

Note that $U(2) = 4U(\sqrt{2}\,)$; that is, $5.5452 = 4 \times 1.3863$. The matrix Q of 1's and point coordinates is

$$Q = \begin{bmatrix} 1 & 0 & 1 \\ 1 & -1 & 0 \\ 1 & 0 & -1 \\ 1 & 1 & 0 \end{bmatrix},$$

combining with P_K to give a matrix

$$L = \left[\begin{array}{cccc|ccc} 0.0 & 1.3863 & 5.5452 & 1.3863 & 1 & 0 & 1 \\ 1.3863 & 0.0 & 1.3863 & 5.5452 & 1 & -1 & 0 \\ 5.5452 & 1.3863 & 0.0 & 1.3863 & 1 & 0 & -1 \\ 1.3863 & 5.5452 & 1.3863 & 0.0 & 1 & 1 & 0 \\ \hline 1 & 1 & 1 & 1 & & & \\ 0 & -1 & 0 & 1 & & 0 & \\ 1 & 0 & -1 & 0 & & & \end{array} \right].$$

The matrix V of target-point coordinates, augmented by 0's, is

$$V = \begin{bmatrix} 0 & -1 & 0 & 1 & 0 & 0 & 0 \\ 0.75 & 0.25 & -1.25 & 0.25 & 0 & 0 & 0 \end{bmatrix}.$$

The vectors $L^{-1}V^{T}$ of coefficients W, a_1, a_x, and a_y are

$$(0, 0, 0, 0; 0, 1, 0)^{T}$$

and

$$(-0.0902, 0.0902, -0.0902, 0.0902; 0, 0, 1)^{T},$$

corresponding to the two rows of V. The coefficients of the first set specify the formula for $f_1(x, y)$, the x-coordinate of the image of (x, y); those of the second set specify $f_2(x, y)$, the y-coordinate.

The meaning of these vectors is as follows. The first corresponds to the function $f_1(x, y) = x$, the identity mapping for the x-coordinate. Indeed, there are no changes of x-coordinate between the left and right configurations of landmarks in Figure 2.2.3 (cf. Figure 7.3.6b), and so all of the terms U have coefficients equal to zero. The function $f_2(x, y)$ is a sum of terms $r^2 \log r^2$ with coefficients that alternate in sign around the square, but that all have the same absolute value. Each term U is unbounded, but the combination as a whole is very delicately balanced, as described in Chapter 2. In the plane of the data, this implies that shifts at large distances out each diagonal are only

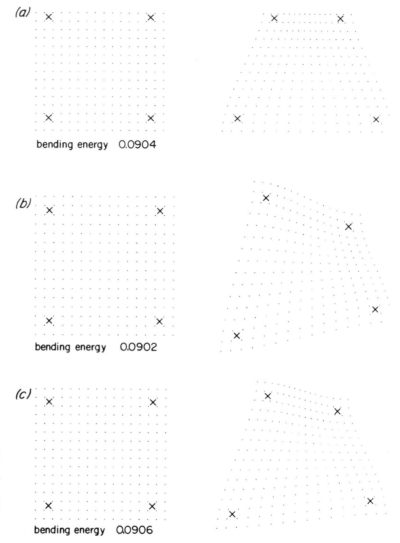

Figure 7.3.6. The purely inhomogeneous shape change as a thin-plate spline in several orientations. These are simple examples of the partial warps to be discussed in Section 7.5.3. (*a*) Along a side of the square, appropriate for Figure 7.3.3*e*: square to trapezoid. (*b*) Along a diagonal (rotation of the grid from Figure 2.2.3): square to kite. (*c*) Bisecting the angle between side and diagonal.

slightly greater than the shifts observed at the landmark locations themselves.

The Cartesian transformation grid of Figure 2.2.3 shows the surface from Figure 2.2.2 conflated with (added back into) one diagonal of the original squared grid. The picture of its effect varies somewhat as a function of the orientation of the grid lines with respect to the direction of the implied "rigid motion" of diagonals. Figure 7.3.6 presents two other typical formats, as the displacement is along a side rather than a diagonal of the original square or halfway between the side and the diagonal. Notice, in Figure 7.3.6*a*, the appearance of a square-to-trapezoid mapping that we have already seen, referred to a different baseline, in Figure 7.2.4*b*.

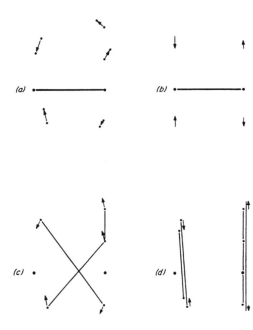

Figure 7.3.7. Modeling the residual from Figure 7.2.9 as a purely inhomogeneous transformation. (*a*) Residuals, magnified 10-fold, from the fitted uniform transformation. (*b*) Summary sketch (cf. Figure 7.3.3*e*). (*c*) Interpretation as motion. (*d*) Better interpretation as a couple. Distances involved in this description are oblique to the principal axes describing the uniform component of the change.

7.3.3. Examples

7.3.3.1. Rat cranial growth. —

Let us return to the uncompleted example of Sections 7.2.5 and interpret, at last, the residual left behind after the uniform transformation that explained more than 90% of the observed mean change. Recall that these are true growth changes in a sample of 21 rats observed at both 7 and 14 days of age (and at six other ages as well). The residuals left behind after fitting the uniform transformation have been redrawn in Figure 7.3.7*a*. Sketched a bit less carefully, as in panel *b*, they are strongly reminiscent of the oblique case of the simple quadrilateral inhomogeneity (Figure 7.3.3*d*). Most of this residual is thus describable with only two additional degrees of freedom as the "vector" of displacement indicated in Figure 7.3.7*c*. This rigid motion, however, has no reality in terms of the biology of the cranial growth that these data are describing. We do better at interpreting the component, having recognized it for the simplest deviation from uniformity that it is, when we pair the vectors of Figure 7.3.7*c* by horizontal position rather than by vector direction. This description, sketched *in situ* in panel *d*, represents a relative excess of horizontal growth at the bottom of the cranium over growth at the top. It will be seen in Section 7.6.4 that *this* interpretation persists through subsequent periods of rat cranial growth long after the growth of the cerebrum, which dominated the observed change over the earliest period, has ceased. The gradient of horizontal growth rate may represent a preadaptation to "orthocephalization," the stiff-

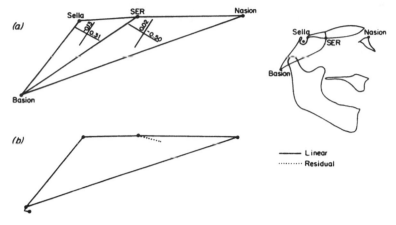

7.3. Pure inhomogeneity

Figure 7.3.8. Anomaly of the cranial base in Apert syndrome. Mean positions of these landmarks are incorporated in Figure 5.4.5. (*a*) Mean tensors for the comparison of $N = 11$ patients to the matched University of Michigan normative means. (*b*) Vectors for the linear and nonlinear components of this change. The latter clearly involves mainly the point SER along the cranial base. The uniform part is clinically and statistically insignificant.

ening of the anterior cranial base to buttress the gnawing that is the rat's lot after weaning. Notice that the vector describing the uniform transformation fitted here is oblique to that describing the inhomogeneous component, and likewise all the derived geometric descriptors lie, in general, obliquely to one another. The successive components of shape change are orthogonal in shape space, not in the two-dimensional diagram of the data. The components we have been describing form a hierarchy of **complexity of description**; they are only rarely geometrically orthogonal upon the form.

7.3.3.2. The cranial base in Apert syndrome. —

We earlier introduced (Section 6.5.3) the craniofacial anomaly that is Apert syndrome or acrocephalosyndactyly. The syndrome is known to have its pathogenesis in the bones of the cranium, in a ring of sutures that begins in the sphenoid bone and passes in a frontal plane up over the vault of the skull. Grayson et al. (1985) analyzed the form of the cranial bases in a sample of these patients (and in samples of other syndromes). Here we reinterpret that analysis in the language of the components of change for quadrilaterals.

For these four landmarks, the general T^2 for significance of the shape change between 11 Apert patients and the age- and sex-matched Michigan normal means is 83, significant at $p < .0001$. Inspection of the mean tensors for a convenient triangulation (Figure 7.3.8*a*) shows a pair of abutting principal axes bearing strains of opposite parity. In the triangle Basion–Sella–SER, distance from Sella toward a point somewhat south of SER are increased from normal by some 30%; in the abutting triangle Basion–SER–Nasion the same directions bear a 50% *reduction* in size from the matched normative mean. We saw such a configuration earlier, in Figure 7.3.2*a*; it is characteristic of purely inhomogeneous transformations.

298

When shape coordinates are taken to the Sella–Nasion baseline, the two components of change may be drawn as vectors attached to the remaining two landmarks. The uniform transformation [$\hat{\alpha} = (0.014, 0.037)$, $F < 0.05$, $p \sim 1.0$, equation (7.2.5)] is represented by vectors proportional to distances from the baseline. In this case, those vectors are very short; the uniform transformation explains less than 1.5% of the change. This component is dominated by the relative change in shape coordinates of Basion – but the triangle Basion–Sella–Nasion shows hardly any shape change, only size change. The residual from this regression, tested by the T^2 of equation (7.2.4), is found to be significant [$F(2, 9) = 40$] at $p < .0001$. Just as the uniform component is mainly due to changes at Basion, the inhomogeneous component mainly expresses changes at SER, the point most collinear with the baseline landmarks. That this separation of components is imperfect (i.e., that the uniform change imputed to Basion is not along its actual direction of shift) owes to correlations between changes of the two shape-coordinate pairs taken into account in the generalized least-squares projection.

The most appropriate biological interpretation of this change is the vector of relative displacement of SER, which is exactly the way we draw the purely inhomogeneous component of change when one landmark is on the baseline. Apert syndrome is a synostosis, a premature closure of cerebral sutures. Subsequent to the synostosis, the infant brain continues to grow, forcing distortions of the bony plates surrounding it, rather than merely pushing them apart as in the usual growth scenario. Landmark SER is the intersection of two shadows on the x-ray (Figure 3.4.3): the greater wing of the sphenoid bone and the anterior cranial base. The pressure of the growing brain apparently has forced the sphenoid wing forward *and* the body of the sphenoid downward. This shape change, then, is not a deformation, but an actual vector of displacement. The two vector components of the inhomogeneous term have *separate* biological meanings. An interpretation of this same shape change as a deformation of the interior of this triangle would gain us very little insight into process.

7.3.3.3. Curving form in Globorotalia. —

In Section 3.4.3.4 we introduced two sets of points on Lohmann's averaged *Globorotalia*: three "corners" that served us well as landmarks in Section 6.5.2 and three pseudolandmarks attempting to record aspects of the curving of the form in between. We may consider each of the pseudolandmarks as combining with its neighboring landmarks to form a fairly skinny triangle. There result three additional triangles representing aspects of the form of these *Globorotalia* in addition to the main triangle of the three "corners" of the form. The shape coordinates of the three additional triangles bear multiple correlations of .738, .470, and .926

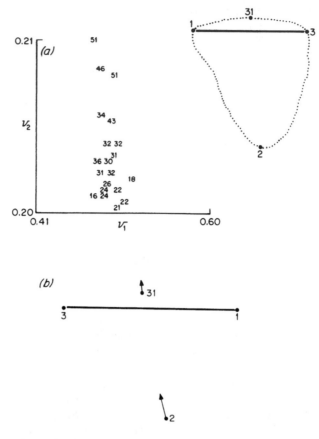

Figure 7.3.9. Analysis of *Globorotalia truncatulinoides* as a quadrilateral. (*a*) Shape coordinates of the triangle #3#1#31 for 20 mean cores, with latitude (°S.) indicated. The correlation with latitude is unexpectedly large. (*b*) Covariances with latitude drawn as vectors of exogenous "displacement" for points #2 and #31 to a #3–#1 baseline.

with latitude. This latter value is startlingly large, nearly as large as for the landmark triangle itself, even though the shape we are now considering lies merely as a curvilinear cap upon one edge of that large triangle.

The dependence of the shape coordinates upon latitude for this triangle of two landmarks and one helping point (Figure 7.3.9) is quite similar to that for the triangle of landmarks only (Figure 6.5.9*a*). The strength of these two correlations with the triangular shapes separately suggests that we combine them into the analysis of the dependence of a complete *quadrilateral* of informative points #1, #2, #3, and #31 upon the single exogenous factor that is latitude. The depiction of these covariances (computed separately shape coordinate by shape coordinate) as vectors of shape-coordinate displacement to a #3–#1 baseline (Figure 7.3.9*b*) indicates (without further computation) that the feature of ecophenotypy previously described, change in the conical parameter, represents only half of the latitude-loading signal. There is an inhomogeneous component of this change nearly as strong as the homogeneous one. Note the comparability of the lengths of the vectors in the figure. The generalized least-squares procedure of Section 7.2.4 does not apply to partitioning this change, as the

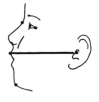

——— Linear
·········· Residual

Figure 7.3.10. The prenatal-alcohol chin effect as an inhomogeneous component. All vectors and components are magnified eightfold.

sample scatter of shape coordinates has a direction of great variance precisely along the latitude factor, which is thereby severely foreshortened (cf. Section 4.3). We partition instead by projecting according to the expected covariance matrix $\tilde{S}$, representing a presumption of circular scatter about the factor prediction by latitude. The projection is likewise invariant under change of baseline for shape space. The linear hypothesis (i.e., geometrical uniformity of the latitude effect) then "explains" 42% of the latitude-related change (cf. Section 7.2.5) by a vector along $(0.024, -0.082)$; the residual inhomogeneity is 58% of the "total." At the same time that the form is becoming less conical with latitude, this side of the chamber is bowing outward. Alternatively, we may interpret this change as an aspect of "rounding up" of the form, associated perhaps with the minimization of surface-area-to-volume ratios associated with growth in colder waters.

7.3.3.4. The alcohol-affected face. —

In the analysis of the alcohol-affected children's faces (Section 7.2.6) we detected a displacement of one landmark that was substantially independent of a uniform change describing displacements for most of the others. The T^2 reported for testing this independence is in fact the T^2 [equation (7.2.4)] for the purely inhomogeneous component (residual from the uniform) applied to the quadrilateral used in the example. Considering that quadrilateral as a whole (Figure 7.3.10), the dominant feature of change remains that nonuniform component, imputed in approximately equal measure to the two landmarks of the vertical landmark pair as they are "displaced" with respect to the other two. We can reject the symmetry of this interpretation in favor of that in Figure 7.2.11b only by recourse to external evidence – the fact that five other landmarks accord with the "residual" assigned to landmark #14 in Figure 7.3.10.

Thus we have finally interpreted the shape change of triangle #14–#19–#23 used to demonstrate the T^2 for mean change in Section 5.4.3. That change is not profitably interpreted as a deformation. It rather resembles a *bending* of the landmarks considered as a linear series. The chin point moves upward-backward independent of the upper pair of points in that triangle, which participate in a uniform transformation involving several other structures.

7.4. THE QUADRATIC COMPONENT AND OTHER GLOBAL NONLINEARITIES

7.4.1. An invariant projection of second-order terms

In Section 7.2.2 we noted that the linear component of the general transformation, though written there in the form $(\Delta\nu_1, \Delta\nu_2) = \nu_2\alpha$, in fact represented the general linear transformation of shape coordinates subject to the constraint that the ends $(0,0)$ and $(1,0)$ of the baseline be left fixed. That is, we were modeling the changes of all shapes coordinates by two polynomials, each linear in the original coordinates,

$$\Delta\nu_1 = f_1(\nu_1, \nu_2), \qquad \Delta\nu_2 = f_2(\nu_1, \nu_2), \qquad f_1 \text{ and } f_2 \text{ both linear,}$$

with the transformed coordinates translated, rotated, and rescaled back to the original baseline. The algebra of the resulting "polynomial" reduced to a single coefficient for each $\Delta\nu$. We reassembled the two coefficients into a single vector that could be scattered over cases or related to the principal-axis constructions in Chapter 6.

It is suggestive to imagine this linear fit as the first in a hierarchy of successive **polynomial components** of change for which the fitting functions f_1 and f_2 are polynomials of successively higher order in the shape coordinates ν_1 and ν_2. The fitting of such models to change or difference data in the absence of prior knowledge (symmetries, exogeneously imposed directions, etc.) requires $(n + 1)(n + 2)/2$ landmarks, where n is the degree of fit; this is practical only for the cases $n = 1, 2$, and perhaps 3.

The most direct interpretation of the higher-order terms is by way of their finite differences. The linear (uniform) fit to an observed mean change of landmark configuration imputes the same specific ratio of change to distances in a particular direction regardless of location. Just as a second-order polynomial has a linear derivative, so the second-order component of a mean change must incorporate linear gradients in the expected divergences of shape-coordinate pairs. The pairs of vectors $(0,0)$ and $(0,1)$, $(0.5,0)$ and $(0.5,1)$, and $(1,0)$ and $(1,1)$, for instance, are altered now not into identical vectors but into a triple of displacement vectors in *arithmetic progression*. The effect on the middle vector is the mean of the effects on the other two.

The **general quadratic transformation** subject to the constraint
of leaving points $(0, 0)$ and $(1, 0)$ fixed is

$$(\Delta \nu_1, \Delta \nu_2) = \alpha(\nu_2) + \beta(\nu_1^2 - \nu_1) + 2\gamma(\nu_1\nu_2) + \delta(\nu_2^2).$$

Here each of α, β, γ, and δ is a vector of two components $[\alpha = (\alpha_1, \alpha_2)$, etc.], and the factor of 2 scaling γ is for convenience in the diagonalization to follow (Section 7.4.2).

There are two linear terms in this expansion. One, that multiplying the vector α, is the same we have already exploited to fit the uniform component. The other, incorporated in the factor multiplying β, is part of the polynomial $x^2 - x$ that has zeros at 0 and 1. [Whatever quadratic we add in ν_1 must still leave the baseline points $(0, 0)$ and $(1, 0)$ unchanged.] This set of functions spans an eight-dimensional subspace of polynomials in which is embedded the two-dimensional subspace of terms in ν_2 only, the space in which the uniform component (Section 7.2) is to be found.

Whenever the number of cases in the data set is comfortably greater than eight, we may fit a "best" member of the class of quadratic transformations to a set of observed changes of shape coordinates by a straightforward generalization of the preceding method. Define patterned vectors

$$\mathbf{V}_3^T = \left(\overline{\nu_{13}^2 - \nu_{13}}, 0, \ldots, \overline{\nu_{1K}^2 - \nu_{1K}}, 0\right),$$

$$\mathbf{V}_4^T = \left(0, \overline{\nu_{13}^2 - \nu_{13}}, \ldots, 0, \overline{\nu_{1K}^2 - \nu_{1K}}\right),$$

$$\mathbf{V}_5^T = \left(\overline{\nu_{13}\nu_{23}}, 0, \ldots, \overline{\nu_{1K}\nu_{2K}}, 0\right),$$

$$\mathbf{V}_6^T = \left(0, \overline{\nu_{13}\nu_{23}}, \ldots, 0, \overline{\nu_{1K}\nu_{2K}}\right),$$

$$\mathbf{V}_7^T = \left(\overline{\nu_{24}^2}, 0, \ldots, \overline{\nu_{2K}^2}, 0\right),$$

$$\mathbf{V}_8^T = \left(0, \overline{\nu_{24}^2}, \ldots, 0, \overline{\nu_{2K}^2}\right).$$

Assemble these, along with the patterns $\mathbf{V}_1$ and $\mathbf{V}_2$ defined in Section 7.2.2, into a design matrix $\mathbf{W}$ of eight rows by $2K - 4$ columns. Then the eight elements of the four vectors α, β, 2γ, and δ are produced (as before) as the entries, in order, of the vector

$$(\mathbf{W}^T S^{-1} \mathbf{W})^{-1} \mathbf{W}^T S^{-1} \Delta \mathbf{V},$$

where $\Delta \mathbf{V}$ is the list of observed shape-coordinate mean changes, and S is the sample variance-covariance matrix of the shape coordinates within groups or, if the design is matched, of the shape-coordinate change scores themselves. Tests for the significance of the fitted quadratic transformation and for the significance of its residual, as well as fractions of mean change "explained," are the same as those given for the linear fit [equations (7.2.2) and (7.2.3)] when degrees of freedom are adjusted appropriately: $q - 2K - 12$.

The coefficients α have been altered from those of the uniform fit. The terms $V_3, \ldots, V_8$ of the design matrix have not been made orthogonal to V_1 and V_2; there can be considerable linear transformation in the term ν_2^2, for instance, if the baseline is chosen on one side of the form rather than passing near to the centroid. In work with the shape coordinates, baselines passing near the centroid are to be preferred for a variety of reasons (recall Section 7.2.3.1).

7.4.2. Interpreting the quadratic component of fit

If the fit of these eight coefficients were analogous to the comparable eight-coefficient fit to a curve, the resulting seventh-degree polynomial would suggest no biological insights whatever. *These coefficients, however, have a geometrical ordering, deriving from their origin in a pair of Cartesian planes.* This dual structure, both spatial and statistical, permits a conversion into a rather useful canonical form that often allows an interpretation of a form comparison as a single spatial gradient or a pair of crossed gradients superimposed over an affine transformation underlying them. The interpretation requires the rearrangement of the net quadratic part of the fit just computed into four coefficients multiplying squared dot products with two unit vectors, as follows.

Let us, for the moment, ignore all linear aspects of the transformation, both the term in ν_2 and the baseline-correction term in $-\nu_1$. There remain a pair of quadratic expressions, one per shape coordinate. Writing

$$\mathbf{A}_1 = \begin{bmatrix} \beta_1 & \gamma_1 \\ \gamma_1 & \delta_1 \end{bmatrix}, \qquad \mathbf{A}_2 = \begin{bmatrix} \beta_2 & \gamma_2 \\ \gamma_2 & \delta_2 \end{bmatrix},$$

we have $\Delta\nu_{1.\text{quad}} = (\nu_1, \nu_2)\mathbf{A}_1(\nu_1, \nu_2)^T$, and similarly for $\Delta\nu_{2.\text{quad}}$. (This notation is the reason for the factor of 2 attached to γ in the original setup.)

By an old theorem (the same underlying the diagonalization of ellipses, Section 6.1.6), any two quadratic forms may be simultaneously diagonalized. That is, there exists a pair of vectors $\mathbf{p}$ and $\mathbf{q}$, which we may take as (not necessarily orthogonal) unit vectors, such that

$$\Delta\nu_{1.\text{quad}} = (\nu_1, \nu_2)\mathbf{A}_1(\nu_1, \nu_2)^T$$
$$= a_{px}[\mathbf{p} \cdot (\nu_1, \nu_2)]^2 + a_{qx}[\mathbf{q} \cdot (\nu_1, \nu_2)]^2,$$

$$\Delta \nu_{2.\text{quad}} = (\nu_1, \nu_2)\mathbf{A}_2(\nu_1, \nu_2)^T$$
$$= a_{py}[\mathbf{p} \cdot (\nu_1, \nu_2)]^2 + a_{qy}[\mathbf{q} \cdot (\nu_1, \nu_2)]^2.$$

There is an alternative characterization of the vectors $\mathbf{p}$ and $\mathbf{q}$ as *conjugates in both forms*, meaning $\mathbf{p}\mathbf{A}_i\mathbf{q}^T = 0$, $i = 1, 2$. The same theorem was used in Section 6.4.2 in the course of proving that triangles sufficed to describe extremes of strain in any comparison of landmark configurations. We shall refer to it again in Section 7.6 in connection with within-group components of variation. Both the computation of the fitted quadratic and its decomposition in this way are included in the program distributed as part of the disk pack for Rohlf and Bookstein (1990).

There are still six free parameters in this reexpression, of course, and the general case is still complicated. It often happens, however, that among the four coefficients a some are considerably smaller than the others. This permits us to construe the general quadratic transformation as a sum of special superpositions in which two or more of the coefficients a are zero. There are thus two important special cases of this general form, as the pair of zeros applies to one of the conjugate directions ($\mathbf{p}$ or $\mathbf{q}$) or to one of the Cartesian coordinates (ν_1 or ν_2). In practice, any of these is an interpretation imposed by inspection of the simultaneous diagonalization. In principle, each may be tested as a specification of reduced rank or of certain elements zero against the alternative hypothesis of a pair of quadratic terms in general form. The test might conveniently be carried out in the form of a likelihood ratio.

7.4.2.1. Special case 1, one quadratic null. —

The most familiar special case is that in which one of the vectors $\mathbf{p}, \mathbf{q}$ is unnecessary. The transformation, apart from linear terms, is then of the form $\Delta \nu_1 = a_x[\mathbf{p} \cdot (\nu_1, \nu_2)]^2$, $\Delta \nu_2 = a_y[\mathbf{p} \cdot (\nu_1, \nu_2)]^2$. Each coordinate is displaced by a multiple of one single quadratic field (Figure 7.4.1a), the squared distance from some line through $(0, 0)$. If the coefficient vector (a_x, a_y) multiplying this term is *perpendicular* to the vector $\mathbf{p}$ (Figure 7.4.1b), then points successively farther from lines in the direction (a_x, a_y) are swept successively farther forward (or backward) along the direction of that line. The effect is that of pure **bending**. The effect of any additional linear term is to change the apparent location of the "axis," the line about which the bending appears symmetric.

If, instead, the coefficient vector (a_x, a_y) is *parallel* to the vector $\mathbf{p}$, then points successively farther out *along* lines in the direction of $\mathbf{p}$ are swept successively farther forward (or backward) along that line; the effect (Figure 7.4.1c) is one version of the classic **growth gradient** introduced by Julian Huxley (1932).

7.4. Quadratic component

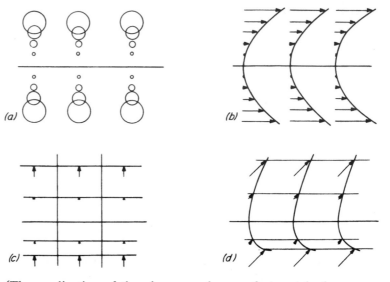

Figure 7.4.1. Special case 1, one square null. (*a*) The quadratic field: squared distance from a straight line. (*b*) Displacement perpendicular to its own coefficient vector: pure bend. (*c*) Displacement parallel to its own coefficients: pure "growth gradient" *sensu* Huxley. (*d*) Composite (here, 45°).

Figure 7.4.2. Special case 2, opposite signs: the bilinear mapping. Three straight lines through each point remain straight. The map is one mathematical model for the purely inhomogeneous component. For its derivative, see Figure 6.6.2.

(The application of the phrase, perhaps unfortunately, has never been restricted to growth studies; it refers in general to any change of proportion along an axis that is itself monotone along that axis.) The superposition of linear changes upon this configuration results, to first order, merely in an apparent shearing of the configuration. The general case of $a_{qx} = a_{qy} = 0$ is the composite of these two cases, as exemplified in Figure 7.4.1*d*.

7.4.2.2. Special case 2, one coordinate linear. —

In a second special case, again two of the coefficients *a* are zero, but now they share a coordinate direction instead of a projected

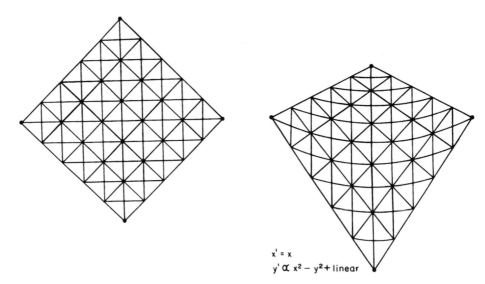

$$x' = x$$
$$y' \propto x^2 - y^2 + \text{linear}$$

306

square. Assume that $\Delta\nu_2$ is purely linear (in ν_2 only), while $\Delta\nu_1$ contains quadratic terms in the form of one or two squares. If one of the quadratic terms can be ignored, we revert to the preceding special case with $a_{py} = 0$. If both are present, the coefficients a_p, a_q may have the same or opposite signs.

If the signs are opposite, the quadratic form factors into a product of two linear expressions. Then, in addition to lines parallel to the ν_1-axis, the transformation leaves two other families of straight lines straight: those parallel to $\mathbf{p} \pm g\mathbf{q}$ with $g^2 = -a_p/a_q$. These maps leaving three families of straight lines straight are the **bilinear** maps reviewed in Bookstein (1985*b*). As can be seen in Figure 7.4.2, the mapping $(x, y) \rightarrow (x, x^2 - x - y^2)$, they incorporate a translation of two landmarks with respect to two others; they thus serve as an alternate mathematical model for the purely inhomogeneous transformation drawn earlier as the thin-plate spline in Figure 7.3.5. **The purely inhomogeneous transformations may usefully be incorporated in the class of quadratic transformations.**

If the signs are not opposite, the lines of this expansion are imaginary. The transformation is better viewed by its effect on ellipses $a_p[\mathbf{p} \cdot (\nu_1, \nu_2)]^2 + a_q[\mathbf{q} \cdot (\nu_1, \nu_2)]^2 = c$. The points of any such ellipse are shifted by c with respect to $(0, 0)$ (Figure 7.4.3). The form is that of an oblique elliptic paraboloid. If $a_p = a_q$, the paraboloid is circular. Additional linear terms in the transformation merely alter the effective angle at which the quadric is "viewed."

7.4.2.3. *Complex* $\mathbf{p}$ *and* $\mathbf{q}$.—

In the preceding special case, for a's of the same sign, the weighting factor g of the lines $\mathbf{p} \pm g\mathbf{q}$ staying straight is not real. But this diagonalization of the quadratic terms can go rogue earlier than that: The vectors $\mathbf{p}$ and $\mathbf{q}$ themselves need not be real. They lie along directions $(-1, X)$ for X satisfying the quadratic equation

$$X^2(\gamma_1\beta_2 - \beta_1\gamma_2) + X(\delta_1\beta_2 - \beta_1\delta_2) + (\delta_1\gamma_2 - \gamma_1\delta_2) = 0,$$

the roots of which need not be real. Consider, for example, the

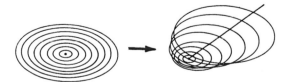

Figure 7.4.3. Special case 2, same signs: The one-component quadratic transformation of positive signature somewhat resembles an off-axis view of an elliptic paraboloid.

307

pair of quadratic forms $\Delta x = x^2 - y^2$ and $\Delta y = 2xy$, matrices

$$\mathbf{A}_1 = \begin{bmatrix} 1 & 0 \\ 0 & -1 \end{bmatrix} \quad \text{and} \quad \mathbf{A}_2 = \begin{bmatrix} 0 & 1 \\ 1 & 0 \end{bmatrix}.$$

Inasmuch as $[a, b]^T \mathbf{A}_1 [b, a] = 0$, the conjugate to a vector (a, b) in $\mathbf{A}_1$ is the vector (b, a). Likewise, the conjugate to (a, b) in $\mathbf{A}_2$ is $(-a, b)$. These two conjugates can be parallel only if $(b, a) \propto (-a, b)$, which entails $a^2 + b^2 = 0$. The pair of vectors we seek, simultaneously diagonalizing $\mathbf{A}_1$ and $\mathbf{A}_2$, must thus be $(\pm i, 1)$, where $i = \sqrt{-1}$. We can check:

$$\begin{bmatrix} 1 & 0 \\ 0 & -1 \end{bmatrix} = -\frac{1}{2}([i, 1]^T [i, 1] + [-i, 1]^T [-i, 1]),$$

$$\begin{bmatrix} 0 & 1 \\ 1 & 0 \end{bmatrix} = \frac{1}{2i}([i, 1]^T [i, 1] - [-i, 1]^T [-i, 1]).$$

It may be difficult to recognize these as directions of growth gradients in tissue!

The situation is as shown in Figure 7.4.4. When **p** and **q** are real, the displacements $a_x[\mathbf{p} \cdot (\nu_1, \nu_2)]^2 + a_y[\mathbf{q} \cdot (\nu_1, \nu_2)]^2$ are di-

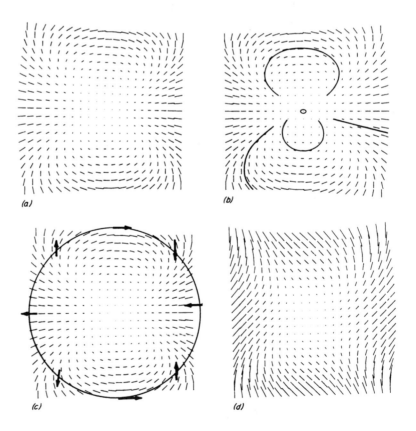

Figure 7.4.4. Example of the complex case: the indefinite quadratic forms $x^2 - y^2$ and xy with principal axes at 45°. The term in x is omitted. (*a*) Displacements. (*b*) (Extrapolated) trajectories. (*c*) A loop of winding number 2. (*d*) Comparison with a case of real **p, q**: $x^2 - y^2$, $x^2 + y^2$ (no winding).

308

rected uniformly to one side or the other of each of a pair of straight lines; that is, their directions are limited to one quadrant of the intersection of lines perpendicular to $\mathbf{p} \cdot (\nu_1, \nu_2) = 0$ and $\mathbf{q} \cdot (\nu_1, \nu_2) = 0$ through their intersection. In the complex case, this alignment of the quadratic displacements does not obtain (Figure 7.4.4a). Instead, the quadratic contribution rotates (by two full turns) as one goes around the outside of the landmark configuration (Figure 7.4.4c). In the case of real $\mathbf{p}$ and $\mathbf{q}$, under indefinite iteration of the transform (which is not biologically meaningful, of course) most trajectories leave the picture. In the case of complex $\mathbf{p}$ and $\mathbf{q}$, the trajectory of landmarks under indefinite iteration is a finite curve, a loop from one baseline point to the other (Figure 7.4.4b).

The complex case occurs only when both $\mathbf{A}_i$ have negative determinants, corresponding to hyperbolas, that is, when both are differences of squares. If we alter the pair in Figure 7.4.4a–c so that the second transformation is positive-definite – the example shows $\Delta y = x^2 + y^2$, so that $\mathbf{p} = (1, 0)$, $\mathbf{q} = (0, 1)$ – we arrive at the scene in Figure 7.4.4d, without loops.

7.4.3. Examples

7.4.3.1. *Growth of 36 normal boys.* —

Section 6.5.1, exploiting only three landmarks, considered the changes in facial shape for 36 normal Ann Arbor boys from age 8 to 14 years. We reuse those landmarks, along with five others, to demonstrate a quadratic component of growth that has often been misinterpreted (cf. the critique in Bookstein, 1981b). The data underlying this example are listed in Appendix A.4.1.

Figure 7.4.5 presents the linear and quadratic fits to this shape change, using a baseline from Sella to Nasion. The coefficients of the fitted polynomial are $\alpha = (0.098, 0.098)$, $\beta = (0.050, -0.009)$, $2\gamma = (-0.100, -0.003)$, and $\delta = (0.050, -0.001)$. The linear term would appear to be a shear somewhat downward and toward the rear of the face; but the baseline here is taken to one side of the form, and so this term cannot automatically be interpreted separately (Section 7.4.1). The linear component $\alpha \nu_2$ is augmented by an additional term $-\beta \nu_1$ (which is considerable smaller in this case). The quadratic part of the quadratic fit corresponds to matrices

$$\mathbf{A}_1 = \begin{bmatrix} 0.0499 & -0.0501 \\ -0.0501 & 0.0494 \end{bmatrix} \quad \text{and} \quad \mathbf{A}_2 = \begin{bmatrix} -0.0093 & -0.0014 \\ -0.0014 & -0.0015 \end{bmatrix}.$$

It is plain by inspection that $\mathbf{A}_1$ is nearly of rank 1 and that $\mathbf{A}_2$ is negligible. By explicit computation, the vectors $\mathbf{p}$ and $\mathbf{q}$ are found to lie along $(-1.0106, 1)$ and $(3.6619, 1)$, with coefficients a equal to 0.0494 and 0.0000 for $\mathbf{A}_1$, and -0.0009 and -0.0006 for $\mathbf{A}_2$.

These data thus fall under special case 1 of the preceding discussion. The vector $\mathbf{q}$ may be ignored, in view of the small size of both its coefficients; also, the vector $\mathbf{p}$ applies only to displacements of the x-coordinate. The quadratic term is, in fact, very nearly the simple form $\Delta x \sim 0.05(x - y)^2$. Together with the linear term, it explains 91% of the generalized variance of this change (in the S^{-1} metric). Its meaning is as follows: In the direction of increasing $|x - y|$ – downward and forward, in this coordinate system – there is steadily increasing steepness of a forward x-shear. Landmarks of low $|x - y|$ – here, only Basion – are shifted relatively *backward*; landmarks of relatively high $|x - y|$, such as Menton and, to a lesser extent, Anterior nasal spine (ANS), are shifted relatively *forward*. The landmarks of middling $|x - y|$, Gonion and Posterior nasal spine (PNS), are left unshifted by $(x - y)^2 - x$, but participate in the remaining linear term, which is the vector $(-0.1\nu_2 - 0.05\nu_1, -0.1\nu_2)$ (our parameter vector α encodes the directions of changes *above* the baseline). The quadratic term thus explicitly accounts for the divergence in directions of shift between the front and back of the face: forward as well as downward at Menton and ANS; backward as well as downward at Gonion, PNS, and Basion. As the vector $\mathbf{p}$ is at 45° to the direction of displacement, the trend observed is neither pure bend nor pure growth gradient, but their hybrid (Figure 7.4.1*d*).

Figure 7.4.5. Six years of growth in 36 Ann Arbor boys: the observed shape change of six landmarks to a Sella–Nasion baseline, and fitted linear and quadratic components. All changes are magnified fivefold. The quadratic term in Δx is approximately 0.1 times the squared distance from the line of slope 1 through Sella, as drawn.

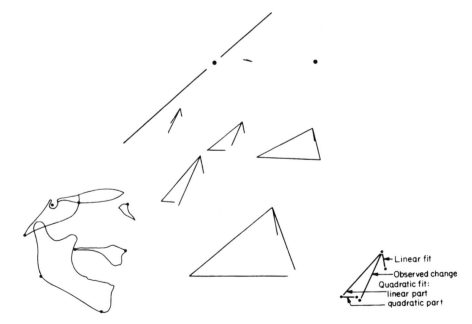

310

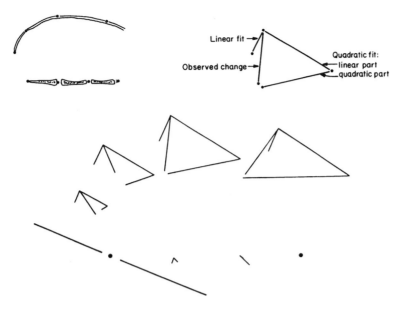

Figure 7.4.6. Calvarial shape change for Vilmann's rats, ages 7 to 150 days. The mean change and the fitted quadratic model are drawn to scale. The straight line through Basion is the locus $3x + 7y = 0$. The square of that term is approximately the quadratic part of the x-displacement.

7.4.3.2. *Vilmann's rat calvaria.* —

Section 4.2.3 introduced the study of the growth of 21 male laboratory rats from 7 days to 150 days of age. Eight calvarial landmarks from x-rays of the rats' skulls were used there to exemplify the interpretation of General Size as the first factor of a matrix of redundantly measured distances. Here we compare the youngest and oldest waves of observations in that data set to provide a geometrical interpretation of the loadings for General Size. The aspect of *timing* that emerged from a consideration of the regression scatter plots will concern us at the end of Section 7.6.

The mean shape change for these rats over 143 days is shown in Figure 7.4.6 to a baseline from Basion to SOS, along the length of the cranial base. As it was for the boys' growth, some 91% of the net generalized distance is "explained" by the quadratic component, whereas relatively little corresponds to any uniform transformation ($R_l^2 \sim 23\%$, representing the general decrease in relative calvarial height; the corresponding coefficient was 91% for the initial period from 7 days to 14 days, Section 7.2.4). The net shape change is quite large (by comparison with other examples in this volume) and yet is subject to rather little individual variation. Hence the residual from the quadratic fit is itself highly significant; nevertheless, we shall concentrate upon the fitted trend. Its coefficients are $\alpha = (0.467, -0.282)$, $\beta = (-0.079, 0.076)$, $2\gamma = (-0.506, 0.004)$, and $\delta = (-0.480, -0.156)$. The quadratic forms of the gradient analysis are thus

$$\mathbf{A}_1 = \begin{bmatrix} -0.0784 & -0.2531 \\ -0.2531 & -0.4810 \end{bmatrix} \quad \text{and} \quad \mathbf{A}_2 = \begin{bmatrix} 0.0754 & 0.0019 \\ 0.0019 & -0.1556 \end{bmatrix}.$$

The vectors $\mathbf{p}, \mathbf{q}$ in this case are not real. (Both matrices have negative determinants.)

We may proceed instead by expressing the matrices $\mathbf{A}_i$ separately as sums of squares of projections. There is no need to compute these exactly; by inspection, we have $\mathbf{A}_1 \sim -(0.3x + 0.7y)^2$, $\mathbf{A}_2 \sim 0.075(x^2 - 2y^2)$. The x-effect is the larger; it is a backward shear proportional to the squared distance from the line $3x + 7y = 0$ in Figure 7.4.6. In comparison with the scheme of Figure 7.4.2, the line of effect zero and the data are both reflected, as is the sign of the leading term in $\mathbf{A}_1$. The net effect is thus the opposite of that in the preceding example: a tendency of the more forward landmarks to be displaced relatively farther *backward* than if the change were uniform. In other words, the baseline is seen to *thrust under* the upper landmarks. This phenomenon is known in the cephalometric literature as *orthocephalization*, the straightening of the face (which "rotates" upward along with the segment Bregma–SES along which it abuts the calva). The quadratic term in y (a vertical drop at the upper landmarks somewhat faster than proportional to their height) is dominated by the linear term, representing a flattening of the entire form by rather more than $\frac{1}{3}$. The x-quadratic is larger both because its coefficients are greater and because in these data the range of the y-coordinate is less than that of the x-coordinate.

The analysis of Figure 7.4.6 is a more organized presentation of the net reconfiguration of these landmarks than the factor analysis of distances reported in Table 4.2.1 in Section 4.2.3. It is clearer graphically than analytically that vertical distances grow more slowly than distances measured horizontally (i.e., they have smaller factor loadings), that of the horizontal distances those along the cranial base have the larger loadings, and that of the vertical distances those measured to Basion and SOS have smaller rates of change than those measured to ISS and SES. All distances along the cranial base appear to grow at nearly the same rate, preserving proportions along this structure and also preserving its straightness, without flexure. Growth there is thus nearly uniform, justifying our choice of this structure for baseline. The quadratic term here is consistent with the purely inhomogeneous residual from the linear term (effect of cerebral growth) for change from 7 days of age to 14 (Section 7.3.3.1). That pure inhomogeneity likewise represented a slowing of growth along the top of the skull relative to that along the bottom. The finding thus represents a continuity throughout this long period of observation. We shall return to these data once more at the end of Section 7.6.

7.4.4. Other global nonlinearities

Beyond these quadratic gradients just illustrated, other global nonlinearities may be identified in the pattern of shape-coordinate

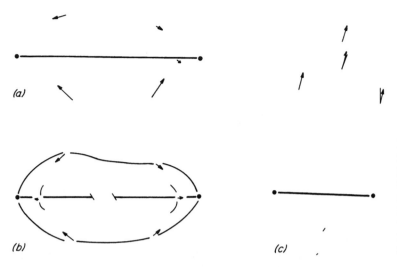

Figure 7.4.7. Difference between two strata of *Veenia* (for landmarks, see Figure 3.4.7). (*a*) To the baseline originally considered. (*b*) Schematic. (*c*) To a baseline restricted to one of the two regions in apparent relative rigid motion, with the fitted rigid motion indicated.

changes Δ**V** by projection onto features having particular biological meanings assigned in advance. Although these are available as a priori models, it is more sensible to treat the task as one of "naming," finding a familiar interpretation for the change that has been seen (without assumptions) in the pattern of displacements at each of a configuration of shape coordinates. Here are two examples.

7.4.4.1. *Rigid motions involving several landmarks.* —

The transformation in Figure 7.4.7*a*, between mean forms for strata 1 and 8 of the ostracode *Veenia* introduced in Section 3.4.3.2, has the appearance of a vanishing point in Renaissance perspective. Landmarks *C* and *D* appear to be shrinking toward the anterior pole *A* of the organism, and landmarks *F* and *G* toward the posterior pole *B*. A bit of reflection suggests the reinterpretation in Figure 7.4.7*b*. The combination of shrinkage toward both ends of the baseline by the same ratio can be modeled as the insertion of additional "space" along the baseline near the middle, followed by renormalization of baseline length. The effect of that additional space is to push the two ends of the form relatively farther apart while lowering the relative scale of the original triangles at the ends.

We can analyze this change more effectively to a baseline that does not straddle these two segments but rather is restricted to one of them (Figure 7.4.7*c*). (Another example of a baseline straddling a pair of components in relative motion was presented in Section 1.2; cf. Figures 1.2.4 and 1.2.6*a*.) With respect to a baseline from *C* to *D*, in one of the "halves," a rigid motion of the other "half" may be estimated by projection onto a basis spanned by the three features $\mathbf{V}_1^T = (1, 0, 1, 0, \ldots, 1, 0)$, $\mathbf{V}_2^T =$

$(0, 1, 0, 1, \ldots, 0, 1)$, and $\mathbf{V}_3^T = (-\bar{\nu}_{25}, \bar{\nu}_{15}, \ldots, -\bar{\nu}_{2K}, \bar{\nu}_{1K})$. The first and second of these span displacements of the second set of landmarks with respect to the baseline (chosen from within the first set), and the third covers (small) relative rotations. The projection is again by generalized least squares, this time with respect to the null-model covariances, as the sample appears to have a strong within-group factor.

The fit to a total of eight landmarks is as in Figure 7.4.7c. It accounts for 85% of the generalized squared length of this transformation by a single biologically interpretable feature: a movement of the anterior pole with respect to the posterior pole without change of shape of either "half." The actual change of shape of the anterior four landmarks is shown here as residual from the model's prediction of no change; the change in shape of the other pole is implicit in the structure of residuals in Figure 7.4.7d. The rigid motion is estimated to have been a shift by the vector $(\Delta\nu_1, \Delta\nu_2) = (0.008, 0.183)$, mainly in the vertical direction, together with a rotation about $(0, 0)$ by 0.025 (about 1.5°). These three quantities are the coefficients of $\mathbf{V}_1$, $\mathbf{V}_2$, and $\mathbf{V}_3$ in the projection of the observed shape change onto their hyperplane. The coefficient for the goodness of fit incorporates the failure of the two additional landmarks A and H on the anterior "half" to stand still; the rigid motion assigns no displacements to them at all. This model, involving three parameters, may be compared to a simple linear model incorporating only two parameters $\hat{\alpha} = (0.033, 0.099)$: a fit to *unequal* shifts, that at each landmark proportional to its distance from the baseline, rather than the same at all the landmarks of the movable "fragment." This fit explains only about 46% of the net configuration. In the linearization to the baseline of Figure 7.4.7a it explains a similar 49% of the net reconfiguration by a vector $(-0.006, -0.106)$ pointing almost straight *toward* the baseline, at an angle of some 45° to the trajectories of all four peripheral landmarks. Notice that a rotation of baseline by about 80° alters the direction of $\hat{\alpha}$ by about 160°, as noted in Section 6.2.2.

Had the changes of landmarks C, D, F, and G been aligned not with lines through the poles but instead with the horizontal, an appropriate feature would instead have been a Huxleyan "growth gradient" cubic in the coordinate ν_1. This extension of the methods previously introduced for quadratic polynomials is left to the reader faced with similar patterns in his or her own data.

7.4.4.2. Spiral parameters. —

Perhaps the first aspect of mathematical biology to succumb to the geometric mode of description was the study of spiral form (Thompson, 1961). A useful series of three generating parameters for forms of this sort was introduced by Raup (1966). Although later workers have concentrated upon this extension to include aspects of the shape of the "generating curve" (cf. Figure 3.4.12*c*), Raup's original parameters still stand as a useful language for comparative architecture. As Figure 7.4.8 shows, changes in each parameter separately may be recognized directly upon the plane of shape coordinates; conversely, one may project observed changes onto ad hoc components **V** one by one, components that represent precisely the effects of changes in a single parameter. In this way, the Raup parameters can *emerge* from the multivariate study of populations of forms (as latent variables, observed differences, ecophenotypic gradients, and the like), rather than having to be guessed at in advance. For an example of this sort of interpretation, see Tabachnick and Bookstein (1990*a*), where Raup's *r* and *θ* are found to express not only sample principal components of landmark configuration in the spiral view but also latent variables explaining the correlations of features of that view with features in the apertural view.

7.4.4. *Other forms*

Figure 7.4.8. Recognizing Raup's spiral parameters in shape coordinates of Tabachnick's *Globorotalia* (Figure 3.4.12). The components of projection are each built by direct computation. I. (*a, b*) A change in *θ*. (*c*) To a baseline from *n* to *n* − 3. (*d*) Vectors of shape-coordinate change. II. (*a, b*) A change in *r* in spiral view. (*c*) To the same baseline. (*d*) Vectors of shape-coordinate change. III. (*a, b*) Change in *t*. (*c*) To a baseline from *s* to a_u. (*d*) Vectors of shape-coordinate change. IV. (*a, b*) Change in *r* in apertural view. (*c*) To the same baseline. (*d*) Vectors of shape-coordinate change. From Tabachnick and Bookstein (1990*a*:Figure 6).

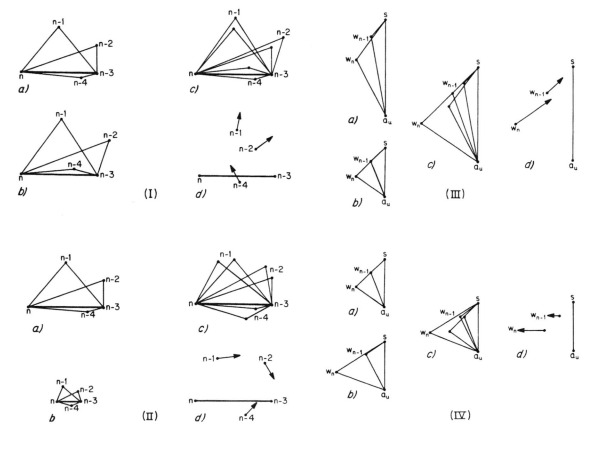

315

7.5. PRINCIPAL AND PARTIAL WARPS: COMPONENTS OF BENDING ENERGY

Much of the material in this section is adapted from Bookstein (1988*a*, 1989*a*). The original idea is due to a suggestion in 1985 from Prof. David Ragozin, Department of Mathematics, University of Washington at Seattle. A program computing these features of shape change is included in the disk pack associated with Rohlf and Bookstein (1990).

7.5.1. Introduction: another shape distance

Growth gradients are familiar aspects of nonuniform shape changes. Nevertheless, they are still *global*, having the same parametric description from end to end of an organism. Likewise, all the other features found by the quadratic polynomial analysis are no more localizable than are the uniform and the purely inhomogeneous components with which we have been working; their second derivatives are the same everywhere. As I mentioned at the outset of Section 7.3, all are regression-based, and none makes much use of the information about the mean form in descriptions, although that form is essential to computation and testing of the "components." An alternate approach to the decomposition of deformations is available, beginning from the thin-plate spline, which supplies a hierarchy of components, the partial warps, that can be "localized"; the hierarchy is in order of "localizability" in a certain technical but very suggestive sense. (But this "localization" is not to the level of individual landmarks, as explained at the end of Section 7.5.4.)

The techniques of decomposition by warps all begin with an eigendecomposition of the bending-energy matrix that represents the mean landmark configuration for the computation of thin-plate splines (Section 2.2). In this section we review the matrix algebra of this decomposition, which produces a set of eigenfunctions I have named the *principal warps* of the landmark configuration to which they pertain. The set of principal warps generalizes the purely inhomogeneous component we found earlier to exhaust the residual from the uniform transformation for quadrilaterals. Principal warps also support a relative eigenanalysis that appropriately localizes within-group shape *variation* (as distinct from between-group shape *difference*) in the setting of landmark data; this is the subject of Section 7.6. Appendix A.1 discusses an extension to deal with a standard problem in image analysis, the task of *distortion correction* (Bookstein, 1990*g*).

The basic themes of these two sections are unfamiliar variants of familiar multivariate strategies: orthogonal decompositions and principal-component analysis. They will, however, look very odd in diagrams, because they both substitute a different distance function, the **bending energy of the thin-plate spline**, for what has been Procrustes distance ρ in the geometry of the printed page (as in Figure 7.1.7). This bending energy, introduced in Section 2.2, has two useful peculiarities. First, it is zero for a large class of shape changes, the *uniform* ones that we already know how to measure by anisotropy. Second, it weights movements of different landmarks differently – that is, it is *not* a "Riemannian [isometric] submersion" of distances from the original digitizing tablet, like the Procrustes distance ρ (Section 5.6.2). Our bending distance is more closely related to "net percentage displacement," displacement as a fraction of the distance to the nearest neighbors (we shall make this concept precise in Section 7.5.2; the interpretation of "localization" will depend strongly on landmark spacing). It remains the case, however, that the bending energy generated by displacing a landmark is not a function of the direction of that displacement.

Given this new shape distance, one can immediately pose two problems the answers to which are the concerns of the remaining two sections. The first problem is to describe the relation between bending-energy distance and Procrustes distance – what kinds of shape changes are given increased weight, what kinds are ignored (relatively or absolutely). The second problem will similarly involve the relation between bending-energy distance and the sample-based Mahalanobis distance between forms.

The answer to the first question corresponds to the diagrams of Figure 7.5.1*b*–*c*: The relation between the two shape distances can be described completely by a certain elliptic cylinder. In the set of shape changes having a given Procrustes magnitude, a given sum of squares for displacements at the optimal superposition, some lie along the axes of the cylinder; these are the pure linear transformations having no bending. Others lie athwart the cylinder; these are the pure bends with no linear component. Both of these come in sets, very difficult to draw, of equivalent distance regardless of direction of displacements. This first question is essentially concerned with the "shape" of this cylinder (we already know the direction of its generators: that direction is the subspace of the uniform transformations). We shall see in this section that the shape of this cylinder is strongly a function of the mean shape of the landmark set. After having complained about its absence from several popular techniques, such as cross-ratio methods and Procrustes techniques, we have at last placed the geometry of the mean landmark configuration squarely at the center of a morphometric analysis. We shall see by the end of Section 7.5 that the axes of the cylinder, the principal directions relating the cylinder to the Procrustes "sphere," are a useful set of features into which to decompose group mean differences.

The second question we can ask about the bending-energy distance relates it to sample variances instead of the Procrustes metric. This question thus involves information from the variation of shapes as well as from the sample mean form. We can find

7.5. Principal warps

Figure 7.5.1. The geometry of bending energy. Each point here is a shape change from a starting form, as shown. The case of no shape change is at the center of each construction. (*a, b*) The starting form is a square. (*a*) A four-dimensional sphere of displacements "equivalent" according to Procrustes distance ρ. There are really two dimensions of circular symmetry for each diameter shown. (*b*) The four-dimensional cylinder of bending-energy distance for the same changes. The circular section corresponds to the circle of the shape changes on the vertical diameter of panel *a*. There are two dimensions of uniform changes packed into each "straight line." The vertical diameters in panels *a* and *b* are the same square-to-kite transformation. The horizontal direction in the diagram shows only one dimension of the uniform subspace, namely, purely horizontal stretching. The oblique diameter of the central circle shows rotations of the simple square-to-kite transformation as in Figure 7.3.6. (*c*) For more than four landmarks, the principal warps are the diameters of circular cross sections of the general cylinder. The figure is in six dimensions; there is only one cylinder, with two perpendicular circular sections shown. The starting form is a sort of a T of five landmarks corresponding roughly to the five-point warp in Figure 7.5.3.

those features of shape that explain the greatest amount of variance per unit bending. In Section 7.6 these will prove the version of principal components most appropriate to landmark data, as they combine "bending at a distance" in exactly the way that ordinary principal-component analysis combines covariances.

In all the analyses to follow, bending energy is, of course, only a metaphor. Neither the actual physics of objects like the plate in Figure 2.2.2 nor the third dimension so casually invoked in that figure has anything to do with descriptions of biological change. The tie between the two contexts, which is ultimately the particular justification of the method of thin-plate splines, is rather that the formalism of bending energy matches our intuitive ideas of biological *localization*. Localization is, in general, a matter of whether or not nearby landmarks appear to move together rela-

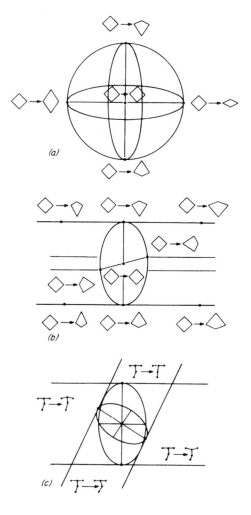

318

tive to those at greater distance. The relative displacement of a pair of landmarks by 1 cm should count for more "distance" if the landmarks are 5 cm apart than if they are 10 cm apart; the shearing of one end of the form with respect to the other end should be described differently than a shearing of the entire form with respect to the wires of the digitizer. The Procrustes distance ρ satisfies neither of these reasonable requirements. Bending energy, in this sense, measures the information *local to proper subsets of the landmarks*. It explicitly omits information about effects that apply equally to all parts of the form; these are the uniform transformations, already measured by anisotropy (ratio of principal strains), as explained in Section 7.2. Also, it is unhelpful regarding the quadratic gradients of Section 7.4, for which the *second* derivative is the same everywhere. (In the purely inhomogeneous transformation and in the thin-plate spline the second derivative is very highly sculpted.) In the metaphor of the thin-plate spline, "bending" is equivalent to "local information" when "information" is measured by the second derivatives of the imputed homology mapping (Section 2.2.4, proposition 2). Other versions of this nonlinear energy are no doubt possible, in which local information would be measured by other aspects of the deviation from linearity or in which the necessary integrals would be taken over the interior of the form, or the polygon of landmarks, instead of over the entire infinite plane. These alternatives would not likely have an algebra as elegant as that of the thin-plate spline.

7.5.2. Eigenanalysis of the bending-energy matrix

We return to the algebra of thin-plate splines. Section 2.2 introduced the so-called **bending-energy matrix** L_K^{-1}, a quadratic form representing the deviation from global linearity that is minimized by the interpolating spline. An example was computed in Section 7.3.2, in the course of visualizing the purely inhomogeneous component, residual from the uniform component for quadrilaterals. That particular matrix is very highly patterned: For a starting form that was square, with the landmarks numbered serially around the perimeter, its numerical value was proportional to

$$\begin{bmatrix} 1 & -1 & 1 & -1 \\ -1 & 1 & -1 & 1 \\ 1 & -1 & 1 & -1 \\ -1 & 1 & -1 & 1 \end{bmatrix}.$$

Thus it is of rank 1, proportional to the dyadic product $(1, -1, 1, -1)^T (1, -1, 1, -1)$. The meaning of this is the following. Patterns of displacement of landmarks of the form

319

$(1, -1, 1, -1)$ – equal and opposite translations applied to the two diagonals – are the only patterns of displacement *not* annihilated by this matrix L_K^{-1}. All other patterns of displacement leave no trace in the nonlinear terms of this interpolation mapping. That is, all other patterns of displacement are in fact *affine*, corresponding to adjustments of the constant and the terms a_x, a_y in f that are not bounded at infinity. This is why the purely inhomogeneous transformation is not localizable "at" a landmark (Figure 7.3.4); it has only one degree of freedom for nonlinearity per coordinate, not enough to specify a location.

The degeneracy of this nonlinear term vanishes as soon as we add any sort of realistic complexity to the interpolation problem posed. Figure 7.5.2 demonstrates the extension by one single additional landmark pair. Now there are five X's on the left and five corresponding X's in a somewhat different configuration on the right. (I find the picture of this deformation, like the other examples of the splines in this volume, rather pleasant and even captivating to contemplate: The thin-plate interpolation behaves visually sensibly even over changes of some considerable magnitude. Of course, like most interpolants, it can be forced to fold.) The form has narrowed considerably from upper right to lower left, not so much from upper left to lower right; and bends have appeared in both "bars," previously nearly straight, of the original T-shaped configuration.

To dissect the features of this and other point-driven deformation efficiently and objectively, we exploit the eigenstructure of the matrix L_K^{-1}. This eigenstructure is coded in Figure 7.5.2 with little lines in the left-hand scene and with certain numbers in the center of the figure. To explain the meaning of these quantities, it will be helpful to have the numerical values of the relevant matrices.

The points on the left, together with the functions $U(r_{ij})$ describing their spatial relations, are encoded in the partitioned matrix

$$L = \begin{bmatrix} 0.0 & 25.4713 & 31.2510 & 1.2938 & 5.8093 & 1 & 3.6929 & 10.3819 \\ 25.4713 & 0.0 & 24.9811 & 18.8511 & 1.9394 & 1 & 6.5827 & 8.8386 \\ 31.2510 & 24.9811 & 0.0 & 7.0360 & 8.6023 & 1 & 6.7756 & 12.0866 \\ 1.2938 & 18.8511 & 7.0360 & 0.0 & 1.4673 & 1 & 4.8189 & 11.2047 \\ 5.8093 & 1.9394 & 8.6023 & 1.4673 & 0.0 & 1 & 5.6969 & 10.0748 \\ \hline & & \text{(sym)} & & & & 0 & \end{bmatrix}$$

for the ordering of landmarks indicated in Figure 7.5.2. This partition was explained in Section 2.2.2. The matrix of landmark coordinates in the right-hand form is

$$V = \begin{bmatrix} 3.9724 & 6.6969 & 6.5394 & 5.4016 & 5.7756 & 0 & 0 & 0 \\ 6.5354 & 4.1181 & 7.2362 & 6.4528 & 5.1142 & 0 & 0 & 0 \end{bmatrix}.$$

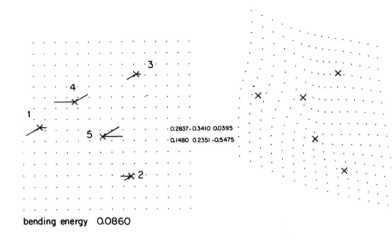

bending energy 0.0860

The vectors $L^{-1}V^T$ of coefficients W and a are

$$(-0.0380, 0.0232, -0.0248, 0.0798, -0.0402;$$

$$1.3552, 0.8747, -0.0289)^T$$

and

$$(0.0425, 0.0159, 0.0288, -0.0454, -0.0418;$$

$$-2.9458, -0.2956, 0.9216)^T.$$

The matrix L_K^{-1} of bending energy as a function of changes in the coordinates of the landmarks on the right is, for this example,

$$\begin{bmatrix}
0.0493 & -0.0023 & 0.0329 & -0.0744 & -0.0055 \\
-0.0023 & 0.0389 & -0.0004 & 0.0439 & -0.0801 \\
0.0329 & -0.0004 & 0.0219 & -0.0485 & -0.0059 \\
-0.0744 & 0.0439 & -0.0485 & 0.1546 & -0.0756 \\
-0.0055 & -0.0801 & -0.0059 & -0.0756 & 0.1671
\end{bmatrix}.$$

This matrix has three zero eigenvalues, corresponding to patterns of landmark displacement that result in affine transformations, and two nonzero eigenvalues, 0.2837 and 0.1480. The eigenvector corresponding to 0.2837 is

$$(0.2152, -0.3265, 0.1346, -0.6554, 0.6320)^T;$$

that for 0.1480 is

$$(-0.4941, -0.2415, -0.3370, 0.4700, 0.6026)^T.$$

Figure 7.5.2. A deformation of five landmarks (large X's). The principal warps (eigenvectors of the bending-energy matrix) are indicated as little vectors of "vertical" displacement at the landmarks; they are drawn in directions counterclockwise from three o'clock in descending order of localizability (ascending order of scale). For the surfaces corresponding to these displacements, see the next two figures. The tables in this and similar figures tabulate the eigenvalue (inverse scale) and vector multiple of each principal warp, smallest to largest scale, the summed products of which make up the actual thin-plate spline mapping shown.

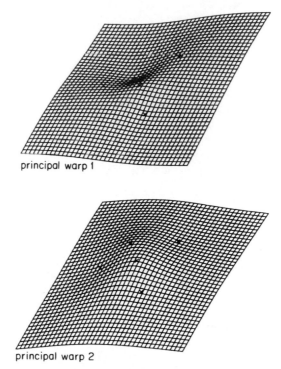

principal warp 1

principal warp 2

Figure 7.5.3. The principal warps for the starting configuration of landmarks in Figure 7.5.1: eigenfunctions of the bending-energy matrix. Top: For the stiffer eigenvalue, 0.2837. Bottom: For the less stiff eigenvalue, 0.1480.

The bending-energy matrix is computed as it applies to patterns of Cartesian displacement of the landmarks in the right-hand frame; but because these eigenvectors are coefficients for the five functions U based at these five landmarks, we may interpret each as the coefficients of a thin-plate spline of its own, attached to a base plane at the left-hand landmarks and horizontal at infinity. That is, each eigenvector can be visualized, and understood, as a pattern of bending (= deformation), a shape change that is distinctive by virtue of having a well-defined geometrical scale and "center." These functions $f_{0.2837}, f_{0.1480}$ are displayed in Figure 7.5.3a–b as lofted into the third dimension – true thin-plate splines – after the fashion of Figure 7.3.5. The height of these surfaces at each landmark is just the corresponding coefficient in the 5-vector expressing it as an eigenvector above.

The surface in Figure 7.5.3a appears to be *more bent* than that in Figure 7.5.3b. To be precise, it requires more bending energy, 0.2837 versus 0.1480, for the same net amplitude of vertical displacement (measured as the sum of squares of coordinate changes at the landmarks). As is plain in the figure, the landmarks whose contrasting changes drive the spline in Figure 7.5.3a lie closer together (i.e., are "more localized"), and so the splined surface must change its slopes at higher rates, thus increasing the quadratic variation that, integrated out to infinity, corresponds to the eigenvalue of 0.2837 reported. That these f's are eigenvectors implies that the coefficients are identical with the displacements

322

given by these f's at the landmarks separately. We may then draw them as well as displacements superimposed over the landmarks in their own plane. In Figure 7.5.2, these loadings were shown as little segments attached to the X's themselves. The loadings of the first eigenvector run left or right, and those of the second, quite arbitrarily, at 30° counterclockwise of these. The segments are signed, so that positive and negative coefficients run in opposite directions out of the X representing the landmark. For instance, the pattern of loadings of the eigenvector $f_{0.2837}$ is absolutely largest, but with opposed signs, at landmarks #4 and #5. It is visualized in Figure 7.5.2 by the opposed horizontal segments attached to those central points. Later, in the technique of partial warps, we shall similarly interpret these as actual deformations in the plane of the data; to do that, we shall assign them an in-plane vector without any arbitrariness at all.

Thus we are interpreting the eigenvectors of the bending-energy matrix L_K^{-1} as a collection of potential **descriptors of deformation**. In that context they provide a canonical description of the modes according to which points may be displaced irrespective of global affine transformations. I have named them (Bookstein, 1989*a*) the **principal warps** of the configuration of landmarks on the left-hand side of figures like Figure 7.5.2. [Note that the principal warps depend only on the landmarks of one form, the "starting" or "mean" form. The second (right-hand) form is involved in finding the vectors by which the principal warps are multiplied to supply the partial warps, as discussed later.] Principal warps are computed features of bending at *successively lower levels of bending energy*; by the identification of bending energy with second derivatives of in-plane displacement, they correspond to features of deformation at *successively larger physical scales*. This is plain in Figure 7.5.3. The first eigenvalue corresponds to a relatively *small* feature – differences in the displacements of the two nearest points of the form, landmarks #4 and #5, with respect to the triangle of the other landmarks at considerable distance. But the last nonzero eigenvalue corresponds to a relatively *large* but still not global (affine) feature – the deviation of landmarks #4 and #5, together, from the average displacement of the three landmarks at the outside "corners." As an affine transformation would move the center of this triangle in accordance with the displacement of those corners, this pair of principal warps may be considered a simple sum-and-difference transformation of the original basis for displacement space (at landmarks #4 and #5 separately). But the *difference* between #4 and #5 has a higher eigenvalue (greater stiffness) than the *sum* of #4 and #5, as it represents a feature at smaller geometric scale.

In this aspect these spline maps deviate greatly from regression-based decompositions of the same landmark correspondences (as introduced in the preceding section). In the regression-based techniques, the effect of an "error of fit" is the same regardless of how close a landmark lies to its neighbors and regardless of the concordance of adjacent "errors." But by its dependence on the matrix K of quantities $U(r)$, functions of adjacency, the principal warps of the spline are inextricable from the geometry of the landmark configuration itself. **The language that is geometrically "natural" for a description of nonuniform shape changes itself depends on the average or typical shape**.

As deformations, these warps (and also their linear combinations the relative warps, to be introduced in the next section) are already in Procrustes-optimal position. In fact, they have no affine part either: They have the same formal properties as the output of any of the affine-Procrustes routines (Section 7.2.3), except that their scale is not controlled. As a deformation, each principal warp has no translational component, no shear, and no rotation. Then each partial warp (as discussed later) represents a "purely inhomogeneous transformation" of its own, with no affine part.

7.5.3. Principal warps and partial warps as features of transformation

To this point the analysis of principal warps has involved only the starting configuration of landmarks; it would be the same whatever the positions of their homologues in the right-hand frame in Figure 7.5.2. Those positions, of course, affect the coefficients W and a we computed.

Let us deal first with the affine part of this map, the function $(x', y') = (1.3552 + 0.8747x - 0.0289y, -2.9458 - 0.2956x + 0.9216y)$. The constant terms merely refer to a shift between the two images (already corrected in Figure 7.5.1); the linear terms may be collected in a matrix

$$A = \begin{bmatrix} 0.8747 & -0.0289 \\ -0.2956 & 0.9216 \end{bmatrix}.$$

The principal axes of this transformation (cf. Section 6.1) are at $+44.9°$ and $-45.1°$ to the horizontal in the starting configuration, and $+53.3°$ and $-36.7°$ in the final form, bearing strains of 1.072 and 0.744, respectively. The factor 1.072 implies some elongation of the form toward the northwest: For instance, the distance from landmark #2 to the midpoint of landmarks #1 and #3 is longer in the right-hand form than in the left. The factor 0.744, which is almost identical with the ratio of decrease in the distance between landmarks #1 and #3, confirms the compression from southwest to northeast.

Turning now to the remaining terms $\Sigma w_i U(|P_i - (x, y)|)$ in the spline formula, we may begin to make sense of these by drawing them out, after the fashion of Figure 7.3.5, as surfaces in their own right, coordinate by coordinate, in Figure 7.5.4. These pictures should now not be considered to represent any particular

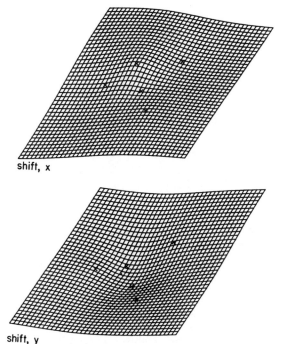

shift, x

shift, y

Figure 7.5.4. Thin-plate splines for the shifts of the coordinates in Figure 7.5.2 separately.

orthogonal projection; the dropping of the affine part of the mapping is equivalent to not knowing "which way was up" in this style of diagram. The X's, as before, represent the points of the surface that are fixed in position; but now there is no way to draw the armature to which to weld them – no "horizontal." Nevertheless, the nature of the bending of the coordinates separately is immediately clear, as is the contrast between them. The nonlinearity in the x-shift appears to be concentrated at landmark #4; that for the y-shift appears to be a larger-scale depression (displacement downward in Figure 7.5.1) of the whole middle of the figure, encompassing both landmarks #4 and #5.

The features of this deformation are expressed in the relationships between Figure 7.5.4 and Figure 7.5.3. Plainly, the surface f_1 of affine-free x-shift in Figure 7.5.4 resembles an inverted version of Figure 7.5.3a, the first principal warp, and the surface f_2 of affine-free y-shift resembles an inverted version of Figure 7.5.3b, the second principal warp. This suggests that we expand the functions f_1, f_2 of the actual thin-plate deformation (Figure 7.5.4) in terms of the principal warps: We have, in fact,

$$f_1 = -0.3410(0.2837f_{0.2837}) + 0.2351(0.1480f_{0.1480})$$

and

$$f_2 = 0.0395(0.2837f_{0.2837}) - 0.5475(0.1480f_{0.1480}).$$

325

These coefficients are ordinary cross-products of the coefficients V, Cartesian coordinates of the right-hand landmarks, by those of the eigenvectors. (For instance, $-0.3410 = 0.2152 \times 3.9724 - 0.3265 \times 6.6969 + 0.1346 \times 6.5394 - 0.6554 \times 5.4016 + 0.6320 \times 5.7756$.) The squares of these coefficients combine with the eigenvalues to make up the bending energy $VL_K^{-1}V^T$:

$$0.2837(0.3410^2 + 0.0395^2) + 0.1480(0.2351^2 + 0.5475^2) = 0.0860.$$

Note that the x-shifts are spatially more concentrated, emphasizing the discrepancy between the displacements of landmarks #4 and #5. (The upper one, #4, has moved considerably to the right between the frames; the lower one, #5, not so much.) The y-shift shows relatively less of this high-energy (small-scale) behavior, but emphasizes instead the displacement of both central points relative to the remaining landmarks: in this case, their joint displacement mainly *downward* – the bending of the previously straight bar (landmarks #1–#4–#3) of the T.

7.5.3.1. Partial warps: vector multiples of principal warps. —

We can make this decomposition even more pictorial by diagramming it back in the original Cartesian plane of the data (Bookstein, 1990*f*). In this approach, to each principal warp corresponds not a picture of a metal plate but a diagram of what the warp represented by that plate does to the positions of grid lines when it alone deforms the starting graph paper by the appropriate vector multiple. I call these **partial warps**, as each except the affine term is a localizable part of the warping actually observed. The three partial warps in Figure 7.5.5, treated as displacements of the five landmarks, add to exactly the net displacements in Figure 7.5.2, and the two at the left in panels a and b add to exactly the negative of those at the right in panel c.

Whereas the display of affine-free shifts, as in Figure 7.5.4, combines the effects of all the principal warps one coordinate at a time, the technique of partial warps displays the effect of one single principal warp on both Cartesian coordinates at once. Each such combination is equivalent to interpreting the principal warp not as a surface but as a pattern of displacements in the plane of the data; the pattern of the principal warp is multiplied by a vector proportional to the pair of relative weights of this principal warp in the shifts of the x- and y-coordinates separately. (Of course, the decomposition is rotationally invariant.) Figure 7.5.5 shows each partial warp twice: on the left, as actual displacements of the landmarks in a fixed (actually, Procrustes-registered) superposition; on the right, as a thin-plate spline map corresponding to the same displacements. The transformation of Figure 7.5.2, a "total warp," is the algebraic sum of the three transformations in Figure 7.5.5.

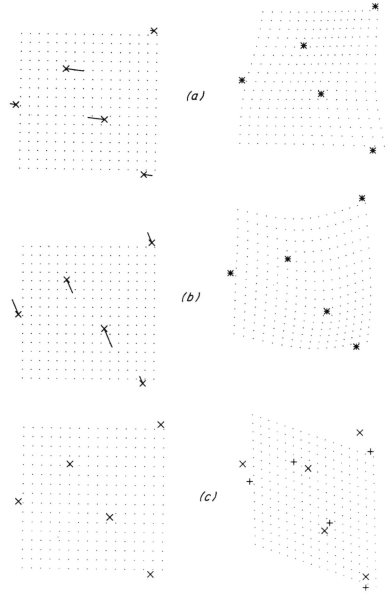

Figure 7.5.5. Partial warps for the transformation in Figure 7.5.4. (*a*) The sharper principal warp (Figure 7.5.3, top) multiplied by 0.2837 times the vector $(-0.3410, 0.0395)$ and added to the original square grid intersection by intersection. As in Figure 7.5.2, each little vector still represents a displacement of the landmark to which it is attached. Unlike the displacements in Figure 7.5.2, these are in-plane. (*b*) The smoother principal warp (Figure 7.5.3, bottom) multiplied by 0.1480 times the vector $(0.2351, -0.5475)$ and added to the same original square grid. (*c*) The uniform term; +, affine transformation of landmarks on left; X, actual locations of landmarks on right; the difference between + and X, landmark by landmark, is the sum of all the little vectors attached to the landmark in the stack of partial warps (*a* and *b*, left).

The comparison of Figure 7.5.3 and 7.5.4 is made quite a bit clearer here. Panel *a* shows the horizontality of the effect at the scale of the sharper principal warp – this grid displacement is mainly horizontal, as are the vectors at the left. In panel *b*, the vectors at left are predominantly vertical, as is the dip in the equivalent grid (right). The vectors at the left in each frame are in mechanical equilibrium (no net translation, no rotation) – this is a consequence of the independence of the affine part of the transformations from that described by the bending energy.

These 2-vector coefficients and the associated partial warps represent the decomposition of single deformations I am recommending as alternative or complement to the global polynomial components of Sections 7.2 and 7.4. Each principal warp specifies a geometrically independent mode of affine-free deformation at its own geometrical scale (which may be taken as the inverse root of its eigenvalue, its "bending energy"). For configurations of three landmarks, all transformations can be modeled as affine, and there are no partial warps beyond the affine term. For four landmarks, there is only one warp, the single eigenvector shown for the case of a starting form that is square in Figure 7.3.5; some possible partial warps are shown in Figure 7.3.6 corresponding to vectors $(\cos 0°, \sin 0°)$, $(\cos 45°, \sin 45°)$, and $(\cos 22.5°, \sin 22.5°)$. For more than four landmarks, the bending-energy matrix has a nontrivial spectrum that can be of great biometric interest.

For describing deformations, this spectrum serves a role analogous to that of the more familiar Fourier spectrum and other orthogonal decompositions in describing single functions (such as pictures or outlines of forms). In the single picture, higher terms of an orthogonal decomposition represent features of progressively smaller scale. Likewise, the higher terms of the bending-energy spectrum represent aspects of deformation of progressively smaller scale: specifications of warping more and more local.

7.5.4. Localizing deformation of many landmarks

The reader may have noticed that both of the principal warps in Figure 7.5.3 somewhat resemble the purely inhomogeneous component for a quadrilateral of landmarks, shown as a thin plate in Figure 7.3.5. When landmarks are spaced with reasonable evenness, this observation extends to any number of landmarks; the principal warps often resemble the four-landmark version (the purely inhomogeneous transformation) at diverse geometric scales, and the largest-order partial warp will usually resemble one of those in Figure 7.3.6.

Consider, for example, the nearly regular hexagon of landmarks in Figure 7.5.6. The eigenanalysis indicates one principal warp rather stiffer than the others (eigenvalue 0.3732, versus 0.1982 for the next stiffest). This most bent eigenvector mainly taps landmarks #1, #2, #4, and #6 – the smallest quadrilateral of landmarks in this scheme, at lower left. From the display of these warps as physical thin plates (Figure 7.5.7), we recognize the discordant-diagonal construction (Figure 7.3.1) of the purely inhomogeneous spline (Figure 7.3.5). Principal warp 2 is a slightly less bent surface, whereas warps 3 and 4, both quite gentle, appear to be permuted versions of one another.

The features of the map in Figure 7.5.6 are combinations of these principal warps given by the details of the reconfiguration on the right-hand form. From the pattern of segments out of

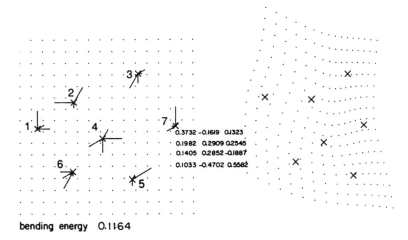

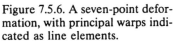

bending energy   0.1164

Figure 7.5.6. A seven-point deformation, with principal warps indicated as line elements.

landmark #7 in Figure 7.5.6, we see that this landmark, so considerably displaced from left to right in Figure 7.5.6, contributes mainly to this last principal warp, which accounts for half of the actual bending observed: $[0.1035 \times (0.4702^2 + 0.5582^2)] = 0.0550$ out of 0.1164. This dominant feature of the deformation is the shift of landmarks #4, #5, and #2 downward-rightward with respect to the others: a relative translation of two diagonals of a square, as in Figure 7.3.5. Because the function f_2 loads mainly

Figure 7.5.7. The four principal warps of the configuration in Figure 7.5.6, each shown as a thin-plate spline.

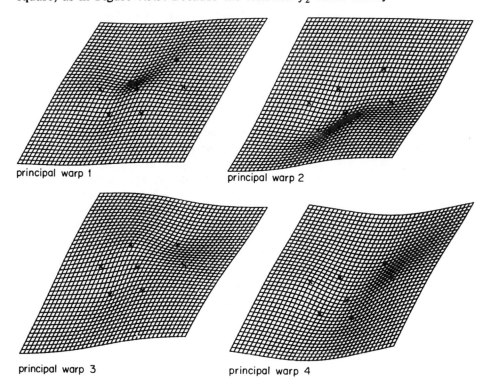

principal warp 1

principal warp 2

principal warp 3

principal warp 4

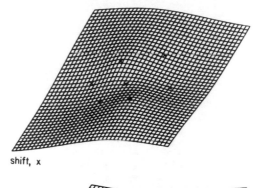

shift, x

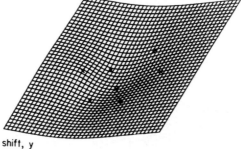

Figure 7.5.8. Shifts of the *x*- and *y*-coordinates separately, shown as thin plates, for the transformation of Figure 7.5.6.

shift, y

on principal warp 4, the thin plate for f_2 (Figure 7.5.8, *y*-shift) strongly resembles that of principal warp 4 in Figure 7.5.7. (The entry 0.5582 dominates the last column of the table in the figure.) The *x*-shift surface is a combination of many different principal warps.

7.5.4.1. *Localization is not landmark by landmark.* —

The meaning of "localization" here is local to *neighborhoods* of at least three landmarks, not to specific single points. If it is known in advance that shape change is affine or even isotropic except at one or two landmarks, the appropriate analysis is of the vectors expressing the positions of those landmarks over a background of those whose shape is known to be unchanging. These vectors are just the residuals from a robust Procrustes fit (e.g., Rohlf and Slice, 1990). Just as in an analysis by global components, the analysis of such a change by warps, either the principal warps of this section or the relative warps of the next, will blur such landmark-specific shape change over most of the spectrum of possible scales. Thus in simulations that manipulate only a few landmarks to change or vary independently of the others, one customarily finds that the diagrams of the warps do not appear to fit the assumptions driving the data. This is quite correct: Assumptions of independence of change at neighboring landmarks are overwhelmingly nonbiological. Outside of the domain of craniofa-

7.5.5. Effect of extremes of landmark spacing

We learn more about the behavior of these spline interpolants by altering the preceding example so as to demonstrate two extremes of landmark spacing. In Figure 7.5.9*a* we have moved landmark #7 quite close to landmark #3 at the upper right and have moved landmark #6 quite distant from all the others, at the lower left.

As indicated in the table within the figure, the spectrum of the bending-energy matrix now ranges over a considerable interval, from 0.0483 to 0.9344. The eigenvector of highest bending energy, sketched at the left with horizontal segments, is apparently a contrast between displacements of landmarks #3 and #7, those closest together (at upper right), together with a small weight for the previously central landmark #4, closest of the others to this pair. Inspection of this first principal warp as a thin plate (Figure 7.5.9*b*) indicates that its principal feature is a slope at the upper right, limited to the region of landmarks #3 and #7. This principal warp specifies mainly the **vertical directional derivative** of the interpolating spline *f* in that vicinity. As tabulated in Figure 7.5.9*a*, the large loading of the *y*-shift upon this highly energetic eigenvector corresponds to the considerable discord between the separation of these two landmarks on the *right* in the figure and the separation implied by the spline based on using one of these points, but not the other, together with the five at a distance. That is, the map with the vertical directional derivative constrained at landmark #3 (or #7), as shown, is highly bent in that vicinity. The pair of points at the upper right is highly informative about bending energy – it is a small-scale feature of the deformation – and, in this instance, there is considerable information at this scale in the *y*-component of the deformation observed.

The second eigenvector of this landmark configuration (Figure 7.5.9*b*) is quite similar to the first eigenvector of the five-point analysis (Figure 7.5.2). It is mainly a contrast of displacements between landmark #4 and landmark #5. Similarly, the third eigenvector of the seven-point configuration is quite comparable to the second eigenvector of the five-point configuration. It represents a central "peak" of its thin plate somewhat broader than the crimp shown for the second eigenvalue – a joint displacement of *both* landmarks #4 and #5 with respect to those surrounding.

Of larger geometrical scale (lower bending energy) than any other deformation is the last principal warp. It is, in fact, the same transformation as the simple nonlinear warp of a square; compare this image to Figure 7.3.5. The form of this surface is clear as well in Figure 7.5.9*a*, where it is coded in the signed lengths of the vertical segments out of the landmarks. In this approximately

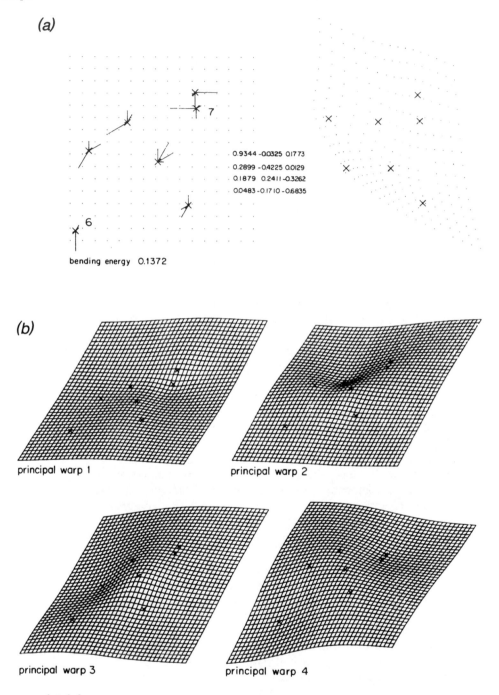

(a)

0.9344 -0.0325 0.1773
0.2899 -0.4225 0.0129
0.1879 0.2411 -0.3262
0.0483 -0.1710 -0.6835

bending energy 0.1372

(b)

principal warp 1

principal warp 2

principal warp 3

principal warp 4

Figure 7.5.9. A seven-point deformation with extremes of landmark spacing. (*a*) The deformation. (*b*) Principal warps.

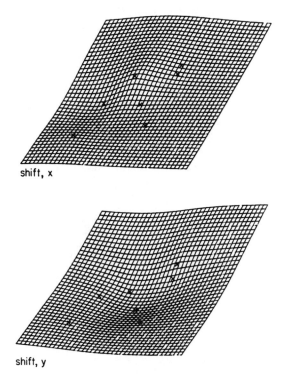

shift, x

shift, y

Figure 7.5.10. Features of the transformation in Figure 7.5.9, coordinate by coordinate.

square configuration, the extremes of one "diagonal" are displaced downward, while all other points, lying upon the opposite diagonal, are displaced upward. In the partial warp here, the direction of shift is reversed (owing to the negative sign on the y-loading of -0.6835). This is the only eigenvector to which landmark #6 contributes to any extent. The large projection of f_2 on this gentlest principal warp owes to the massive upward translation of this landmark between left and right configurations.

The displays of affine-free coordinate shifts (Figure 7.5.10) confirm that, as tabulated in Figure 7.5.9, the y-shift is a superposition of principal warps 1, 3, and 4 at roughly equal energies ($0.1773^2 \times 0.9344 = 0.0294, 0.3262^2 \times 0.1879 = 0.0200, 0.6835^2 \times 0.0483 = 0.0226$). The x-shift is mainly a multiple of principal warp 2 (principal warp 1 from Figure 7.5.3), just as it was before augmentation of the scene by landmarks #6 and #7.

7.5.6. Example: the upper face in Apert syndrome

Examples earlier in this book (Sections 5.4.3.2 and 7.3.3.2) introduced the congential craniofacial deformity that is Apert syndrome: underdevelopment of the maxilla, apparently consequent upon abnormalities of the sutures of the sphenoid bone and calvarium. In this section I analyze the change of mean configuration of eight upper facial landmarks, stripping off the wholly global affine component of the change and then interpreting the loadings upon the various principal warps. This analysis supersedes that in Bookstein (1987a), which used finite-element methods instead.

Figure 7.5.11 shows the deformation in question. It involves eight landmarks (operational definitions in Section 3.4.2) observed in the University School Study (USS) lateral films and in 14 cases of Apert syndrome (Ap) from the Institute for Reconstructive Plastic Surgery, New York University Medical Center. The spline was fitted just as described in Chapter 2.

Figure 7.5.11. Thin-plate spline, with vector loadings of the principal warps, for interpretation of mean Apert upper facial form (right grid) as deformation of the appropriately age- and sex-weighted University School Study normative mean (left grid); Nas, Nasion; Sel, Sella; Orb, Orbitale; InZ, Inferior zygoma; PtM, Pterygo-maxillary fissure; SER, Sphenoethmoid registration; ANS, Anterior nasal spine; PNS, Posterior nasal spine.

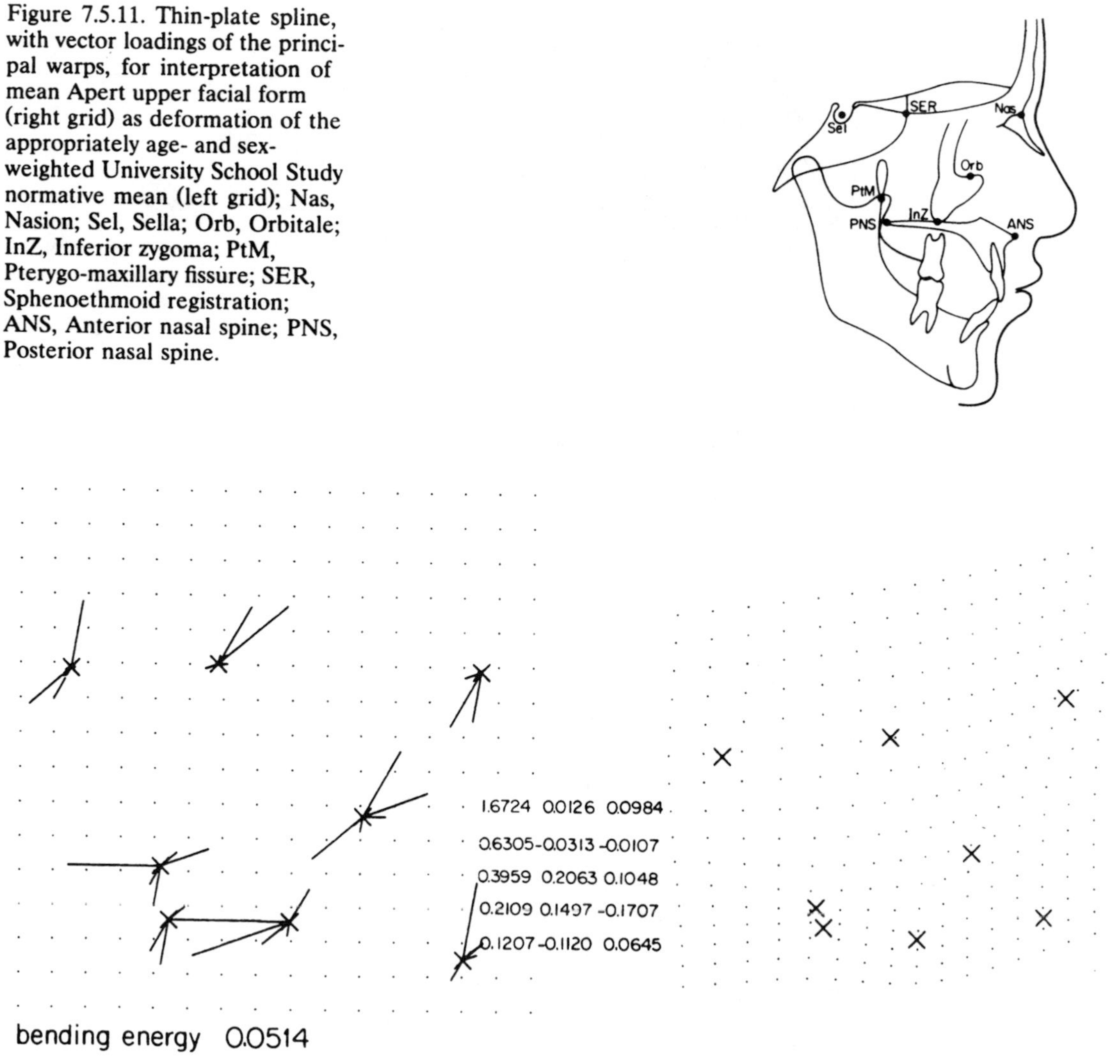

1.6724 0.0126 0.0984
0.6305 -0.0313 -0.0107
0.3959 0.2063 0.1048
0.2109 0.1497 -0.1707
0.1207 -0.1120 0.0645

bending energy   0.0514

334

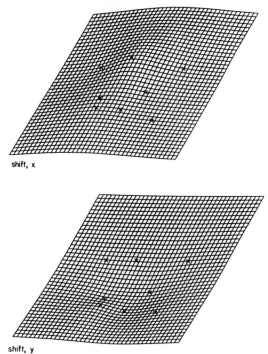

shift, x

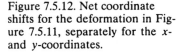

shift, y

Figure 7.5.12. Net coordinate shifts for the deformation in Figure 7.5.11, separately for the x- and y-coordinates.

The affine part of the mapping is

$$x_{\mathrm{Ap}} \sim 0.8493 x_{\mathrm{USS}} - 0.0000 y_{\mathrm{USS}},$$
$$y_{\mathrm{Ap}} \sim 0.1375 x_{\mathrm{USS}} + 0.7167 y_{\mathrm{USS}},$$

having principal strains of 0.882 and 0.690 in directions respectively along and perpendicular to $(0.937, 0.350)$ on the left, and $(0.902, 0.431)$ on the right. This represents a change of proportion by some 21% involving compression aligned along a direction through ANS passing somewhat anterior to SER. The general appearance of this affine transformation is hinted at toward the upper right corner of the right-hand grid of Figure 7.5.11. It conforms to that reported previously in a subsample of these data (Bookstein, 1984*b*).

The deviations of the observed data from this uniform change – that is, all the remaining terms in the spline formulas – are shown in Figure 7.5.12 by one thin-plate spline for the x-coordinate and another for the y-coordinate. The dominant feature of x-nonlinearity is the "upward" deviation at landmark SER (its relative displacement *forward*, as observed in Section 7.3.3.2). The y-nonlinearity appears to have a crimp in the vicinity of PtM–PNS and a dip (relative motion of landmarks *downward*) posterior and superior to ANS.

The objective decomposition of this deformation into local features afforded by principal warps is the roster of vector multiples listed in Figure 7.5.11 for the five principal warps shown in Figure 7.5.13 (by plates) and Figure 7.5.14 (by partial warps). The bending energies associated with these principal warps, products of the eigenvalues by the summed-squared loadings, are 0.0166, 0.0006, 0.0212, 0.0108, and 0.0020, totaling 0.0514, as noted in Figure 7.5.11. For instance, $0.0166 = 1.672 \times (0.0126^2 + 0.0984^2)$, the numbers from the first written line in the middle of Figure 7.5.11.

It is helpful to deal first with the warps of *lowest* observed signal, the second and the fifth. As displayed in Figure 7.5.13, the second may be seen to be flat (i.e., in accord with the global affine term) except for the three lateral maxillary landmarks Orb, InZ, and PtM; it thus represents shape change localized to this structure alone. The vanishing of the partial warp corresponding to this principal warp implies that no such localized effect is observed in this shape comparison – the effect of the Apert deformation on this triangle may be expressed wholly in terms of its involvement in gradients of larger scale. The fifth principal warp is by now quite familiar to us (cf. Figure 7.3.5) as the "pure inhomogeneity" so often found as the largest-scale component of nonlinearity. Here it explains little of the net bending energy, indicating that the change is not usefully considered to incorporate any aspect of

Figure 7.5.13. The five principal warps for the configuration of eight landmarks in Figure 7.5.11. Eigenvalues, in order: 1.672, 0.631, 0.360, 0.211, 0.121.

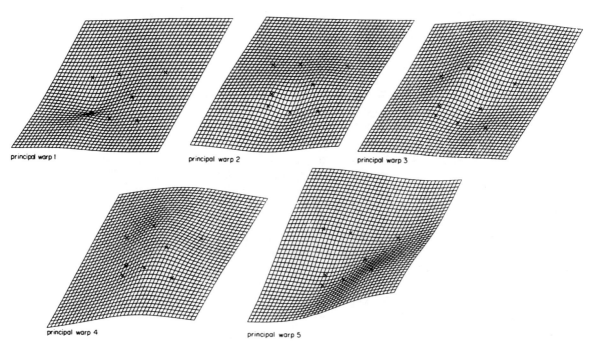

principal warp 1

principal warp 2

principal warp 3

principal warp 4

principal warp 5

the rigid shift of one diameter of the structure with respect to the other landmarks.

The meaning of the principal warp of smallest scale, warp 1, is clear by comparison with the corresponding warp in Figure 7.5.9*b*. The most local feature of deformations of the set of landmarks here is the relative displacement of the pair at closest separation: PtM and PNS. In this example, that principal warp incorporates a signal primarily in the vertical direction (loadings 0.0126 : 0.0984, as written in Figure 7.5.11). Plainly this pair of landmarks is considerably closer together in the Apert cephalogram than in the normative. This does not correspond to any commensurate reduction of distance in the solid skull, as landmark PNS lies along the midline, whereas PtM represents a pair of structures lying somewhat laterally. This is not a difficulty of the method of principal warps per se, but rather a limitation of two-dimensional cephalometric data, resolvable in principle by recourse to landmark locations in three dimensions.

There remain for consideration the principal warps of intermediate geometrical scale. Principal warp 3, explaining the most observed bending $[0.3959 \times (0.2063^2 + 0.1048^2) = 0.0212$ unit out of a total of $0.0514]$, represents our familiar "pure inhomogeneity" applied to the anterior part of the scene: landmarks SER and ANS (and a bit of PNS–PtM as well) translated with respect to the line Sel–Orb–InZ in between them. As it happens, whereas SER is involved in such an apparent displacement in Figure 7.5.11, ANS is not, for ANS participates "equally and oppositely" in the compensating effect of principal warp 4. Graphically, the general topography of *x*-nonlinearity in Figure 7.5.12 may be imagined to be a weighted sum of the sharper ridge of warp 3 (Figure 7.5.13) with the gentle dome of warp 4. The general facies of the *y*-nonlinearity in Figure 7.5.12 is, apart from the clamped derivative at PtM–PNS, a weighted *difference* of these surfaces.

As can be seen from the vicinity of point ANS in Figure 7.5.13, ANS contributes substantially to bending energy only through principal warp 5, which describes very little of the deformation observed in this case. Because ANS is at a good distance from these neighbors, and because it lies at a sharp convexity of the hull of the configuration, this adjustment would require relatively little bending energy even if it were needed. In effect, the spline formalism takes into account the existence of all that space around ANS (Figure 7.5.11) across which the steel plate can adjust itself to asymptotic flatness.

In respect of these eight projected landmark locations we have expressed the deformity that is the sample mean Apert syndrome as the combination of four processes of deformation, separated out in Figure 7.5.14: a general affine term (panel *f*) representing compression along an axis at about 60° clockwise of the cranial base; a highly localized change (panel *a*) in the (projected) relation between PtM and PNS; and two localized relative displace-

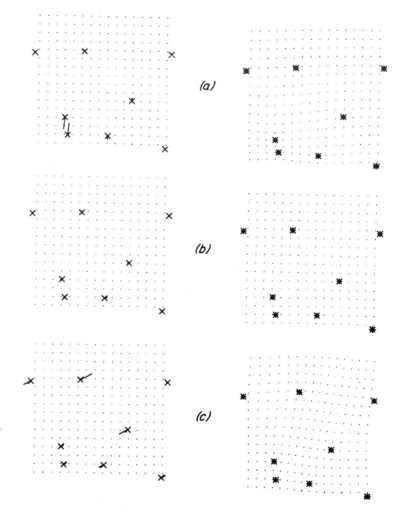

Figure 7.5.14. Partial warps for the transformation in Figure 7.5.11: projections of Figure 7.5.13 into the plane of the data, together with the uniform term. *a–c*: Partial warps 1, 2, and 3. *d–f*: Partial warps 4 and 5 and the uniform term. For notations, see the legend for Figure 7.5.5.

ments, SER to the right with respect to its neighbors (panel *c*), and SER and Orb to the right and downward with respect to their neighbors (panel *d*). The landmark ANS participates in these regional contrasts and in the overall affine transformation, but otherwise represents no particular local modification of the global scene. This summary may be contrasted with that in Bookstein (1987*a*), which found that ANS and PNS participated equally in displacements with respect to the positions they would have been expected to adopt under relative translation and scale change of the lateral maxillary triangle, without deformation. In the analysis by principal warps, the unchanging shape of this triangle is the accidental cancellation of competing processes: a global shear together with the composite of local bends. In light of the severe problem of foreshortening of the distance PtM–PNS, any further analysis probably ought to be carried out in three dimensions.

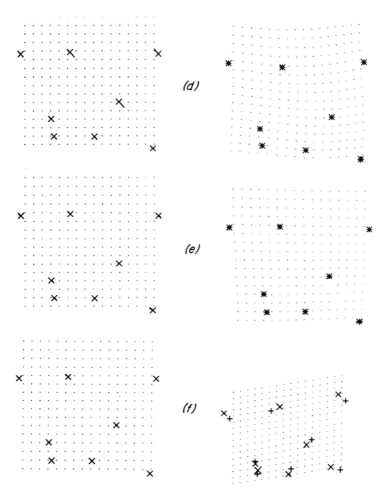

Figure 7.5.14. *Continued.*

7.6. RELATIVE WARPS: COMPONENTS OF WITHIN-SAMPLE VARIATION

We saw in the preceding section how a change of landmark configuration could be decomposed into a global linear term together with features each representing a distinct nonlinearity having a certain location, scale, and form (square-to-kite, square-to-trapezoid, or straight-to-bent-segment). More precisely, what was "decomposed" was the bending energy $WP_K W^T = VL_K^{-1} V^T$ of the pair of thin-plate splines representing the transformation as a deformation. The expression of the $2 \times K$ matrix V of coordinate changes in terms of the $K - 3$ partial warps partitions its net bending into a collection of features drawn from an orthogonal spectrum of purely inhomogeneous terms. Each of these usually depends mainly on a small number of landmarks and may be assigned a geometrical scale indexed by the reciprocal of the square root of the bending energy.

339

In Section 5.3.3 we identified a single factor in the shape variation of a single triangle whenever the distribution of its shape coordinates deviated from circular form. We could do this because the circle described equivalent amounts of shape difference (anisotropy) in all directions independent of the basis chosen for the shape coordinates. We have not hitherto described any extension of this strategy to data involving more than three landmarks, as we have not yet introduced any equivalent of the circle – the quadratic form calibrating magnitude for shape variation in diverse directions – likewise invariant against changes of basis for the shape coordinates. The principal warps, diameters of the cylinder in Figure 7.5.1, supply just such an invariant basis against which we may calibrate observed variation within samples of more than three landmarks.

7.6.1. Components relative to bending energy

In the usual development of principal components for a "measurement vector" of scalar variables X_i, one computes **eigenvectors** of their covariance (or correlation) matrix. The first of these is the vector $\{a_i\}$ – the variable $\Sigma a_i X_i$ – corresponding to the maximum of the ratio $\Sigma\Sigma a_i a_j \text{cov}(X_i, X_j)/\Sigma a_i^2$. The numerator of this expression is the variance of $\Sigma a_i X_i$; the denominator represents the set of linear combinations of the X's as a sphere upon which all directions are equally weighted. To optimize the variance of $\Sigma a_i X_i$ for fixed Σa_i^2 is to declare one patch of the sphere just as good as any other as a direction for this optimum. Recall Section 2.3.2; this vector, scaled up to its eigenvalue, is the best rank-1 fit to the whole covariance matrix of landmark displacements about the mean form. The second principal component maximizes this ratio subject to the condition of being orthogonal to the first; the first and second together supply the best rank-2 approximation to the covariances of landmark displacements; and so on.

We have no access to such a sphere of directions in the space of shape coordinates as soon as the number of landmarks exceeds three. Different bases for the space give rise to different patterns of covariance among the shape coordinates, patterns that share no particular geometry. We cannot define "even coverage" of shape space by any specification of simple shape variables (ratios of distances, angles, or other measures of triangles). Without such a prior notion of evenness, any principal component of a set of manifest variables is arbitrary.

But by recourse to the bending-energy matrix, such a system of coordinates for shape space, a system invariant against changes of shape basis and yet not a function of the observed covariance structure, may be supplied *by ignoring the linear parts of transformations*. We may use the bending energy itself as a unit for making *nonlinear* changes commensurate in different directions.

Just as the distance δ/h in shape space supplied a unit for scaling diverse simple shape variables in the vicinity of a single mean triangle (Section 6.3.2), so the bending energy supplies a metric for diverse nonlinear changes in the vicinity of a single mean configuration of four or more landmarks. As the transformations are made up of a uniform part and a nonuniform part, we ultimately arrive at a composite metric that is **non-Archimedean**, an assemblage of two incommensurable portions. Certainly it does not much resemble the Procrustes form of Section 7.1. Changes between points closer together are weighted more sensitively than changes between landmarks farther apart, but only to the extent that the changes are not shared by the penumbra of points neighboring both; and if changes are shared affinely throughout the entire configuration of landmarks, there is no possible "localization," no bending term at all.

This separation of two incommensurate aspects of shape change, global and local, has already been diagrammed in Figure 7.5.1. It is the difference between the generators and the cross sections of the cylinder shown there. No "rotation" can get us from one set of directions to the other, can change bending energy from zero to something nonzero. Rather, one measures distances along the generators by one formula (net strain ratio, anisotropy) and distances within the cross sections by another formula (bending energy), with no exchanges possible. There is ample precedent for this sort of separation in mathematical physics. In Newtonian mechanics, for instance, space is measured in centimeters, and time is measured in seconds; and there is no possible rotation between the two. (Einstein changed this, of course, but the new version is much less relevant to biology!) This corresponds to an interpretation of Figure 7.5.1 with time along the generators and space laid out along cross sections. For the history of this idea, the so-called Galilean model, see Yaglom (1979).

For the subspace of uniform features of shape change, the appropriate metric is anisotropy, and the appropriate analogue to principal components has already been introduced in Sections 1.2, 5.3.3, and 6.5. The analogue for the complementary part of shape space, the nonuniform part, is introduced here. Because there is no useful single metric for all of shape space, there is no useful single set of "principal components" for a sample of shapes. Rather, components come in two incommensurate sets: one set of two for the uniform part, and another set of $2K - 6$ (twice the number of principal warps) for the nonuniform part. The description of shape change does not require that these aspects be separated (e.g., we could describe a change by a quadratic fit that combined linear and nonlinear terms). That choice is precluded for describing within-sample shape variation: I know of no alternative to the method described here. For an explanation of the unexpectedly subtle role of the thin-plate spline formulas in this decomposition, see Section 8.3.2.2.

7.6.1. Relative eigenvectors

7.6.1.1. The geometry of relative eigenvectors. —

The matrix-algebraic technique appropriate to this goal of decomposing within-group nonlinear shape variation is the technique of **relative eigenanalysis**. This is the same matrix algebra as pertains to ordinary principal components, but referring to a criterion of "reference length" different from the sphere $\Sigma a_i^2 = 1$ of the more familiar version. The matrix being decomposed is the same in either case – the variance-covariance matrix of the landmark coordinates – but it is referred to bending energy instead of to a reference of 1's down the diagonal.

Geometrically, the techniques of eigenanalysis and relative eigenanalysis differ only trivially. The relation of orthogonality that characterizes the eigenvectors that are ordinary principal components is actually a geometric constraint that can be expressed for ellipsoids as easily as for spheres. That the eigenvectors with respect to a sphere are orthogonal may be rephrased as follows: At the point of intersection of any eigendirection with the sphere, the tangent plane incorporates (is spanned by) all the other eigenvectors. Such a set of directions is referred to as **conjugate** with respect to the sphere. For the sphere, of course, tangent planes are normal to diameters; hence the interpretation as orthogonality. The principal components of an observed variance-covariance matrix are the sets of directions that are conjugate, in this sense, *both* upon the sphere and upon the ellipsoid representing the matrix. This set comprises the axes of the ellipsoid together with a set of orthogonal diameters of the sphere. The same set of edge directions give rise to a cube for the sphere, a brick for the variance-covariance matrix.

When the sphere is replaced by a more general ellipsoid, the concept of "orthogonality" is replaced by the *same* notion of conjugacy already applying to the variance-covariance ellipsoid. In two dimensions the generalization to **simultaneous diagonalization of two quadratic forms** – we have seen this twice before, in Sections 6.4.2 and 7.4.2 – is as shown in Figure 7.6.1. We seek a pair of directions that form a conjugate set in respect of both ellipses. *In both forms,* each direction must lie parallel to the tangent to the ellipse at the point of piercing by the other. (This criterion replaces that of "starting and ending at 90°" for the case of one ellipse a circle.) If one ellipse is a circle, the construction reduces to the ordinary extraction of principal axes of the other. Because affine transformations preserve tangency and parallelism, they preserve the relation of conjugacy among directions. Then all sets of conjugate directions upon an ellipse are produced by affine transformation of sets of perpendiculars (themselves conjugate directions) upon a circle. Hence the algorithm in Figure 7.6.1c.

For the application to high dimensions, this results in the most direct algorithm for simultaneous diagonalization of two quadratic forms $\mathbf{E}_1, \mathbf{E}_2$: Transform one ellipsoid $\mathbf{E}_1$ into a circle by a change

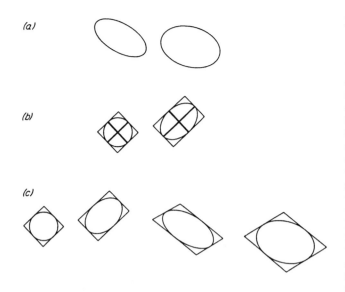

Figure 7.6.1. Sketch of relative eigenanalysis for an arbitrary pair of ellipses. (*a*) General case (two ellipses). (*b*) One ellipse a circle (principal-component analysis). (*c*) Algorithm for the general case: Reduce one ellipse to a circle by affine transformation; find the axes of the other after the same transformation; undo the transformation. In the application to principal warps, the ellipse on the left in each pair will represent bending energy, and that on the right, sample covariance. All analysis will be in the space of the warps only, without any affine components. (For instance, for the case of four landmarks, these have only two dimensions, i.e., they really *are* ellipses.)

of basis $\mathbf{A}_1$ (computed by way of its own principal axes); transform the other ellipsoid $\mathbf{E}_2$ by this same change of basis $\mathbf{A}_1$; compute the ordinary principal axes of the transformed second ellipsoid, together with the corresponding diameters of the circle that was $\mathbf{E}_1$; and then apply the inverse $\mathbf{A}_1^{-1}$ to both sets of axes, so that these directions can be reported in the original coordinate system. The **relative eigenvalues** of such a set of directions upon the ellipsoid $\mathbf{E}_2$ (in this case, that representing the observed variance-covariance matrix of a group of landmark configurations) are the same as the *actual* eigenvalues of the axes upon the ellipsoid in Figure 7.6.1*b*; as they are the ratios of lengths in corresponding directions between the two ellipsoids, they are left unchanged by all affine transformations.

7.6.1.2. Interpretation. —

When $\mathbf{E}_2$ is the covariance matrix of landmark locations and $\mathbf{E}_1$ is bending energy, the interpretation of these relative eigenvectors parallels what one is used to for principal components. If we restrict our attention to cross sections of the cylinder in Figure 7.5.1, we are dealing with two finite ellipsoids. The largest component of within-group shape variation, corresponding to the largest relative eigenvalue (ratio of sample variance to bending energy), is the nonlinear shape feature of largest "energy-specific variance." Geometrically, this is the diameter of the cylinder that is the smallest multiple of the corresponding diameter of the covariance ellipsoid. Ordinarily it will represent a bending-energy form of *small* intrinsic energy, hence a most global feature of shape variability, exactly as we would wish. Usually this "relatively least

343

bent variance" approximates some square-to-kite variation spanning landmarks all across the configuration. In that case it will have an effective "direction," like the vectors generating the partial warps of Figure 7.3.6. The *next* relative eigenvector is the direction of shape variability having greatest relative variance among all those that are energy-orthogonal to the first: all those for which the energy of the sum with the first component is the sum of the energies. The third has the largest relative variance subject to energy orthogonality to the first two; and so forth. The later components tend to be at smaller physical scale, as they represent aspects of shape variation that, other things being equal, tap energy modes of higher intrinsic bending.

Thus far we have treated the variation of one shape coordinate, ν_1 or ν_2, at a time. But there are two Cartesian coordinates involved in shape space, and although the bending-energy formalism L_K^{-1} is uncoupled (*x*- and *y*-shape coordinates bend separately), observed changes of shape coordinates may certainly be *correlated*. What we mean by bending energy is really the $(2K - 6) \times (2K - 6)$ matrix that has the bending-energy matrix *twice* down its diagonal, and zeros elsewhere. The relative eigenvectors, which I have called **relative warps**, will now tap correlated aspects of change in *both* shape coordinates and will exploit their correlation to decrease the relative bending energy of the succession of relative eigenvectors. Then the first two of these might both be square-to-kite transformations, in directions at about 90°; or they might include substantial fractions of more local principal warps as well (cf. MacLeod and Kitchell, 1990).

Each component so extracted is a purely nonlinear transformation with features of its own – inconsistent linear tendencies in different regions of the form, quadratic gradients, whatever. It may be visualized, just as factors were visualized for triangles, by the effect of its coefficients on one single set of shape coordinates. Because the essence of these features is localization, however, we do better to draw them out as displacements at each landmark in the original coordinate system. Like the corresponding picture for the principal warps (Section 7.5.3.1), these figures are automatically at the optimal affine-Procrustes superposition, up to scale: They are normalized for translation, shear, and rotation. When each ν is regressed on the component by a simple regression, its regression coefficient is given by the corresponding coefficient of the relative eigenvector. We draw out the component as the shape difference between the mean form and the form predicted at a conveniently *low* or *high* value of the component. In this way the component is interpreted as a deformation in its own right, so that the "features" reviewed elsewhere in this chapter may be applied, as it were, recursively.

Relative warps are like partial warps in attributing a little segment of relative displacement to each landmark separately. They may be thought of as principal components of the set of all partial warps for a whole sample of forms as each is derived by deformation from the mean shape. (In this "equivalent" principal-component analysis, each partial warp must first be scaled by the inverse of its energy, not its geometrical length.) The relative warps differ from the partial warps, however, in that the little displacements are not in general parallel – no single vector multiple of a scalar bent plate is, in general, sufficient to describe them. Also, whereas a partial warp is part of the relation between a particular pair of forms, and thus has a particular magnitude, a relative warp is only a pattern of proportionality among directed landmark displacements; to characterize a transformation requires a scale (a "score") as well (cf. Figure 7.6.3d or 7.6.4b).

Relative warps supply a useful description of patterns of changes correlated all across the form. But if instead the null model of Chapter 5 applies – landmark locations distributed around their means by i.i.d. circular variation – then the matrix $\mathbf{E}_2$ of the text is approximately a multiple of the identity, and the eigenanalysis results simply in the eigenanlysis of $\mathbf{E}_1$, the bending energy, with the usual principal warps now emerging in reverse order. The first two relative warps would then represent the principal warp of largest scale, multiplied by an arbitrary pair of orthogonal 2-vectors, and both relative eigenvalues, up to sample variance, would represent the reciprocal of the eigenvalue of that last principal warp. The next two relative warps similarly would be an arbitrarily rotated pair of vector multiples of the next-to-last principal warp, and so on. Deviations of relative warps from this pattern represent deviation of the data from the null model. I have no statistical tests of this deviation to offer at this time; their development is overdue.

7.6.1.3. Scale dependence of bending energy. —

As we have seen (Section 2.2), the bending energy of any thin-plate spline, such as the relative eigenvectors here, is an inverse-squared function of geometric scale. Any deformation of a configuration of landmarks has just four times as much bending energy as the same displacements applied to the same configuration scaled up by a factor of 2. The relative eigenvalue corresponding to a sample relative eigenvector thus scales *directly* as the square of physical scale: The smaller it is, the smaller-squared a fraction it is of the bending energy appropriate to that scale.

But the cardinality (available count) of warps at smaller scale increases, too, as approximately the inverse square of the physical scale. (Compare Figures 7.3.5 and 7.5.5: There were four times as many principal warps covering a set of quadrilaterals each about half the size of the whole configuration.) These two scale factors cancel: To a good approximation, the total "magnitude" available for features of within-group variation represents the same amount of "potential relative bending energy" at every physical scale. This is the morphometric equivalent of the "improper flat prior" dear to every Bayesian statistician at the beginning of an analysis of more ordinary spaces of variables. The word "improper" here, of course, is not intended to disparage.

Such a uniformity seems sensible in morphometrics as well. Systematic and other biologists are accustomed to finding discriminatory features at nearly any physical scale of observation, from overall shape down through small details of minuscule regions of forms. In the representation of variation or difference by sums of principal warps, the magnitude of the "net information" available at any scale of feature extraction is approximately constant, corresponding to the biologist's flat prior much as it does to the statistician's.

In another phrasing, intended to be highly suggestive, the formalism here declares that bending energy may be expected to behave as a **fractal** (Mandelbrot, 1982). The total amount of this energy increases indefinitely as the scale of observation decreases. The fractal character of shape change could be studied efficiently by considering hundreds of homologous points changing position over time. These would then be not named landmarks but sheets of cells identified by pigmentation patterns or particles of adherent carbon black followed over periods of rapid embryonic growth. Pursuit of this aspect of growth modeling is, however, beyond the scope of this book.

7.6.2. Algorithm

The computation of the relative warps proceeds in eight steps. Let there be K landmarks.

1. Select a suitable pair of landmarks to serve as baseline, and compute the sample means of the shape coordinates of the other landmarks to this baseline.

2. Compute the $K - 3$ nontrivial principal warps corresponding to the configuration of mean landmark locations. As explained in the preceding section, this is by eigenanalysis of the bending-energy matrix L_K^{-1}, which is K by K, with respect to the identity matrix (representing Procrustes distance ρ in the subspace of affine-free transformations).

3. Scale each principal warp as a deformation to have bending energy 1. (That is, divide its formula through by the square root of the corresponding eigenvalue.)

4. Construct a basis of $2K - 6$ dimensions for the nonlinear part of shape space as the Cartesian sum of $K - 3$ two-dimensional subspaces, one for each principal warp. The subspaces can be spanned by using the coefficients of the scaled warps to multiply first all the x-coordinates ν_1 of shape, and then all the y-coordinates ν_2. These are the "circular sections" of the cylinder in Figure 7.5.1.

5. Compute the variance-covariance matrix Σ of the original coordinates (*not* the shape coordinates) in any convenient alignment, such as is typically used for conscientious digitizing. Baselines should *not* be scaled; if scaling is required, it should be by Centroid Size.

6. Using the covariance matrix from step 5, compute the covariance matrix, $2K - 6$ by $2K - 6$, of the $2K - 6$ linear combinations, spanning the subspace of nonlinear shape variability, erected in step 4.

7. Extract the conventional principal components of this covariance matrix. (The computation, like all the other eigenanalyses in this book, must be "unscaled," referring to covariances, not correlations.) These principal components are the **relative warps** of the data with respect to bending energy.

8. The eigenanalysis yields expressions of the relative warps to the basis from step 6, consisting of the principal warps for x- and y-shape-coordinate subspaces separately (that is, the relative warps have been expressed in terms of their own partial warps). These should be reexpressed in the original coordinate system as vectors of displacement at the mean positions of each of the original K landmarks or at the corresponding mean shape coordinates (including baseline points). In that form, these patterns of displacement are automatically at optimal Procrustes superposition in respect of position, orientation, and shear. That is, the transformations indicated have no affine part.

Why does this work? The dimensions of shape space we are extracting here annihilate (zero-out) translations, and so we can deal with uncentered data, which yield the correct configuration of landmark means in any case. Because rotations are also linear transformations, they too are annihilated by the principal warps to a sufficient degree of precision in the vicinity of any consistent alignment, such as is supplied by an unscaled baseline orientation (cf. Appendix A.4.5). Whether or not Centroid Size is adjusted out of the data affects only the relative weights of specimens in the principal-component analysis at step 7. If specimens vary widely in size, they might be standardized before analysis; if they do not vary widely, the effect of not standardizing is hardly detectable.

A program computing the relative warps by this algorithm is included in the disk pack associated with Rohlf and Bookstein (1990). As of this writing, Rohlf has just released an improved implementation (TPSRW) that is considerably easier to use.

7.6.3. Example: rat calvaria

I exemplify these computations using the youngest rats from Appendix A.4.5 (Figure 7.6.2). The principal warps of their mean configuration have bending energies of 8.34, 6.17, 3.31, 1.40, and 1.08; the first two are most local, the last two most global. The

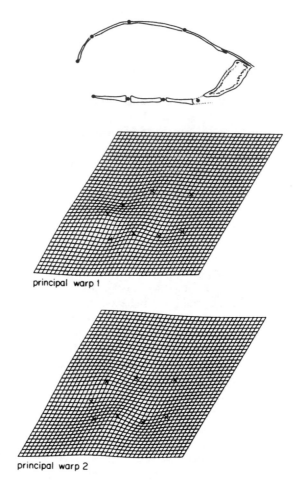

principal warp 1

principal warp 2

Figure 7.6.2. Principal warps of the mean landmark configuration for 21 male rats aged 7 days.

principal components of covariance corresponding to the normalized principal warps for abscissa and ordinate have relative eigenvalues $0.000147, 0.000091, 0.000037, \ldots$. These are not the same numbers reported in Bookstein (1989*b*); those were mistakenly computed with baseline landmarks fixed.

The two dominant relative warps are diagrammed in Figure 7.6.3 (where they are scaled rather arbitrarily, I am afraid). They are both closely aligned with the last principal warp, the largest-scale geometric aspect of nonlinearity for these landmarks. [That is, the last principal warp account for the bulk of the first *two* relative warps. Compare Figure 7.3.6*a* to the effect of going from the X's in Figure 7.6.3*a* or 7.6.3*b* to a form having its landmarks at the ends of the segments shown.] Here, as usual, that warp is just another version of the familiar square-to-kite transformation. Its vectors of loadings for the dominant pair of relative warps (step 7 of the algorithm) are $(0.87, 0.36)$ and $(-0.44, 0.79)$, far larger than for any of the other principal warps and nearly at 90° themselves.

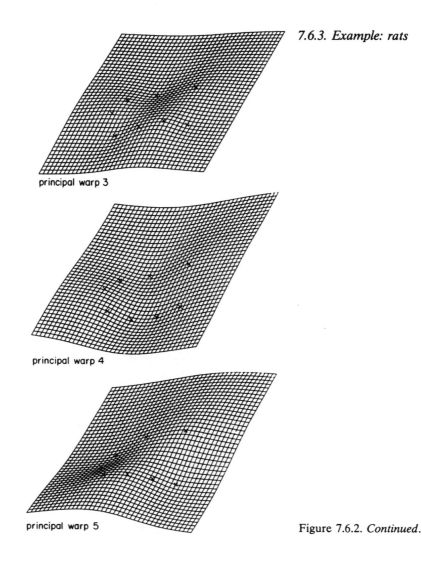

principal warp 3

principal warp 4

principal warp 5

Figure 7.6.2. *Continued.*

The first of these represents a generalized lengthening of upper cranial structures with respect to the lower border (the cranial base), one of the diagrammatic forms of the pure nonlinearity introduced in Section 7.3. In accord with Moss's functional-matrix hypothesis, this process would appear to represent biological variability of net neural mass independent of the size of the sphenoidal bone underlying that growing mass. The second relative warp, explaining about two-thirds as much scaled bending energy as the first, represents a relative rotation of the cranial vault about the cranial base. It approximates a different multiple of the last principal warp, perpendicular to the first as a vector. In this orientation it would be interpreted as a relative tilting of the vault with respect to the cranial base. Features of bending at

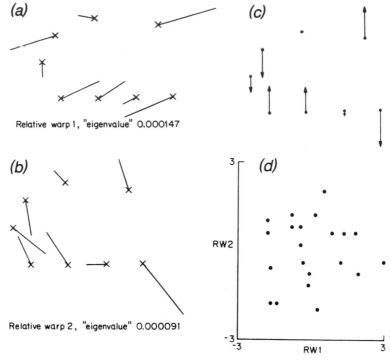

Relative warp 1, "eigenvalue" 0.000147

Relative warp 2, "eigenvalue" 0.000091

Figure 7.6.3. Within-group components of affine-free shape variation for 7-day-old rats. (*a, b*) The first two relative warps at the Procrustes superposition (step 8 of the algorithm of Section 7.6.2). (*c*) The largest-scale principal warp of the bending-energy matrix (algorithm steps 2 and 3) in the same format. The first two relative warps here are both predominantly 2-vector multiples of this one principal warp. (*d*) Sample scatter of relative warps 1 and 2 for 21 rats.

smaller geometric scale, such as of the vault or the cranial base separately, are not observed to bear any sample variance.

The ratio of the first two relative eigenvalues here, 147:91, is consistent with the origin of this pair in random spinning of multiples of the last principal warp, the finding under the null model as explained at the end of Section 7.6.1.2. Nevertheless, this relative warp is *not* "null." For instance, it is aligned with the nonlinear part of the mean change from age 7 to age 14 for these

Table 7.6.1. *Loadings of first two relative warps, 8 landmarks, 21 rats, 8 ages (see Figure 7.6.4a)*

Landmark	Component 1 (0.001995)		Component 2 (0.000065)	
	ν_1	ν_2	ν_1	ν_2
Basion	0.275	0.076	−0.023	0.129
Opisthion	−0.143	−0.121	0.203	−0.237
IPS	−0.318	−0.168	0.125	−0.243
Lambda	−0.039	0.092	−0.100	0.111
Bregma	0.426	0.130	−0.130	0.248
SES	−0.355	−0.215	0.330	−0.405
ISS	−0.092	0.016	−0.124	0.065
SOS	0.246	0.190	−0.280	0.332

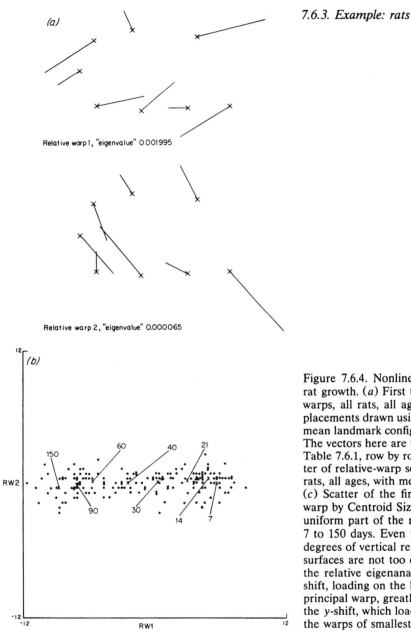

(a)

Relative warp 1, "eigenvalue" 0.001995

Relative warp 2, "eigenvalue" 0.000065

(b)

Figure 7.6.4. Nonlinear part of rat growth. (*a*) First two relative warps, all rats, all ages, as displacements drawn using the grand mean landmark configuration. The vectors here are those of Table 7.6.1, row by row. (*b*) Scatter of relative-warp scores for all rats, all ages, with means by age. (*c*) Scatter of the first relative warp by Centroid Size. (*d*) Nonuniform part of the net change, 7 to 150 days. Even though the degrees of vertical relief of these surfaces are not too different, in the relative eigenanalysis the *x*-shift, loading on the largest-scale principal warp, greatly dominates the *y*-shift, which loads mainly on the warps of smallest scale.

data, and so it may serve as a factor for "timing" (cf. Figures 7.6.3*a* and 7.3.7*d*).

When this analysis is repeated for the full sample of 164 rats having complete data, the relative eigenvalues emerge as 0.001995, 0.000065, 0.000051, ... The first two relative warps are listed in Table 7.6.1 and are diagrammed in Figure 7.6.4*a*. Scores and their means by age are displayed in Figure 7.6.4*b*. These two relative warps are nearly the same as those we extracted in Figure

351

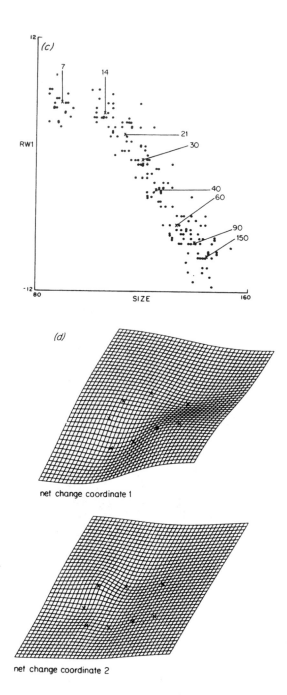

Figure 7.6.4. *Continued.*

net change coordinate 1

net change coordinate 2

7.6.3 for the youngest age group alone. But their shares of bending-specific variance have changed drastically. The first (relative lengthening or shortening of the vault) now explains 13 times as much variance as formerly; the second (tilt of the vault) has, if anything, less leverage than before. The first shows a strong age-related trend, whereas the second just drifts. We saw evidence

352

of this trend in the change from the 7-day mean form to the 14-day mean in Section 7.3.3.1. We see it as well in Figure 7.6.4*d*, where the large-scale bending appears to be restricted nearly to the *x*-direction. This relative-warp analysis is clearly significant (i.e., the first two relative eigenvalues, in a ratio of 30:1, are clearly distinct) over the full age range. Because the first relative warp of the analysis of the 7-day-old sample alone (Figure 7.6.3) is the same, we have another reason to consider it meaningful in spite of its apparent consistency with the null model when studied in isolation.

7.6.4. Juxtaposing the linear part

Recall that the bending-energy matrix is of deficient rank. Three of its eigenvectors are of zero eigenvalue: those corresponding to shifts of the Cartesian coordinates of the landmark by terms that are linear in the coordinates of the mean landmark positions. These directions would appear in the relative eigenanalysis, had they not been intentionally nullified, as directions having zero length with respect to the bending-energy matrix but having positive length (variance) with respect to the actual covariance matrix of the shape coordinates. We already know how to extract this uniform part of the shape variation in factor form; a convenient estimate was introduced in Section 7.2.3.

By combining this uniform factor with the relative warps, we arrive at a composite analysis accounting for all the large-scale features of a distribution in shape space. Within-group shape variation is a composite of two sorts of components (Bookstein, 1990*e*). One part comprises the first few relative warps of the sample variance-covariance matrix with respect to bending energy. The other is a single vector of length 2 estimating the uniform factor for shape difference about the mean. The linear factor may covary with any or all of the nonlinear components, and both may covary with size.

7.6.4.1. Example: Vilmann's rats, last computations. —

As a final example, consider now all the shape information for the 21 rats at eight ages; this is the combination of Figures 7.6.4*c* and 7.6.5*a*. Analysis of this same data set by conventional multivariate methods (Section 4.2.3) found three ordinary principal components that could be interpreted as one dimension of nonlinear allometry; but we were not able to describe what processes were unfolding over that dimension. In Section 7.4.3.2 we extracted a quadratic component of this same change, from 7 days to 150, without reference to intermediate forms – but surely no one would assert that growth over that interval is temporally homogeneous. We have now a complete analysis of all the data exactly parallel-ing the factor analysis of all possible distances but residing in the shape space of 12 shape coordinates instead of the unnecessarily extended space of 28 distances. As these analyses are of exactly the same data, we ought to be able to report the same phenomena by inspection of covariances among the descriptions of the full sample of 164 forms in the various feature subspaces of the data set out in this chapter. The combination of the arch of Figure 7.6.5*a* and the horizontal trend in Figure 7.6.4*d* yields the summary model of Figure 7.6.7, "accounting" for most of the features in Figure 7.6.6 and thus for all the panels of Figure 4.2.2. The

Figure 7.6.5. Estimated uniform components for Vilmann's rats (using the grand mean shape, Figure 7.6.4*a*) to a Basion–Bregma baseline (Section 7.2.3). (*a*) Scatter at all ages, with means by age. (*b*) Scatter of the first uniform coordinate by relative warp 1. (*c*) First principal component of the uniform factor (here, horizontal, representing shear along the Basion–Bregma direction), scattered against Centroid Size.

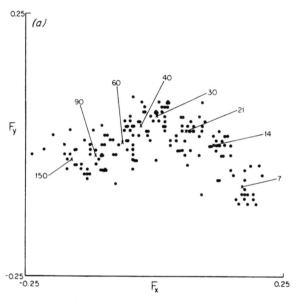

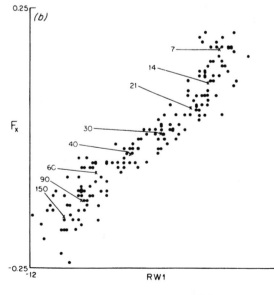

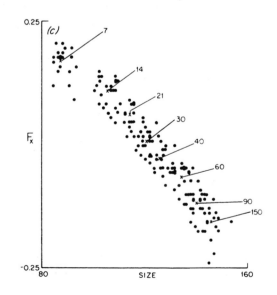

meaning of all these coefficients and components is plainly visible in the mixed parabolic-cubic arching of the paths of means in Figure 7.6.6. In my view, it is the pattern of deviation of these curves from linearity and parallelism, not the regression lines of Figure 4.2.2, that best describes both global and regional aspects of "timing" in this growth process. The vault rolls first backward, then forward, relative to the cranial base, all the while steadily reducing its relative scale in spatially graded fashion.

We can usefully summarize the growth of these rat skulls by reference to periods in which all three of these descriptors (size, the dominant horizontal component of the uniform factor, and the first relative warp) are mutually linear. These periods certainly include the age range from 30 through 150 days, the last five means in Figure 7.6.6. From age 7 days to 14 days, the uniform change lies well off this dominant allometry: This is the time of growth of the cerebrum, which drives the uniform change in a different direction, already analyzed in Section 7.2.5. The change in relative warp 1 over this period, however, is in the same allometry that will continue to apply. In fact, the pure inhomogeneity we identified for this earliest period in Section 7.3.3.1 seems to be an invariable part of growth between any pair of ages.

There is a suggestion in Figure 7.6.5b that the cerebral forcing function applying to the uniform component persists, decaying, through age about 30 days. We can summarize this entire period of growth, then, in two "stages." The earliest is dominated by cerebral growth having principal directions at 45° to the cranial base. This is smoothly replaced by a superposition of processes

7.6.4. Linear term

Figure 7.6.6. Mean shape trajectories, 21 rats, eight ages, to the Basion–SES baseline. Horizontal at bottom: Baseline. Vaults at top: Mean changes at each age, connected from IPS forward to Bregma. "Vertical" lines: Trajectories of single mean shape-coordinate pairs, ages 7 through 150 days. Squiggles under baseline: The same for SES and ISS (illegible).

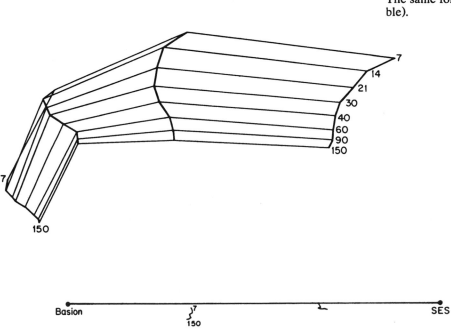

355

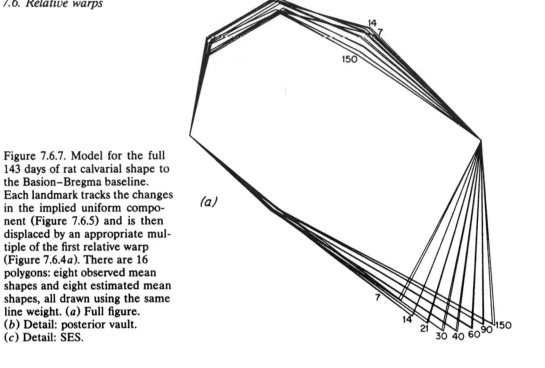

Figure 7.6.7. Model for the full 143 days of rat calvarial shape to the Basion–Bregma baseline. Each landmark tracks the changes in the implied uniform component (Figure 7.6.5) and is then displaced by an appropriate multiple of the first relative warp (Figure 7.6.4a). There are 16 polygons: eight observed mean shapes and eight estimated mean shapes, all drawn using the same line weight. (a) Full figure. (b) Detail: posterior vault. (c) Detail: SES.

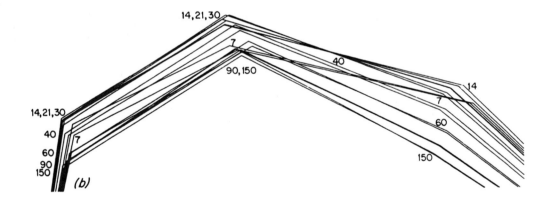

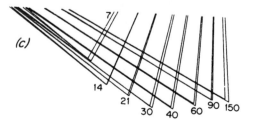

356

that run jointly to the end of the growth period: a continuing uniform change, now with principal axes at 48° counterclockwise and 42° clockwise of the direction Basion–Bregma, and a constant extension along the first relative warp – the relative lengthening of the cranial base vis-à-vis the vault in the horizontal direction. The fit of modeled to observed mean forms is adequate (Figure 7.6.7). Note especially the match between model and data in handling the exceptional behavior of the 7–14 change from landmark to landmark.

For another example of this study of many feature subspaces at the same time, see Tabachnick and Bookstein (1990b). Another example of the use of relative warps, this time in connection with size allometry, is presented in MacLeod and Kitchell (1990). The two incommensurate metrics of these analyses, anisotropy and bending energy, can be combined artificially by an arbitrary multiplier to produce "relaxations" compromising between different sources of information for image-processing applications (Bookstein, 1990a).

7.6.4. Linear term

8

Retrospect and prospect

Chapter 1 set out four principles that I claimed would underlie all the tools and tactics of this treatise. By now, many exhaustively worked examples later, those principles have been fairly thoroughly exploited. In these closing comments I would like to remind the faithful reader of what has been covered so far, but mainly I want to touch on what this tool kit has produced – what seems to me to be temporary scaffolding, and what I believe to be built in stone, to last. Though I am proud of the masonry, it is the scaffolding that interests me most. Its struts and lacework jump across many conceptual gaps in the metrological discipline laid out here. Behind the façade lie many open questions at the joint frontier of algebra and mathematical biology for these techniques. As Chapter 3 emphasized, the locations of landmarks are conveniences for the attachment of biological explanations to form. Different explanations leave their traces in form in different ways; our statistical algebra and geometry must be free to adapt appropriately.

8.1. FIRST PRINCIPLE: LANDMARK LOCATIONS

8.1.1. Routine procedures

The first step in any landmark-based morphometric analysis is to collect well-placed landmarks (Chapter 3). As a configuration, they must encompass the trace in tissue of the biomechanical or other determinants of form the covariances of which are to be unearthed by the morphometric analysis. They should provide reasonably even coverage of the form; they should appear to correspond both geometrically and biologically from specimen to specimen; and they should be of Type 1 (discrete juxtapositions of tissues) in preference to Type 2 (extrema of curvature), and of Type 2 in preference to Type 3 (extrema of single coordinates), whenever feasible. Landmarks should be collected carefully and conscientiously, guided by an explicit table of operational definitions. Examples according with this discipline are rapidly increasing in number – not only those in this volume and in Rohlf and Bookstein (1990), but many more currently in preparation, in manuscripts and theses, for both rigid structures (mammalian skulls and scapulae, shark teeth, etc.) and flexible structures (e.g., the wings of rays).

8.1.2. Open questions

The preceding paragraph mainly advises imitation: If your problem looks like one of mine, then do as I do. The fundamental "open questions," then, have to do with other sorts of problems than more or less clearly defined point locations on rigid, biomechanically constrained organs.

8.1.2.1. Vagueness of homology. —

Landmarks can be "missing" in two ways. In one sense (excluded from the examples in this volume, by deletion of cases as necessary) their locations are unobservable in occasional specimens owing to patternless defects of development, breakage of parts, or blurring of the image from which they are digitized. Data missing for such capricious reasons may be estimated case by case according to regression upon the rest of the landmark locations, or they might simply be "splined in" from the average shape.

But other problems with missing landmarks are topological, and more stubborn. As pointed out in Chapter 5 of Bookstein et al. (1985), the appearance or disappearance of landmarks, or their identifiability, may itself be information. Sometimes landmarks merge or split; sometimes extrema of curvature are annihilated as an S-curve straightens or one bulge engulfs another; sometimes there is genuine ambiguity regarding which point of one structure corresponds to a clearly characterizable landmark of a closely, even ontogenetically related form. Beyond these logical problems, there are algebraic problems whenever landmarks "almost" violate the deformation model. All the geometric techniques have trouble with landmark pairs at distances having too high a coefficient of variation, as when, for instance, all interlandmark distances change by ratios between 0.5 and 1.5, except for distances to one landmark, which quintuple. With shape changes so extreme, regressions may curve, the splines may fold, the principal warps become unstable, and all the linear approximations of Chapters 5 through 7 tend to become unreliable. We need "robustification" of the landmark methods in all these aspects.

Landmarks represent some kinds of form in very inconvenient ways. On the surface of the human neural cortex, for instance, homology goes according to the homunculus (the part of the larger organism projecting to that cortical column). Unfortunately, that information cannot be read in the cortical anatomy per se. Of the demarcations between gyri of the normal cortical surface, most are accidents of intracranial folding during embryogenesis; only a few are of value for a neurometric "endophrenology." At about as great a phenetic distance from this example as one can get is the general problem of plants. The entire botanical kingdom seems characterized by a variability of form that, though topologically well controlled, appears to frustrate any scheme of well-defined points in a well-characterized graph of adjacencies. Whereas the function and form of many animal organs are tightly associated, so that selection on function bears implications for the expected form, in plants form and function are much more likely to be decoupled, especially for leaves, so that hardly anything about life history can be expected to constrain form to any linear subspace of shape. A similar problem applies to attempts at extending the concept of a landmark to a form that is a bag of organs (protists, larvae, etc.). A different sort of problem with the notion of landmark arises in structures that are intrinsically multiple: landmarks in organisms with rotational symmetry, for instance. In colonial organisms, some landmarks lie upon two specimens at the same time: How does one construct a feature space for such patterns?

8.1.2.2. Differential landmarks.—

In many of these "difficult" cases, collectively of far more interest than landmark-rich forms like the mammalian skull, differential geometry sometimes supplies pseudolandmarks expressing patterns in the curving of the form in the absence of any legible information regarding homology. We have already reviewed the role of the symmetric axis in supplying centers of curvature at extrema of curvature of two-dimensional outlines and in locating plausible candidates for the "branch points" of forms with lobes. But texts of differential geometry usually dismiss the two-dimensional case in one short chapter. In two dimensions, the only local descriptor is curvature or its reciprocal, which can generate only two kinds of privileged points (vertices, which are extremes of curvature, and inflections, which are zeros of curvature). Aside from these, and points of the symmetric axis (aspects of curvature averaged "across" the form), there is not much differential geometry to exploit for plane outlines.

The prospect is more favorable for enriching the punctate language in three dimensions. The classic differential geometry of surfaces is an elegant branch of nineteenth-century mathematics the implications of which are familiar to anyone who has seen the reflection of sunlight in a circular bowl of water. In contrast to two-dimensional biological form, three-dimensional form may suggest a richness of local and regional geometric descriptors that

360

often matches our intuitive sense of how biological forms are usefully compared. In three dimensions, landmarks arise not only as points having characteristic curvature properties (tips of structures, "depths of saddles" like the bridge of the nose) but also as the touching points of *lines* with optimal properties – "asymptotic lines" around which the surface can roll, parabolic lines across which the surface changes from convex to concave. Other types of loci, likewise recognizable by eye, are defined by peculiarities of higher-order fits, such as the "ruffles" and "gutter points" drawn by Koenderink (1990) where osculating cylinders or cones have special properties; and there are many other distinctive differential species. Bookstein and Cutting (1988) suggested one experimental invocation of differential geometry that would extract "ridge curves," loci locally edgelike (the line of the jaw, the lip commissure, the orbital rim), then search for new point landmarks upon these substructures.

The factor limiting the study of curving form via landmarks is not the need to express the curving in punctate form – we have already seen how the symmetric axis creates new points to record features of the large-scale assembly of parts – but the need to discern a quantitative descriptor of the surface for which the extreme point reliably exists and actually tracks the intended effects upon the form. After speculating in the abstract on these matters, I often turn to an old volume of artistic advice by Wolchonok (1959). In the quantitative descriptive systems suggested by Wolchonok's figures can be found equivalents of most of the classic terminology of comparative anatomy. For the next edition of this book, surely some of these will have been converted to pseudolandmark points specifying reliable aspects of surface bending. We shall thereby have examples of covariances involving the shapes of foreheads, cheekbones, breasts, and heartbeats in humans, and their analogues for a great variety of functional and evolutionary investigations in other species.

8.2. SECOND PRINCIPLE: SHAPE COORDINATES

8.2.1. Routine procedures

Chapter 5 has shown how the scheme of *shape coordinates* – reduction of landmark configurations to sets of triangular shapes represented by single two-dimensional points – supports all the conventional tests and descriptive purposes of biometrics as applied to samples of landmark configurations. Ordinarily one selects a single baseline – an axis of symmetry, a long diameter connecting relatively reliable endpoints, a biomechanical strut – to which all the other landmarks are referred. The first steps in any analysis, after the shape-coordinate pairs are actually computed, are explicitly concerned with these coordinates. Pair by pair, their

361

sample scatters are to be inspected for outliers, for elliptical evidence of factors requiring interpretation, for ordination or overlap of a priori groupings, and so on. Often one can understand most of the regularity of one's landmark data without procedures any more multivariate than these bivariate plots and their enhancements by information on size or group. For shape data of modest range, such as are typified by the examples of this volume, the statistics of the joint distribution of the shape coordinates or their descriptive features are nearly invariant to choice of this baseline.

The mathematical statisticians who have attended to this problem agree that there is one unique statistical space for the analysis of large samples of landmark location data (cf. Goodall, 1991, and the discussion following it) and that the shape coordinates span that space. No technique can be more efficient at detecting shape changes of unspecified (i.e., geometrically unrestricted) structure than analysis of the shape coordinates. Some techniques, such as Goodall's (1991) generalized Procrustes approach or the maximum-likelihood procedure of Mardia and Dryden (1989b), are equivalent to this analysis; but within this group the shape coordinates seem to have the simplest algebra and graphics. Many other techniques (some of them unfortunately fashionable), from finite-element techniques through "Euclidean distance matrix analysis" to the conventional schemes of ad hoc distances and angles, are demonstrably less efficient and should be abandoned except for the diagramming of particular interpretations of morphometric findings after analysis is completed. All this is a matter of theorems (Bookstein, 1989a; Chapter 5 of this volume), no longer even worth arguing about.

Within the family of fully efficient analyses, it is the main advantage of the shape coordinates that they supply convenient access to the many a priori subspaces of features. For instance, the linear component, fitted in the Procrustes family of computations (cf. Rohlf and Slice, 1990) as a nuisance parameter, is displayed here as a single composite shape coordinate (Section 7.2) corresponding to a regression or factor estimate; its sample statistics are thereby much more clearly visualized. Whether or not viewed by shape coordinates, the important subspaces of the shared shape space are inaccessible to the conventional multivariate techniques, which involve no metric beyond that of the covariance matrix. Then whenever landmark locations are available there is good reason not to reduce one's data to distance measures prior to their statistical analysis. Compare the complete analysis of the growth of the rat skulls by analysis of multiple distances (Section 4.2) with analysis of exactly the same information by landmark-specific procedures (Section 7.6). The landmark procedures, *because they have recourse to the information about the mean form and the subspaces it determines*, produce a much greater variety of alternate views of these ontogenies, and much more clearly separate them into interpretable features and stages.

8.2.2. Open questions

The representation by shape coordinates of the shape space held in common among my implementation, Goodall's, and Kendall's is likely to be a permanent fixture of morphometric praxis. In the metaphor opening this chapter, it is part of the masonry, not the scaffolding. Yet, at root, the construction of shape coordinates, a matter of complex affine ratios, is remarkably elementary; as stonework, it is rather rude. The advances to come, though potentially numerous, are likely to be quite a bit more technical. There is room for improvement in our understanding of the exact distribution of the shape coordinates for data more complicated than triangles and in suitable models for their global covariance structure. The probability model of Chapter 5, for instance, implies a covariance matrix among shape coordinates to be expected if all landmark coordinates are distributed independently and identically around their means. This pattern is hardly ever seen in data. Can the bending-energy form of the thin-plate spline (Section 7.5) be developed into a more realistic alternative to this "null model"?

There is also considerable work to be done in the graphics of the three-dimensional extension. A proper scheme of shape coordinates for three dimensions augments the two-dimensional complex number by three more parameters, one additional point in space (e.g., in the lower-triangular representation of Goodall, 1991). The scheme I suggested in Section 5.4 for purposes of visualizing covariances of three-dimensional shape uses eight coordinates per tetrahedron: a considerable degree of redundancy. We need schemes for visualizing the variability of tetrahedra in order to erect the three-dimensional equivalents of the figures of Section 5.4. The simplest probability model for landmark locations in two dimensions yields a circle in shape coordinates; a diagram is needed for presenting the tetrahedral case with an equivalent degree of symmetry. I do not know how to do this, either for the Procrustes metric or for an anisotropy metric.

8.3. THIRD PRINCIPLE: THE FORM OF QUESTIONS

8.3.1. Routine procedures

The routine procedure for biometrical investigations recommended throughout Chapters 5 and 6 and the first half of Chapter 7 is to apply appropriate conventional linear statistical machinery

8.3.1. Procedures

within the vector space of shape coordinates taken to any convenient baseline. Centroid Size plays the role of an exogenous covariate in these analyses. The shape coordinates support unambiguous tests for group mean differences in shape, for correlations of shape with size or with aspects of function or environment exogenous to the landmark data, for the statistically significant presence of particular features in the analysis of shape, and for the correlation of shape *with* shape, as when one form is predicted by its own earlier observation. In all this the shape coordinates support not only the usual questions about "significance" on various more or less unrealistic null models of covariances of shape with group, size, or other factors but also a specialized series of questions about features peculiar to morphometric data. Section 7.2, for instance, shows how to ask whether there is a "linear component" to a particular comparison of shapes, and whether within the noise of the residuals there is a "nonlinear component" as well. Section 7.4 demonstrates machinery for inquiring whether there is a statistically significant Huxleyan growth gradient, a rigid motion relating two samples of otherwise identical assemblages of two parts, a "growth center" from which most landmarks are displaced radially, and the like.

These questions deal either with the existence of unspecified differences in mean location or predicted locations in shape space or with the specification of those differences in terms of features that are functions of the mean form alone. Still more specialized landmark statistical machinery supports another set of questions regarding the morphometric equivalent of principal components, factors, and similar summaries of sample variation: questions that invoke a *geometric* metric as well as a statistical one. It is the presence of this a priori spatial ordering of the data alongside the empirical ordering via a covariance matrix that most clearly distinguishes morphometrics from other biological applications of multivariate analysis. The statistically equivalent approaches to shape space that are the subject of the Second Principle diverge on this point in content and especially in notation. Any appropriately paired "geo-metrics" for shape (e.g., anisotropy and bending energy) are much more easily discriminated and diagrammed via shape coordinates than via the equivalence classes of Kendall's shape space. There the relations between configurations of landmarks are represented by a "natural" metric that is actually natural only for lower-triangular matrices, not for the world of biological processes (cf. my discussion following Goodall, 1991).

The interaction of multivariate analysis with biological geometry in the extraction of features of shape comparison is the pervasive concern of Chapter 7. For the nonlinear part of shape space there are a priori principal components, the principal warps and their vector multiples the partial warps, that characterize the inutility of the Procrustes metric by the "energetics" – patterns of adjacency between landmarks – that the former does not take into account.

The computation and testing of single or group mean differences in shape ought to be followed by reexpression in terms of the partial warps; usually it is much easier to understand them in those graded diagrams than when they are laid out separately shape coordinate by shape coordinate. The principal warps, in turn, underlie the computation of relative warps, a posteriori principal components of the nonlinear subspace over a sample of forms (Section 7.6). The corresponding components of the "linear part," precisely two in number, are the ordinary principal compnents of the estimated uniform factor in its two-dimensional plane (Section 7.2). Then the description of the variability of a sample of shapes requires component extraction in these two incommensurate subspaces, together with a variance in the one-dimensional subspace of Centroid Size; the set of three components is tied together only by a covariance structure, not by algebra (Section 7.6). Procrustes analysis, which uses only one metric at a time (Section 7.1), seems unsuited to problems of feature extraction and should be considered instead either as an alternative to the shape coordinates for the specific statistical fitting or testing of diverse "null hypotheses" or as a variety of graphical display averaging over many different sets of shape coordinates at the same time.

8.3.2. Open questions

There are at least three gaps in this series of questions. One gap involves some technical concerns about new sorts of optimality apposite to the descriptors that are generated, and another involves some alternatives to the particular thin-plate splines exploited here. More generally, some biomathematically important questions arise from the formalism of landmarks as it interacts with algebraic or statistical spaces of distributed biological process.

8.3.2.1. Statistical issues of optimal description. —

Some additional tactics of modern exploratory data analysis ought to be adaptable for landmark data. One might ask, for instance, about the equivalent of "stepwise multiple regression" for landmarks. For a given landmark set (e.g., the 13 landmarks of the brain-scan data shown pictorially in Appendix A.1.3), what subset of the landmarks leads to the most precise descriptions of covariances with complex exogenous data bases, such as gray-scale imagery, metabolic function, or mentation? For evolutionary data, how does one best describe ecophenotypy? Regression by the method of Goodall and Lange (1990), using the Procrustes metric for residuals, appears unjustifiably arbitrary. Indeed, conventional approaches to the problem of multiple dependent variables, whether via canonical correlations or by Partial Least Squares, do

365

not seem to extend to the separation into linear and nonlinear feature subspaces of shape. Should an ontogenetic trend or ecophenotypy be computed separately in these two spaces, then combined? Or should it be computed once, and the canonical variates of shape decomposed into their projections into the two spaces?

A similar problem of optimal description arises in connection with the generalization of the linear component of shape change from triangles to configurations of any number of landmarks. Section 6.3 shows how any mean change in a triangle of landmarks can be interpreted as the ratio of a particular pair of transects of the triangle, and Section 7.2 shows how change or variability in any configuration of landmarks can be reduced to a single linear component or scatter of linear components. It would be very convenient if these themes could be combined. In principle we ought to be able to construct a "principal cross" – a ratio of distances between pairs of constructed landmarks at an angle averaging 90° – for these more complex linear terms and for principal components of this term in within-population scatters. But I do not know how to combine all the landmarks of a configuration into an estimate of "length in a particular direction" having optimal sample precision, nor how to combine two of these into a ratio of perpendicular distances itself having optimal precision. It must matter how closely this principal cross is aligned with the principal moments of the mean landmark configuration. Likewise, how would one visualize the uncertainty of a fitted growth gradient? And what ratio of parallel or collinear distances would best characterize it for the discrimination of two samples, or for diagnosis of specimens as they vary around a mean form?

A somewhat different problem of optimal description arises in one version of the extension of the landmark techniques to treat curving form. Appendix A.1.3 demonstrates the use of the splines to average entire images by standardizing the positions of the landmarks they contain. When the images also contain information about edges, then naturally the edges get "averaged" as well. One can imagine two different ways of using the unwarping based on the landmarks to drive a computation of the "average outline." In one approach, one would locate the edges separately case by case using the ordinary maneuvers of medical image processing, warp these edges onto the average image by image according to the superposition given by the landmarks there, and then average the positions of the nearly overlapping edges in the coordinate system of the mean shape into which every image is warped. This averaging of curves could be carried out by taking means of intercepts along nearly shared local normals. In another approach, one would average the pictures first, and then extract a consensual edge only once, in the averaged picture, where presumably its locus is a bit smoother or more generic. (The same pair of procedures could be imagined to apply to three-dimensional data, for the extraction of either curving surfaces or space curves.) Under what reasonable models for the distribution of location and sharpness of samples of edges is one of these protocols to be preferred to the other? The sharpness of the edge in the averaged picture (cf. Figure A.1.11) is a convolution of the sample distribution of edge locations and their separate localizations by the derivatives of the transverse gray-scale gradients. Is this sum of variances a reasonable statistic for the "net precision" of the location of that outline in the sample average? What role is played by the uncertainty of landmark locations parallel and perpendicular to nearby edges in calibrating this procedure? Under what circumstances, in particular, will the *omission* of landmarks from the registration procedure improve the sharpness of edges? A technology for the interaction of outlines with spline-based unwarping by modeling of the images that are their common source might provide the long-sought formal tie between the analysis of biological outlines and the analysis of landmarks (cf. Rohlf and Bookstein, 1990).

8.3.2.2. Why this particular spline?—

The sense in which we have separated global from local features of shape – the separation of the linear term from the localizable residual – is induced by the thin-plate spline technology used for interpolating homology maps between landmarks. It is not the only decomposition possible, because the thin-plate spline here is not the only interpolant appropriate to our notions of biological correspondence and the localizability of morphometric descriptors.

The discoverers of the thin-plate spline interpolant we are exploiting, Duchon and Meinguet, introduced it as only the first in a series of interpolating splines satisfying extremal conditions on integrals of squared partial derivatives of progressively higher order. That the features of Sections 7.5 and 7.6 are all interpretable as having a location and a scale follows ultimately from the fact that the spline minimizes an integral of this sort – the function $U(r)$ of the formulation ultimately is generated by the calculus of this functional minimization. The thin-plate spline of Section 2.2 minimizes the integral of summed-squared second derivatives. It decomposes shape space into a manifold on which all those derivatives are zero (the affine transformations), plus the interesting residual space of localizable shape phenomena explored in Sections 7.5 and 7.6. The value at the minimum of the integral being minimized provides the metric for the "localizable part" of shape difference, whereas a metric for the global part had to be supplied by geometry of another sort (e.g., the log anisotropy, Section 6.2).

The next spline in the hierarchy models the homology map as a quadratic function (cf. Section 7.4) together with sums of multiples of the function $U = r^4 \log r$ that is a fundamental solution of

367

the *triharmonic* equation $(\partial^2/\partial x^2 + \partial^2/\partial y^2)^3 U = \delta_{(0,0)}$, rather than the *biharmonic* $(\partial^2/\partial x^2 + \partial^2/\partial y^2)^2 U = \delta_{(0,0)}$ satisfied by $U(r) = r^2 \log r$. [Thus, the only aspect of the formula for $U(r)$ that is arbitrary is the exponent.] Such an interpolant (which even for two-dimensional data requires six landmarks for its computations – the principal warp of largest scale now involves *seven* landmarks) would supply the deterministic component of a spline in the form of a quadratic map rather than a linear map. For configurations of seven or more landmarks, the feature space of shape change or shape variation would thereby be decomposed into a quadratic part – a growth gradient having second derivatives constant – together with a residual more localizable than the one introduced in Section 7.3. [For instance, the "purely inhomogeneous term" of that section, along with all the $(r^2 \log r)$-based principal warps for sets of six or fewer landmarks, would be considered global in such an alternative decomposition.] At present the main obstacle to this development is the unavailability of any natural metric for the quadratic part that serves to generalize the elegance of anisotropy distance (Section 6.2 and Appendix A.2) for the linear map. The decomposition of quadratic fits in Section 7.4 is not a metric for the study of within-population variation, but applies only to the extraction of features from between-population comparisons one at a time. The anisotropy metric permits the extraction of principal components of the affine part in a very natural-seeming way; we would need an equally natural metric for quadratic gradients before it would be worthwhile to inspect the $(2K - 12)$-dimensional space of their residuals.

Among the set of quadratic forms that annihilate (assign "length" zero to) the space of linear transformations, there are many others besides the actual bending-energy metric used for the relative eigenanalyses of Section 7.6. Within the space of residuals from affine transformations, for instance, one might replace bending energy by a reference metric spherical in Procrustes distance. Under what circumstances, under what probability models would this lead to the computation of biologically more reasonable features? The interested reader may experiment with this possibility by manipulating the parameter α of Rohlf's program TPSRW.

8.3.2.3. The geometric ordering of form as one ordering among many. —

Perhaps the deepest and most biological questions that will ultimately be supported by the tools of this volume are independent of the technology of splining, but instead explore the very foundation of the idea of landmarks. Biological homology, as I mentioned in Chapter 3, is not properly a matter of description via geometrical points at all. It is rather concerned with *parts*. One sort of question asks what distinguishable parts an organism appears to have across a particular ecological or evolutionary range. This is the great question of *morphological integration*, the previous literature of which invokes mainly matrices of correlations of the usual disconnected variables of a multivariate study. The decomposition of a transformation into its partial warps (Section 7.5) supports a new quantification of morphological integration quite different from the older methods (e.g., it applies to samples as small as two forms, and it represents integration in "spacetime" as a function of both geometrical scale and ontogenetic age). Miriam Zelditch and I are preparing some exemplary analyses of this sort for ontogeny in the cotton rat, *Sigmodon*. At root, questions about integration pursue details of the match between the geometrical regulation of function or development and the statistical geometry of landmark locations as separated points. Such analyses go much better when the geometrical information about the mean landmark locations is preserved by the methods of this book.

The question of integration is the first in a series of mixed questions relating the geometry of shape space for landmarks to the geometries of other sorts of biological descriptions. The only tool this book offers for such mixed questions, Partial Least Squares (Section 2.3), though respectful of the symmetries of shape space, does not exploit its ordering by geometrical scale. It would be very useful to be able to phrase questions about the interrelations of the geometrical ordering of landmarks with other frequently encountered biological orderings: beyond ontogenetic time, the one-dimensional ordering by cyclic time, as in respiration, heartbeat, and reproduction by budding; for black-and-white images, the different one-dimensional ordering by a scalar field of image intensity (or such simulated gray scales as labeling ratios in tissue sections). There are also interesting higher-dimensional orderings to consider, for instance, the two-dimensional ordering of map coordinates (three-dimensional, for jungles and soils) or the two-dimensional ordering by an alien coordinate system (the "homunculus" I have already mentioned, or the retinotectal map in the vertebrate visual system). There are also orderings by strong theory from other fields, as by the torques or the tensor fields of material strain as they overlie Cartesian coordinates of muscle origins and insertions. At present, the confrontation of such competing orderings with the geometrical ordering of landmark locations is wholly ad hoc; it would be fine to have some heuristics, or even one good worked example. In precisely the opposite mood, the approach to analysis of random walks in Appendix A.3 needs to be generalized further to test for the presence of random walks (versus stasis or trend) on shape space, in a data-analytic counterpart of the origins of Kendall's (1984) shape-space theory in processes of diffusion.

8.4. FOURTH PRINCIPLE: THE FORM
OF ANSWERS

8.4.1. Routine procedures

In the same way that the form of morphometric questions can be made sensitive to the peculiar riches of landmark data – geometrical ordering a priori according to the mean locations, decomposition of features by geometrical scale – the form of answers should likewise express this richness. That is best achieved by *diversity*: Answers are to be presented in displays (not tables) following more than one of the available orderings (statistical, geometrical, or biological) in more than one of the available feature spaces. This volume has exercised a great variety of graphical and diagrammatic devices to communicate the findings the tools have unearthed. We have seen depictions of patterns via ordinary one- and two-dimensional statistical scatters and their enhancements, and via stacks of those scatters into "small multiples," including the Procrustes plot of Figure 7.1.6 and also assorted shape-coordinate trajectories. We have considered diagrams of simple finite elements (triangles) and complex finite elements (smooth interpolations over polygons more complex than triangles), with the imputed principal strains drawn either as ellipses or as ratios of finite distances. We have drawn transformations as vector fields, but also as extended deformations, and further as stacks of the special deformations, partial warps, that embody the eigenfunctions of bending energy. We have drawn shape changes as if they involved displacement out of the picture and also as displacements within the picture in which the data were collected. And we have represented patterns and regularities of shape change or its measurement with almost every geometrical element of classic analytic geometry – lines, perpendiculars, circles, ellipses, and their higher-dimensional equivalents. (Recall the six-dimensional ellipsoidal cylinder in Figure 7.5.1!)

8.4.2. *The* open question: morphometric visualization

Most of these figures display vectors, whatever their orientations within the feature space of the shape coordinates and whatever their semiotics on the printed page. Yet in the most satisfying versions of morphometric analysis, answers to questions take the form of *forms per se*: not vectors, but actual shapes of possible organisms representing averages or deviations from averages according with particular doses of factors. (Many of the figures in Section 3.4 would have been of this genre, for example, had the outlines been traced back over the landmarks after they were statistically displaced. Cf. Appendix A.1.2.) Because this book *is* a book, it has had to present these abstractions via ink on paper: static graphics drawn after the data have been analyzed. The next great surge in morphometrics will involve the superb new technology of "high-speed workstations," those machines for three-dimensional visualization as currently marketed by Silicon Graphics, Stardent, Apollo, and others. These units can be programmed to display changes of form, in two or three dimensions, *in real time*. One "moves" a landmark (usually by dragging it via a mouse), and the form's image on the screen deforms to keep pace (cf. Bookstein and Jaynes, 1990). In this way one will be able to *sculpt* real forms, individual specimens or observed means: to visually extrapolate observed processes to arbitrary extents, and combine them in arbitrary ad hoc combinations, so as to "see what happens." Under the guidance of a theory of osteogenesis, for instance, one might stress a neonatal mandible by various combinations of muscles, just to (literally[1]) see how it would grow; or one might evolve a horse, or a human, or a dairy cow, for another few thousand generations, to see (literally) which orthogenesis becomes dysfunctional first. One could simulate many different parameters of reconstructive facial surgery and tune them jointly for the most subjectively "beautiful" resulting form, skin and all. The greatest ultimate advantage of the morphometric tools this volume offers will be the routine display, at very high speed, of their common base of biometric information as the consequences for visualized form that ensue from covariance with any other information, measured or simulated, within or outside the limits of natural variability.

8.5. ENVOI

These tools for landmark data, and the extensions I expect to be developed over the next decade, make it possible to visualize effects upon form as if they were forms themselves. In this respect the new morphometric technology at last encourages the analyst of biological forms, their regularities and the processes controlling them, to rely upon the same scientist's retina as was used. to apprehend the original data. Contemporary morphometrics thus can lead the way to a recombination of biometrics with natural history, remedying the intellectually calamitous schism that arose early in this century when data were first tabulated in columns separated from the organic forms that bore them. The new morphometrics severely modifies the fundamental metaphor of biometrics, that organs or organisms be represented by vectors in a feature space or arbitrarily many freely rotatable "dimensions." Throughout this tool kit, that vector space has been tightly bound to the physical space occupied by the organism generating the data, so that the questions asked of the data in its space unite the statistical geometry of covariance with the physical geometry of

[1] The word "literally" is inappropriate here, but the English language does not really offer an equivalent for vision: perhaps "eidetically"?

371

8.5. Envoi

the Euclidean plane or Euclidean space that we share with our specimens. The answers to morphometric questions properly reside not in statistical space but back in the actual two- or three-dimensional visualizable space of the biologist's inquiries: the space of organisms and the patterns of their parts, their growth, and their evolution.

Only with the same two eyes Adam used to name the animals (Genesis 2:20) can we hope to decode the traces of evolutionary and developmental processes encoded within every realized biological form. To "name" the beasts, in the sense of measuring them, is to explain the features wherein they differ. To name them in this sense is to understand how causes and consequences of form are implicate with the notations of space and time, the geometrical-statistical descriptions of processes that account for form in its own terms. It is my hope that the tools of this treatise will become a permanent part of the calligraphic art by which those names are written.

Appendices

A.1. MORE ON THIN-PLATE SPLINES

A.1.1. A Fortran listing

The following code executes the thin-plate spline interpolation introduced in Section 2.2. The calling program first calls TPSOLV with arguments as follows:

IDIM – number of dimensions of the data: 1, 2, or 3

NPTS (passed in common /FORMS/) – number of landmarks

POINTS (passed in common /FORMS/) – Cartesian coordinates of the landmarks. First subscript is Cartesian coordinate, second landmark number, third the form (1 or 2). Here, dimensioned to a maximum count of 50.

The subroutine returns the coefficients w_i and a_1, a_x, a_y in entries TPCOEF (1 ... NPTS) and TPCOEF (NPTS + 1 ... NPTS + 3), separately for each coordinate of the data. The net integral bending energy is also returned in the value SCORE.

The subroutine TPSOLV is essentially a setup and loop over calls to a linear equation solver. That incorporated here is from the package LINPACK; one may substitute other matrix inversion routines as convenient.

Once the coefficients TPCOEF have been computed, the effect of the spline mapping on any point PT of the starting image is computed by calling TPEVAL with arguments IDIM and TP-COEF copied from TPSOLV and input point PT as shown. The image of the argument point is returned in EVAL.

A.1. Thin-plate splines

```
      SUBROUTINE TPSOLV(IDIM,TPCOEF,SCORE)
C
C     thin-plate spliner for one-, two-, or
C        three-dimensional landmark data
C
C        Fred L. Bookstein
C        Center for Human Growth and Development
C        University of Michigan
C        May 1985
C
C     algorithm from notes of conversations with
C        David Ragozin
C
      COMMON /FORMS/ NPTS, POINTS(3,50,2)
      DIMENSION TPS1(54,54),SVEC(54,2),TPCOEF(54,3)
      NP4=NPTS+4
C
C     rows and columns of tps1, and columns of tpcoef, are:
C        NPTS coefficients of terms |arg-points(**1)|
C        coefficients of 1, X, Y, Z
C
C     rows of tpcoef are:
C        before statement 250: Cartesian coordinates of
C           homologous landmarks in the other form
C        after statement 300: coefficients of the splines
C           for the i-th Cartesian coordinate, i=1, ... .
C
      DO 60 I=1,NP4
      DO 50 J=1,NP4
50    TPS1(I,J)=0.
      DO 60 J=1,IDIM
60    TPCOEF(I,J)=0.
      DO 200 I=1,NPTS
      DO 100 J=I,NPTS
      IF (I.EQ.J) GO TO 100
      GO TO (70,80,90), IDIM
70    TPS1(I,J)=ABS(POINTS(1,I,1)-POINTS(1,J,1))**3
C     the one-dimensional case: |r|³
      GO TO 100
80    X=
     1 (POINTS(1,I,1)-POINTS(1,J,1))**2 +
     2 (POINTS(2,I,1)-POINTS(2,J,1))**2
      TPS1(I,J)=X*ALOG(X)
C     the function U = r² log r² of Section 2.2
C        for the i-th and j-th landmarks
      GO TO 100
90    TPS1(I,J)=SQRT (
     1 (POINTS(1,I,1)-POINTS(1,J,1))**2 +
     2 (POINTS(2,I,1)-POINTS(2,J,1))**2 +
     3 (POINTS(3,I,1)-POINTS(3,J,1))**2 )
C     the three-dimensional case: |r|
100   TPS1(J,I)=TPS1(I,J)
      TPS1(I,NPTS+1)=1.
      TPS1(NPTS+1,I)=1.
      DO 160 K=1,IDIM
      TPS1(I,NPTS+K+1)=POINTS(K,I,1)
      TPS1(NPTS+1+K,I)=POINTS(K,I,1)
160   TPCOEF(I,K)=POINTS(K,I,2)
200   CONTINUE
250   CALL SSICO
     1 (TPS1, 54, NPTS+1+IDIM, SVEC, RC, SVEC(1,2))
```

374

```
      DO 300 K=1,IDIM
300   CALL SSISL
     1 (TPS1, 54, NPTS+1+IDIM, SVEC, TPCOEF(1,K))
C
C     equation solver, here, via UDU-decomposition
C         these routines are from LINPACK
C
      SCORE=0.
      DO 400 I=1,NPTS
      DO 400 J=I,NPTS
      IF (I.EQ.J) GO TO 400
      GO TO (310,320,330), IDIM
310   X=
     1 ABS(POINTS(1,I,1)-POINTS(1,J,1))**3
      SCORE=SCORE+X
     1 * (TPCOEF(I,1)*TPCOEF(J,1))
      GO TO 400
320   X=
     1 (POINTS(1,I,1)-POINTS(1,J,1))**2 +
     2 (POINTS(2,I,1)-POINTS(2,J,1))**2
      SCORE=SCORE+X*ALOG(X)
     1 * (TPCOEF(I,1)*TPCOEF(J,1)+TPCOEF(I,2)*TPCOEF(J,2))
      GO TO 400
330   X=SQRT (
     1 (POINTS(1,I,1)-POINTS(1,J,1))**2 +
     2 (POINTS(2,I,1)-POINTS(2,J,1))**2 +
     3 (POINTS(3,I,1)-POINTS(3,J,1))**2 )
      SCORE=SCORE+X
     1 * (TPCOEF(I,1)*TPCOEF(J,1)+TPCOEF(I,2)*TPCOEF(J,2)
     1 + TPCOEF(I,3)*TPCOEF(J,3))
400   CONTINUE
      SCORE=2.*SCORE
      RETURN
      END
      SUBROUTINE TPEVAL(IDIM,TPCOEF,PT,EVAL)
      COMMON /FORMS/ NPTS, POINTS(3,50,2)
      DIMENSION TPCOEF(54,3), PT(3), EVAL(3)
      DO 100 K=1,IDIM
      X=TPCOEF(NPTS+1,K)
C     coefficient of 1.0 (constant)
      DO 20 L=1,IDIM
20    X=X+TPCOEF(NPTS+1+L,K)*PT(L)
C     coefficients of X, Y, Z (linear term)
      GO TO (30,50,70), IDIM
30    DO 40 L=1,NPTS
40    X=X+TPCOEF(L,1)*ABS(PT(1)-POINTS(1,L,1))**3
      GO TO 100
50    DO 60 L=1,NPTS
      Y=
     1 (POINTS(1,L,1)-PT(1))**2 +
     2 (POINTS(2,L,1)-PT(2))**2
60    IF (Y.NE.0.) X=X+TPCOEF(L,K)*Y*ALOG(Y)
      GO TO 100
70    DO 80 L=1,NPTS
80    X=X+TPCOEF(L,K)*SQRT (
     1 (POINTS(1,L,1)-PT(1))**2 +
     2 (POINTS(2,L,1)-PT(2))**2 +
     3 (POINTS(3,L,1)-PT(3))**2 )
100   EVAL(K)=X
      RETURN
      END
```

375

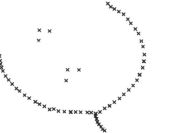

Figure A.1.1. A pair of simulated botanical scenes.

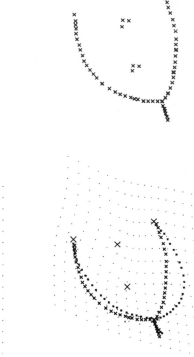

Figure A.1.2. Result of applying the splined mapping of Figure 7.5.2 to Figure A.1.1. Large X's, "landmarks"; medium-sized X's, edge "data"; small X's (right), images of left-side edges under the splined mapping.

bending energy   0.0844

A.1.2. Differential constraints and relaxation

The material in this section previously appeared in Bookstein (1989*a*). The landmarks of the scene analyzed in Figure 7.5.1 were extracted from the pair of simulated edge images (actually, doodles on a desk pad) shown in Figure A.1.1. (The width of the X's at each digitized point is presumed to encode the uncertainty of edge location.) If these were botanical data, the landmarks would be the "stem" of the flowers, the ends of the two "petals," and the upper left corners of the pair of "seeds." When the warping function of Figure 7.5.2 is applied to every point in the left-hand image, there results the warped image shown in Figure A.1.2. Here, the large X's locate the five landmarks used to drive the thin-plate spline. The edge points of Figure A.1.1 are copied into this diagram by middle-sized X's. Finally, the small X's in the right-hand image represent the edge points of the left-hand flower after transformation by the splined map $f = (f_1, f_2)$ based on these five landmarks.

It is apparent that this map fails to do justice to the form of the flowers; the petals on the right do not overlie the images of the petals on the left. We may begin to remedy this failure by somewhat arbitrarily selecting points along the petals near the

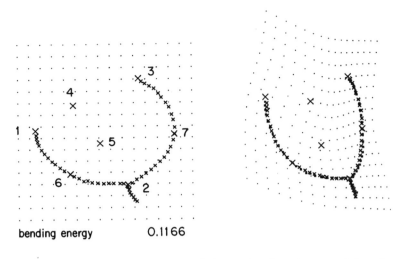

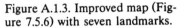
bending energy 0.1166

Figure A.1.3. Improved map (Figure 7.5.6) with seven landmarks.

middle of their arcs, left and right, and using them to drive the seven-landmark spline mapping shown in Figure A.1.3, a map seen earlier (to a slightly different digitization) in Figure 7.5.6. This augmentation of the data greatly improves the apparent goodness of fit of the warped left image to the actual right image, at little cost in bending energy (net deformation). The units of this quantity, as printed under the grid, are arbitrary, a function of the scale of my digitizing tablet.

A.1.2.1. Deficient landmarks. —

In passing from Figure A.1.2 to Figure A.1.3 we have augmented our store of information about the correspondence of points between the two forms, but we have inserted a bit of misinformation as well. We do not know precisely which point of the curve between landmarks #1 and #2 on the right should be considered to correspond to the landmark #6 we selected on the left, and likewise which point of the arc from #2 to #3 corresponds to landmark #7. I shall refer to landmark #7 in explaining the procedure by which such ambiguities are resolved.

Landmark #7 on the right could have been chosen to be any point of the appropriate arc. As the "best" point (in a sense to be explained in the next paragraph) is likely not too far from the point actually chosen, we can model this "freedom of choice" as the freedom of point (x_7', y_7') to vary along the line tangent to the right-hand curve near the starting guess. For ease of exposition, take this tangent line to be vertical; then the "data" are limited to the x-coordinate x_7' of landmark #7, and the y-coordinate y_7' may be set subject to any reasonable criterion. Because the digitized location of landmark #7 on the right has only one valid Cartesian coordinate, not two, I refer to it as a **deficient landmark**.

In the context of these splines, a criterion that immediately suggests itself is to place the point (x'_7, y'_7) so that *the net bending energy of the resulting spline is least*. In effect, we are using the energy of the spline as a measure of information content (measured by squared second derivatives) of the deformation as it deviates from the affine condition, the map with all second derivatives zero. We seek the representation of the map that has the least information consistent with what we actually know about the data (in this case, the coordinate x'_7, but not the coordinate y'_7).

The computation to be performed may be intuited graphically. Figure 7.5.8 presented the thin plates corresponding to the complete nonlinear (affine-free) part of the transformation in Figure A.1.3. We see there that the y-shift is bent somewhat upward at landmark #7; therefore, its relaxation toward a state of lowered bending energy will push it downward. Landmark #7 loads most heavily on principal warp 4 (Figure 7.5.7d), and secondarily on principal warp 2 (Figure 7.5.7b). Its movement downward rapidly decreases the bending energy associated with principal warp 4, but also increases, albeit more slowly, that associated with eigenvector 2 (because it is already tacked down by that landmark: Figure 7.5.5b). At the computed optimum of this shift, the amount of downward displacement of the coordinate y'_7 will just balance the decrease in bending energy of the fourth principal warp against the increase in bending energy of the second (each squared, then weighted by its eigenvalue).

Similarly, we may inquire as to the possible effect on the bending of the spline of allowing landmark #6 on the right to slide along the tangent line there. A glance at Figure 7.5.8 indicates that we are not likely to move it too far: This landmark tacks both coordinate sheets *down*, and by roughly the same amount. The direction of the tangent line, along which we must move this landmark, is $(-1, 1)$; then any improvement in flatness of the x-sheet induced by a shift will be obviated by increased bending of the y-sheet, and vice versa. Because these contributions go as the squares of the projections on the eigenvectors, the effect of freeing landmark #6 to slide will very likely be null.

To accommodate this relaxation procedure in algebra, we must slightly extend the usual spline formalism in a direction somewhat different from that of statistical splining (cf. Wahba, 1990). Deficient landmarks are allowed to vary along straight lines. That is, the homologue (x'_i, y'_i) of (x_i, y_i) may be any point of the form

$$(x'_i, y'_i) = ([x'_i]_0 + t_i r_i, [y'_i]_0 + t_i s_i),$$

where $([x'_i]_0, [y'_i]_0)$ is the point actually digitized, now merely representative of its tangent line; r_i and s_i are direction cosines of the line along which (x'_i, y'_i) is varying; and t_i is the amount of shift along the tangent line, determined so as to minimize the net bending energy. If k homologues are freed to slide along lines in this way, the matrix V actually covers an affine k-flat (k-dimensional vector subspace shifted away from the origin):

$$V = V(t_{j_1}, \ldots, t_{j_k})$$

$$= \begin{bmatrix} x'_1 & \cdots & [x'_{j_1}]_0 + t_{j_1} r_{j_1} & \cdots & [x'_{j_k}]_0 + t_{j_k} r_{j_k} & \cdots & x'_n \\ y'_1 & \cdots & [y'_{j_1}]_0 + t_{j_1} s_{j_1} & \cdots & [y'_{j_k}]_0 + t_{j_k} s_{j_k} & \cdots & y'_n \end{bmatrix}.$$

As the t_{j_l} vary, the integral $I_f = I_f(t_{j_1}, \ldots, t_{j_k}) = V(L_n^{-1})V^T$ varies about a nonnegative minimum as a positive-semidefinite quadratic form in $t_{j_1}, \ldots, t_{j_k}$. The minimizing of $I_f(t_{j_1}, \ldots, t_{j_k})$ is numerically very tractable for $k \le n - 3$.

The result of this relaxation in the current example is shown graphically in Figure A.1.4. The previous locations of landmarks #6 and #7 at the right are shown with large + signs. When each is freed to slide along the tangent line indicated, the computed positions of least bending energy are shown by the new large X's on the right. As expected, landmark #7 has moved considerably downward, whereas landmark #6 has hardly moved at all. The

Figure A.1.4. Locations of landmarks #6 and #7 after a relaxation to minimize bending energy; +, previous positions; new large X's, relaxed locations.

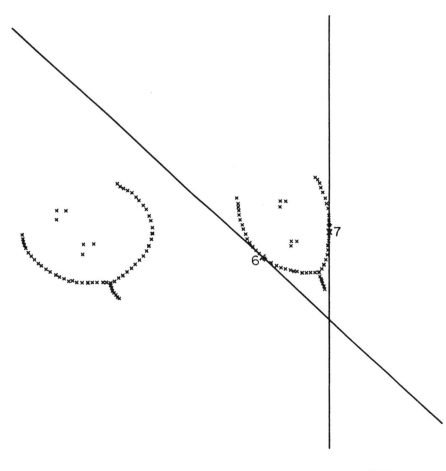

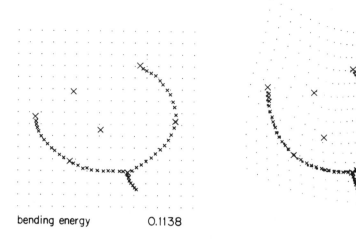

Figure A.1.5. Splined mapping corresponding to the relaxation of Figure A.1.4.

bending energy   0.1138

spline map that results is shown in Figure A.1.5; it is no less consistent than Figure A.1.3 with the information we actually have about biological homology, but its bending energy is only 0.1138. We have "saved" unnecessary bending induced by the passage from five landmarks to seven.

A.1.2.2. Iterative refinement of deformations. —

In Figure A.1.5 there is a systematic deviation of the tangent to the right-hand form below landmark #7 from the image of the tangent in the left-hand form. We may attempt to further refine the mapping in this region by choosing yet another intermediate landmark. In Figure A.1.6 I have added, arbitrarily, a landmark #8 slightly below #7 on the left and a bad guess at a homologue for it on the right. The addition of the eighth landmark pair adds 0.0096 unit of bending energy to the computed spline – not an

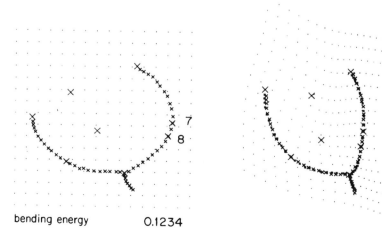

Figure A.1.6. Attempt to align direction of tangent through landmark #7.

bending energy   0.1234

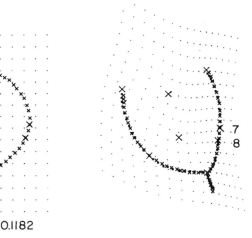

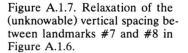

bending energy   0.1182

Figure A.1.7. Relaxation of the (unknowable) vertical spacing between landmarks #7 and #8 in Figure A.1.6.

inconsiderable amount. Although the deviation of tangent direction below landmark #7 has been corrected, this warping function is obviously inappropriate in the vertical direction. The grid lines of the right-hand form are bent apart in between landmarks #7 and #8; the directional derivative has been specified inappropriately. Again, we have allowed ourselves to be misled by the pairing of Cartesian coordinates. About landmark #8 on the right we know only that it lies on a nearly straight line through point #7, but we do not know which point of that line it is. What we know, in fact, takes the form of a constraint on the directional derivative of f at landmark #7. Specifically, the direction into which the map takes the tangent to the curve on the left at landmark #7 is known – the ratio $df_2/ds : df_1/ds$ along the homologous arc of the left-hand flower – but not the magnitude of the derivative in this direction.

Landmark #8 must be freed to relax so that the projection on the eigenvector of highest bending energy (the constraint on the directional derivative; cf. Figure 7.5.8*b*) is close to zero, where its square will be balanced by increasing contributions to all the other, less stiff eigenvectors. The result of freeing both this landmark and (again) landmark #7 is shown in Figure A.1.7: The additional bending energy required is reduced from 0.0096 unit to 0.0044.

The right-hand petals still fail to line up just above the "stem," because the angles at the stem have changed considerably beyond what is consistent with the curving of petals farther away. We can fix this by incorporation of two landmarks near the stem on opposite sides, both freed to slide. (The effect is to specify the effect of the affine derivative on angles, but not to constrain its effects upon lengths.) The addition of this local feature "costs" 0.0056 more bending (Figure A.1.8). The net effect on the outline of relaxing all five intercalated landmarks along the petals is to

381

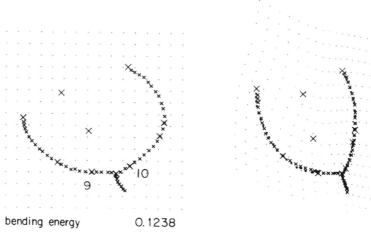

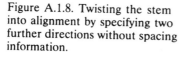

Figure A.1.8. Twisting the stem into alignment by specifying two further directions without spacing information.

bending energy   0.1238

somewhat sensitively estimate the homology map *along* those arcs consistent with the pairing of petal ends and stems and otherwise yielding the minimum of bending over the whole picture given the positions of the seeds. This is a distinct improvement upon the treatment of the same problem in Bookstein (1978), where it was required that homology be linear in arc length between adjacent landmarks of a boundary arc.

Further adjustment of the warping function to match the scales of the seeds to each other costs another 0.0760 unit of bending energy (Figure A.1.9), comparable to all the bending in Figure A.1.1. The shrinkage of the scale of the seeds is massively inconsistent with the behavior of the map all around the periphery of the flower, and it is not helpful to model it as a deformation of the area in between the seeds and the petals, where there are, after all, no data. One might choose to relax *this* part of the spline by allowing rotation without change of scale.

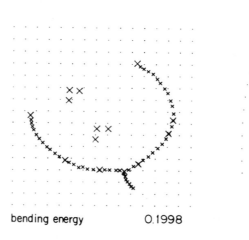

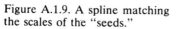

Figure A.1.9. A spline matching the scales of the "seeds."

bending energy   0.1998

A.1.3. Picture averaging

Another application of the splines to image analysis is the provenance of averaged pictures for the summary and discrimination of categories. A procedure we have found useful at Michigan averages gray-scale medical images by standardizing landmark locations. The computation proceeds in four steps, as follows:

1. Landmarks are extracted for each of a series of homologous images, like the midsagittal magnetic-resonance images in Figure A.1.10.

2. The landmark configurations are averaged (Section 5.4).

Figure A.1.10. Two of a set of 14 MRI sections for UCLA medical students who were "otherwise normal." The form at right is missing two landmarks; its interpolation is based on the others. Top: Original images. Bottom: Unwarpings to the sample average shape coordinates. Data from Dr. John Mazziotta; landmarks digitized by Daniel Valentino; execution in X Windows on a Stellar GS1000 by William Jaynes.

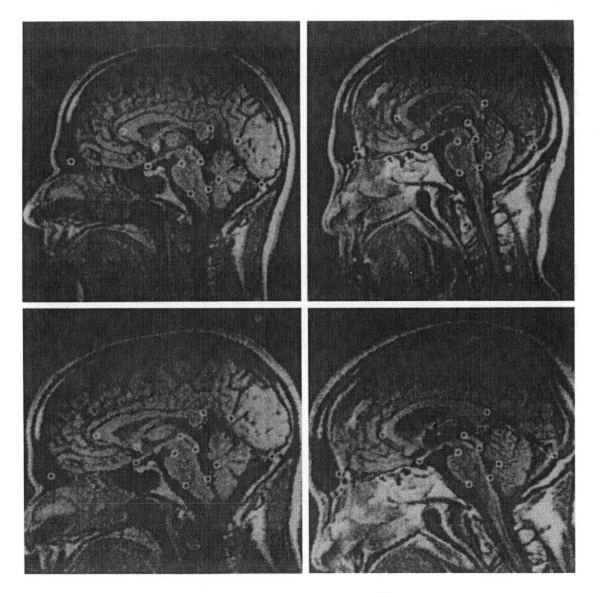

A.1. Thin-plate splines

3. A suitably sized grid of pixels around the averaged landmark set is warped *back* to each picture in turn. For each pixel of the "standard" image, the interpolated pixel for the specimen image is ascribed to the locus in the standard form.

4. These imputed pixel values are averaged over the images of the series. A composite photograph (Figure A.1.11) has thereby been produced rigorously. As in this example, there can be considerable information in the composite beyond the specific features normalized via the landmark standardization. See Bookstein (1991).

Figure A.1.11. Averaged mid-sagittal sections, 14 students. Landmarks were lacking in the midface and at the top of the skull; hence the images are out of registration there. But many contours of the midbrain emerge with unexpected sharpness.

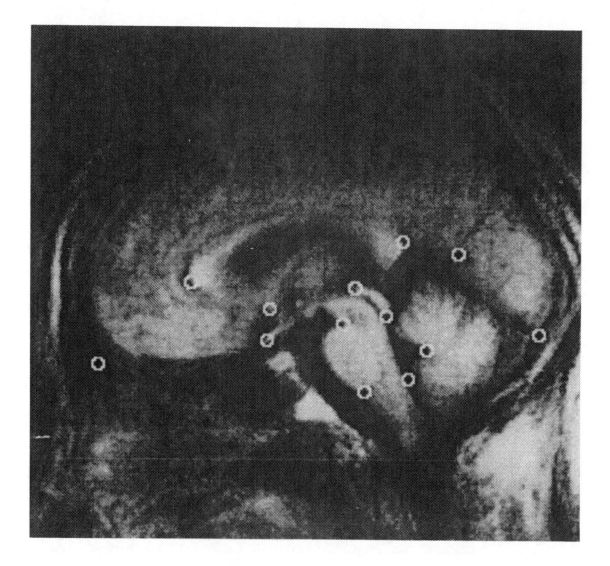

A.2. ANISOTROPY AND THE POINCARÉ GEOMETRY OF TRIANGLES

The statistical methods for triangles of landmarks introduced in Chapters 5 and 6 were all declared "approximately" invariant against changes of the choice of baseline underlying scatters of shape coordinates. The quality of this approximation, I often averred, was to be inferred from exact results that dealt with sets of points at arbitrary finite separations in the space of shape coordinates. This appendix sketches the classic nineteenth-century geometry that governs these computations. Most of the unfamiliar terms are explained in the auxiliary readings about non-Euclidean geometry surveyed in Section 2.5.3.2

This geometry is *not* that of David Kendall's shape space (Section 5.6). The geometry of that space is that of the Procrustes metric (Section 7.1) it incorporates; for triangles, the metric has constant positive Riemannian curvature (Kendall, 1984), so that Kendall's "shape space" accords with a patch of a sphere. The geometry with a function of anisotropy as metric, as hinted at in the approximation in Figure 6.2.9, exemplifies the other classic non-Euclidean geometry: the **hyperbolic plane** in its implementation via the **Poincaré model** (cf. Coxeter, 1965:sect. 14.8). This appendix shows that the usual hyperbolic metric of that space is the same as the logarithm of the anisotropy measure with which we are already familiar, and it sets forth in detail the connection between non-Euclidean diameters of shape scatters and the accuracy of the invariances asserted throughout Chapters 5 and 6.

Recall from Section 6.2.6 that any collection of data equivalent to second-order tensors – elliptical inclusions in rocks, or second-order moments of extended features – may be interpreted as a collection of "triangles" generated by applying the feature, interpreted as a deformation, to one standard triangle. Thus all of the geometric constructions in this appendix apply to oriented elliptical inclusions, such as records of physical strain or summaries of texture, as well as to triangles of observed landmark locations.

A.2.1. Straight lines and distance

The formula for anisotropy of a change of triangular shape is one version of the most fundamental construct underlying projective metric geometry (Busemann and Kelly, 1953), the notion of a **cross-ratio**, a ratio of ratios, here taken among four concyclic points of the plane. According to the classic Cayley-Klein approach, projective metrics take the form of logs of cross-ratios. (Oddly, the principle was first discovered in the measure of angle, by Laguerre. Euclidean angle is the log cross-ratio of two lines in respect of the lines of slope $\pm \sqrt{-1}$ through their intersection.) It is by reason of this equivalence that log anisotropy is the natural

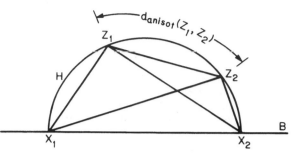

Figure A.2.1. Anisotropy as a log cross-ratio $d_{\text{anisot}}(Z_1, Z_2)$, equation (A.2.1). This value is the hyperbolic distance between the triangles having shape coordinates Z_1 and Z_2.

measure of size-free strain among homologously labeled triangular shapes.

Let us set up two triangles in the usual two-point registration (Figure 6.2.1). Write X_1 and X_2 for the intersections with the baseline B of the circle H passing through Z_1 and Z_2 and centered upon the baseline. For the transformation from $X_1 Z_1 X_2$ to $X_1 Z_2 X_2$ shown in Figure A.2.1, the anisotropy is the ratio of change in the distance to one of the X's divided by the ratio of change in the distance to the other. Explicitly, this is the cross-ratio

$$\frac{|Z_2 X_2| \div |Z_1 X_2|}{|Z_2 X_1| \div |Z_1 X_1|} = \frac{|Z_2 X_2| \div |Z_2 X_1|}{|Z_1 X_2| \div |Z_1 X_1|}. \tag{A.2.1}$$

The log of this ratio of ratios will be denoted $d_{\text{anisot}}(Z_1, Z_2)$.

A.2.1.1. *"Straight lines" in shape space are Euclidean circles.* —

Suppose three points Z_3, Z_1, and Z_2 lie, in that order, on the circle H perpendicular to B shown in Figure A.2.2. We have

$$d_{\text{anisot}}(Z_3, Z_2) = \log \frac{|Z_3 X_2| \div |Z_2 X_2|}{|Z_3 X_1| \div |Z_2 X_1|}$$

$$= \log \frac{|Z_3 X_2| \div |Z_1 X_2|}{|Z_3 X_1| \div |Z_1 X_1|} + \log \frac{|Z_1 X_2| \div |Z_2 X_2|}{|Z_1 X_1| \div |Z_2 X_1|}$$

$$= d_{\text{anisot}}(Z_3, Z_1) + d_{\text{anisot}}(Z_1, Z_2).$$

Hence Z_1, Z_2, and Z_3 lie on a "straight line" according to the metric d_{anisot}. The purpose of taking the *logarithm* of anisotropy is

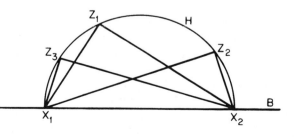

Figure A.2.2. Three triangles on a hyperbolic straight line (cf. Figure 6.2.3).

386

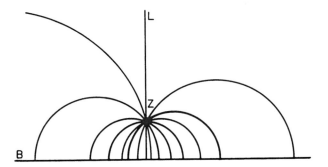

Figure A.2.3. Some hyperbolic straight lines through a point Z.

essentially the provenance of this addition formula. **The "straight lines" of this hyperbolic geometry are circles like H, perpendicular to the baseline.** Figure A.2.3 shows a sample of some of these incident upon a single point (triangular shape) Z. One actually looks straight: the line L through Z perpendicular to B. Here, as in Figure 6.2.2, it plays the role of a "circle" of infinite radius.

On the right in equation (A.2.1), the cross-ratio has been rearranged so that Z_2 appears only in the numerator, and Z_1 only in the denominator. The logarithm of this ratio, the **log anisotropy** of the strain, is then

$$\left| \log \frac{|Z_2 X_2|}{|Z_2 X_1|} - \log \frac{|Z_1 X_2|}{|Z_1 X_1|} \right| = \left| \Delta \log \left| \frac{Z - X_2}{Z - X_1} \right| \right|,$$

the change in absolute value of a function defined upon the Z's one at a time. (At the right in the preceding equation, the notation $|Z - X|$ in place of $|ZX|$ refers to the points of the figure as complex numbers.) The formula is not yet particularly helpful, as X_1 and X_2 are functions of the Z's.

For points Z and $Z + dZ$ separated by a small shape displacement dZ, we have

$$d\left(\log \frac{Z - X_2}{Z - X_1} \right) = \left(\frac{d}{dZ} \log \frac{Z - X_2}{Z - X_1} \right) dZ$$

$$= \frac{X_2 - X_1}{(Z - X_1)(Z - X_2)} dZ.$$

The modulus of the complex coefficient of dZ is $1/\text{Im } Z$ – ratio of baseline to twice the area of triangle $X_1 Z X_2$ – and of course the product is real for dZ along the circle H, the direction that leaves X_1 and X_2 fixed. In this direction,

$$d_{\text{anisot}}(Z, Z + dZ) = \left(\frac{d}{dZ} \log \frac{Z - X_2}{Z - X_1} \right) dZ = \frac{|dZ|}{\text{Im } Z}.$$

This "extraordinarily simple result" (Klein, 1928:301) was demon-

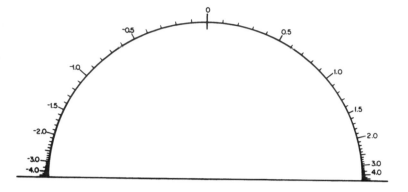

Figure A.2.4. The hyperbolic ruler (not a protractor!). This device does not have the kinematics of an ordinary ruler, which you are free to translate and rotate arbitrarily on your paper, but the relative scale of which you may not change. The hyperbolic ruler may be translated, but only along the baseline, and may be rescaled, but does not rotate. (In practice, one rescales implicitly by printing the ruler on transparent plastic to all magnifications at once; see Figure A.2.7.) The scale marked is log anisotropy to the base e. For instance, triangles having as shape coordinates the points marked as "0" and "1" differ by a uniform transformation of anisotropy $e^1 = 2.718$.

strated by Euclidean geometry alone in Section 6.2.4. We see that the global quantity being approximated in Figure 6.2.10 is actually not anisotropy minus 1 but *log* anisotropy.

A.2.1.2. The global appearance of log anisotropy. —

Figure A.2.4, using logs to the base e, indicates the scale of distance d_{anisot} on various straight lines through Z, as in Figure A.2.3. Because all triangles on X_1 and X_2 inscribed in H are right triangles, the ratio of distances to the two intersections of the circle with the baseline is the tangent (or cotangent) of the angle between either of those segments and the baseline. By a theorem of Euclid, this angle is half the angle at the center. Hence the *distance* function plotted here is $\log \tan \theta/2$, where θ is the (Euclidean) *angle* measured at the center of the circle between the radius vector and the baseline. The particular scale in Figure A.2.4 measures anisotropy distance from the isosceles right triangle (hypotenuse down) represented by the vertex of the semicircle.

Near the baseline B, the scale approaches a constant offset from $\pm \log y$, increasing in absolute value by 1.0 for every reduction by a factor e in distance to the baseline. Along the "circle" L in Figure A.2.3 – the Euclidean line perpendicular to the baseline – the scale of distance is $\log y$ throughout. The baseline is at infinite distance from all proper triangles. In Cayley-Klein language, it serves as the **Absolute** of this projective metric (Klein, 1928; Busemann and Kelly, 1953). The fact that triangles of zero area are infinitely far away (cannot be grown allometrically into triangles having a proper interior) forces us to eschew the Procrustes metric in the context of measuring shape change (cf. Bookstein, 1986a:rejoinder).

A.2.1.3. Extrapolation. —

In Euclidean geometry, we extrapolate changes by executing the same translation of coordinates over and over. A change from Z_0

to Z_1, for instance, is extrapolated to $Z_t = Z_0 + t(Z_1 - Z_0)$ for $t > 1$, interpolated for $0 < t < 1$, and reflected (extrapolated backward) for $t < 0$. For exponential extrapolation, one would replace the Cartesian coordinates by their logarithms and proceed in the same manner. A similar procedure is possible in the hyperbolic geometry of shape space for triangles. Figure A.2.5 shows the application of the ruler, Figure A.2.4, to mark off series of equally spaced shapes. Biologically, these have the meaning of *iterations of allometry*: Huxleyan growth by unvarying specific rates along both principal directions at the same time. These directions are presumed held constant by explicit inscription upon the form, and the landmarks are merely borne along.

A.2.1.4. *"Circles" in shape space are likewise Euclidean circles.* —

Let Z_1 represent a starting form (i.e., let $X_1 Z_1 X_2$ be a starting triangle, for some X_1, X_2 on B), and consider the set of forms derived from Z_1 by strains all of the same anisotropy δ but with various principal crosses. This will be called a d_{anisot}-*circle of radius δ*. Because distances d_{anisot} in the direction of B, the fixed line, increase faster than distances d_{anisot} in the direction away from B, one would expect that d_{anisot}-circles around any point (triangle) Z_1 would not look the same as Euclidean circles; they should be lopsided.

This expectation is subtly in error. In fact, d_{anisot}-circles *are* Euclidean circles; it is just that their centers have shifted. As Figure A.2.6 indicates, the set of "straight lines" through the point Z is perpendicular to another set of Euclidean circles. The d_{anisot}-circles about Z are the circles of this other set, perpendicular to H and to all the other "straight lines" through Z. The point Z is called the **hyperbolic center** of each of these circles. Whereas the smallest d_{anisot}-circles are indistinguishable from Euclidean circles centered at Z, the larger ones are progressively more and

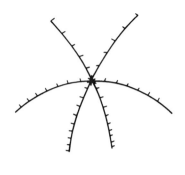

Figure A.2.5. Equally spaced series of points on straight lines: a model for extended allometric growth.

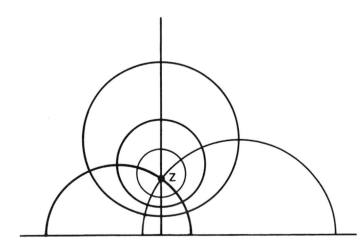

Figure A.2.6. Hyperbolic circles around a point Z of shape space, together with three of the hyperbolic straight lines (two Euclidean circles and a Euclidean line) to which they are perpendicular.

more severely offset to avoid cutting the baseline. This orthogonality is a theorem in Euclidean geometry dealing with so-called **conjugate pencils** of circles. The pencil in Figure A.2.3 is elliptic; that in A.2.6, hyperbolic. For details, see Schwerdtfeger (1962: 30–1, 67).

The identification of triangular shapes with points of this classic non-Euclidean geometry permits the reinterpretation of many Euclidean constructions in terms of anisotropy, allometry, and shape comparison. For instance, the intersection of two circles perpendicular to the baseline, each extrapolating one pair of observed triangular forms, represents the shape that is common to the two allometric sequences. But not all circles intersect; some pairs have a unique pair of points of closest approach, whereas still other pairs are "parallel." These topics, though charming, are beyond the scope of this appendix.

A.2.1.5. The diameter of a scatter in hyperbolic space.—

One measures the diameter of a Euclidean point set by rotating a grid of parallel lines to the position of maximum span by the set. The equivalent to the grid for this hyperbolic geometry is the set of rays shown in Figure A.2.7. The template, panel a, should be imagined a large sheet of transparent plastic. In use, it is slid along the baseline of the Poincaré plane (no vertical displacement, no rotations; this sliding is the non-Euclidean equivalent of rotating a Cartesian grid). At each position, the observer notes the separation of extremes of the scatter, reading this distance, of course, according to the $\log \tan \theta/2$ scale of the ruler. For panel b, we are using the spring of the circle from the baseline for an "infinitely large" template centered "infinitely far away": In the vertical direction, hyperbolic distance is the ordinary logarithm of

Figure A.2.7. The graphical computation of hyperbolic diameter. (a) Template. (b–d) Applications to a single scatter rotated into (b) vertical, (c) horizontal, and (d) oblique orientations. The measured diameters are all the same, about 0.60.

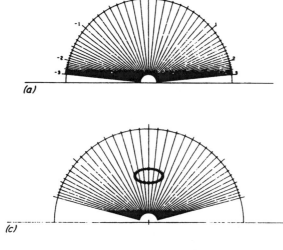

(a)

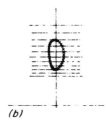

(b)

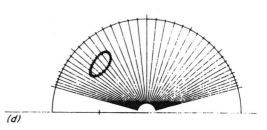

(c)

(d)

390

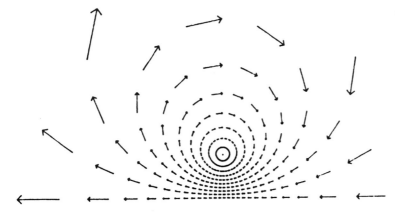

Figure A.2.8. A hyperbolic rotation. The baseline (the straight line at the bottom of the figure) is moved along itself.

ratios of Euclidean distance from the baseline. The major diameter of the scatter is the largest of these separations and represents the actual hyperbolic length of a circular arc (of center upon the baseline) connecting the two extreme points of tangency. There is a minor diameter as well, the smallest of these spans. For scatters that are approximately ovoid, the two circular arcs involved intersect at approximately 90°.

A.2.2. Diameter of scatters and the accuracy of approximations

When the baseline for construction of shape coordinates is changed, the scatter changes according to a nonlinearity that is generally rather mild. The effect of this nonlinearity upon the multivariate statistical analyses that ordinarily follow may be typified by its effect on one single derived quantity, the sample centroid.

The effect of change of baseline is in fact a hyperbolic *rotation* (cf. Figure A.2.8). Centering the change at the point $i = (0, 1)$, this is a transformation of the form $z \rightarrow (kz + 1)/(k - z)$ for some real number k. (That formula represents a Möbius transformation that takes the real line onto itself and leaves $\pm i$ invariant; Schwerdtfeger, 1962:69.) One may calibrate the effect of these rotations on the location of the Euclidean centroid by appealing to one simple distribution: the sample spaced with hyperbolic uniformity along a line (Figure A.2.9). (To the Euclidean eye, the spacing looks logarithmic, of course.)

If the hyperbolic length of this distribution is $2r$, then the centroid (computed Euclideanly) is the point on the same line at ordinate

$$\frac{1}{2r} \int_{-r}^{+r} e^s \, ds = \frac{e^r - e^{-r}}{2r} = 1 + \frac{r^2}{6} + \frac{r^4}{120} + \ldots$$

(from the power series). A reasonable upper limit on r is approxi-

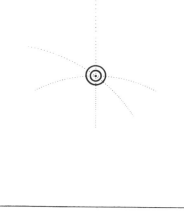

Figure A.2.9. Euclidean centroids of hyperbolic rotations of the anisotropy-uniform distribution on a line segment. The large circle shows the distribution of the centroids for rotations of the hyperbolic segment as drawn $(r = \frac{1}{2})$ in three orientations (cf. Figure A.2.5); the smaller, its middle 71% $(r = 0.35)$.

mately 1, corresponding to a sample range of $e^2 \sim 8$ in anisotropy. For r in this range, the upward bias of this centroid is approximately $r^2/6$.

To ascertain the directional dependence of this bias, we might consider rotating the hyperbolic line by 90° (Figure A.2.9). The distribution previously vertical now lies about the vertex of a Euclidean semicircle, where its angular width is $\tan^{-1}r$. The Euclidean centroid now has ordinate approximately

$$\frac{1}{2r}\int_{-r}^{+r} \cos s \, ds = \frac{\sin r}{r} = 1 - \frac{r^2}{6} + \frac{r^4}{120} - \cdots.$$

According to its leading term, this quantity is biased just as far *below* the center of rotation as the previous centroid was biased *above* it.

We may proceed to compute the same centroid for every other relative rotation of the line distribution. Figure A.2.9 summarizes these: They lie very nearly on a circle (hyperbolic or Euclidean) about the hyperbolic center of rotation, a circle of radius $r^2/6$. Note that the two centroids we just computed lie at opposite ends of a diameter: Axes of linear variation at 90° correspond to displacements of the centroid that are equal and opposite. Hence for empirical scatters, the radius of nutation of the centroid is proportional to the *difference of squares* of diameters at 90°. We have already encountered this difference of squares in the small: It is the variance explained by the single-factor model for elliptical shape distributions (Section 5.3.3). For circular scatters (the null model of Chapter 5), the leading term of this dependence vanishes: The centroid of a circular scatter in shape space, though a "biased" estimate of the center of the distribution (Mardia and Dryden, 1989a), is virtually invariant against changes of baseline.

> **The sensitivity of shape centroids to baseline indeterminacy is circular, with radius on the order of one-sixth of the largest difference of squares of the scatter's diameters in two perpendicular directions.**

A.3. A NEGATIVE COMMENT ON MORPHOLOGICAL ''DISTANCE''

The material in this appendix was originally published in slightly different form in Bookstein (1987*c*, 1988*b*). Section 4.3.4 indicated that distances measured among landmarks could not be exploited as predictors (i.e., in any technique based on multiple regression or matrix inversion) if one hoped to make biological sense of the resulting coefficients. In this appendix I argue a similar theme for a different application of morphometric variables: the measurement of net intersample "distance" (dissimilarity) by multivariate summaries such as Mahalanobis's D^2, followed by clustering or similar phenetic or phylogenetic reinterpretations. Here the difficulty is not our ignorance of the true factor structure of the data, as it was in Chapter 4, but instead the unexpectedly great variability of those differences *as we sample possible variables out of the space of alternative size and shape measures*. These standard errors, paradoxically, are *not* a diminishing function of population size. They can be made manageable only by taking a number of variables approaching the counts of base pairs used in molecular analyses; in practice, we never have access to that many independent measures of morphology.

A.3.1. The random-walk hypothesis and the range statistic

Many evolutionary data sets show a structure consistent with an underlying model of **random walk** applying to all morphometric characters simultaneously. Its goodness of fit to one data set, for instance, is demonstrated in a reanalysis of Bell's *Gasterosteus* data (Bookstein, 1988*b*). This null hypothesis, however irritating to the evolutionist (as it claims that evolutionary "rates" generally do not exist, and therefore cannot be tested against zero by regression methods), actually appears to the systematist somewhat congenial. For random walks, the variance of divergence from the initial state is *linear in time*; then morphological "distance" in squared units may be expected to serve as an unbiased measure of divergence time, and analysis of these "distances" might be expected to support a quantitative reconstruction of evolutionary trees just as if they measured branch lengths directly.

A.3. "Distance"

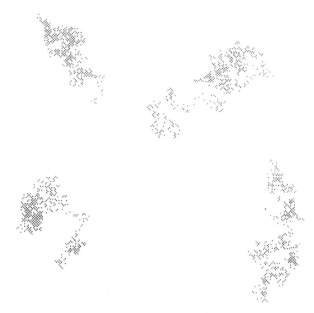

Figure A.3.1. Four separate bivariate distributions of widely divergent structures.

In practice, whenever it is attempted, the reconstruction is found to be an excessively labile function of the choice of characters. This difficulty is intrinsic to the method: It follows from a distributional property of the range of random walks that is little known outside of probability textbooks. The coefficient of variation of morphological "distance" measures is so large as to effectively eliminate them from serious consideration as sources of data for classification or taxonomic reconstruction.

For example, Figure A.3.1 presents four separate bivariate distributions manifesting diverse combinations of clusters, intercluster divergences, and remnants of putative evolutionary experiments with extreme types. *None of this structure has any meaning.* The distributions of Figure A.3.1 are merely traces of the two-dimensional random walks of Figure A.3.2. In fact, all four of these walks realize the same underlying process. Rudnick and Gaspari (1987) cite simulations showing that the typical covariance matrix of such a two-dimensional walk has eigenvalues in the ratio of $2.3 : 1$, quite sufficient to wholly misleadingly suggest high reliability of the long axis.

In the present context, the discussion of reliability of morphological "distance," we would like to establish a model for the distribution of a "net distance" based on a set of characters undergoing simultaneous random walks. These walks must be held to be independent. Otherwise, their correlation structure would involve "factors" representing either ecophenotypy or morphological integration. The former would destroy the equivalence of "distance" with divergence time and would also force a recursion of the problem (now one of measuring change in the factors), and either would reduce the number of effective characters (of which

394

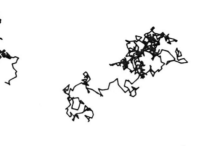

Figure A.3.2. Origin of the data in Figure A.3.1: four random walks with identical generating parameters. The x- and y-coordinates of these points are executing separate 2,500-coin walks independently. Every fifth point is shown. The coordinates plotted are the running excesses of heads over tails in the two-coin series.

it will be seen that we come up very short anyway). We shall estimate net evolutionary excursion by measuring the *maximum* mean difference from the starting mean over entire evolutionary sequences from one epoch to another. (After all, it is near such extremes that new species are likely to be declared.)

To compute the coefficient of variation of such a measurement, we need some notation. A **symmetric random walk** is the cumulative sum of an arbitrarily long series of **independent, identically distributed** elementary steps for which the probability of any positive deviation is the same as the probability of the corresponding negative deviation. For flips of a coin, these steps might be coded $+1$ for "heads" and -1 for "tails." Denote the elementary step of the walk by the variable X taking sample values $X_1, X_2, \ldots, X_k, \ldots$; then the random walk is the series $0 = S_0$, $X_1 = S_1, \ldots, X_1 + \ldots + X_k = S_k, \ldots$. For our purposes the variable X will be taken to have a finite variance σ^2; then X has expected value (population mean) zero.

The random walk $\{S_k\}$ is not to be confused with two simpler, more familiar structures that it incorporates. One is the underlying distribution of X, the elementary step (for evolutionary data, the difference between means for successive generations). Whenever the central limit theorem applies, the large-scale consequences of the distribution of X are functions mainly of σ, which is observable (in principle). The other substructure, familiar from the elementary statistics of independent samples, is the distribution of the value $S_n = \Sigma X_k$ of the walk at the nth step. Whenever X has a variance σ^2, S_n has mean zero and standard deviation $\sigma\sqrt{n}$. The "mean" and "standard deviation" here do not pertain

A.3. "Distance"

to the n replications of the sampling of X, but to replications of the entire walk, the summation of n independent samples of X each time.

We shall use the sample range $\max_{1 \le k \le n}|S_k|$ as a measure of "distance" character by character. It is convenient to study this feature in the form of its probability distribution $P(\max_{1 \le k \le n}|S_k| \ge x\sigma\sqrt{n})$ for various values of x. Figure A.3.3 demonstrates this **range statistic** by applying it to a random walk previously published in Bookstein (1987c): the running lead of heads over tails for 20,000 simulated flips of a fair coin. The maximum excursion of this walk from zero is to the positive side, achieved at about step 18,000 (which location is not unexpected – Bookstein, 1987c). The state of the walk at this maximum happens to be 191 (the accumulation of 191 more heads than tails). In the case of the coin flips, we know the standard deviation, 1.0, of the individual flip, and we can compute the final-step standard deviation directly as $1.0(20,000)^{1/2} = 141.4$. In the case of evolutionary time series, this standard deviation must be estimated instead from the elementary increments. Its value is their root sum square: Whether the speed of the series is constant or variable, we have

Figure A.3.3. The range statistic x, exemplified using a random walk of 20,000 steps. The horizontal band entraps the maximum excursion of the walk from the starting value. Along the vertical line at the right is graphed, toward the left, the distribution of the expected final state S_n of the walk: normal around zero with standard deviation $\sigma\sqrt{n}$ (estimated by the root sum square of all the elementary steps of the walk) indicated by the spacing of the tick marks. To the right of this vertical is shown the distribution of the statistic x in units of that final-state standard deviation. The upper tail of this distribution (2.25 for a 5% cutoff) may be considered to suggest *anagenesis* (directionality or trend) as an evolutionary interpretation; the lower tail (0.62 for a 5% cutoff), representing walks improbably constrained, corresponds to the evolutionary finding of *stasis*. The null model of random walk is seen to separate these two findings. For the example, we compute $x \sim 1.35$, corresponding to a cumulative probability of 0.65; the walk here is apparently quite typical. After Bookstein (1988b).

$$\mathrm{est}\left(\sigma\sqrt{n}\right) = \left[\Sigma_k(S_k - S_{k-1})^2\right]^{1/2},$$

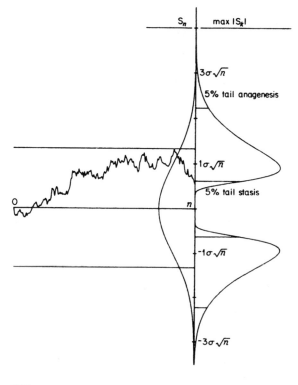

396

in which form it can be very easily supplied by any statistical package.

In Figure A.3.3, the curve to the left of the vertical line is the normal distribution of mean zero and standard deviation $\sigma\sqrt{n}$: approximation to the distribution of S_n according to the central limit theorem. To the right of this same vertical line is drawn the theoretical distribution of the sample range statistic

$$x = \max_{1 \leq k \leq n} |S_k| / \sigma\sqrt{n},$$

the observed range as a multiple of the standard deviation imputed to the final step. It is drawn in duplicate, once for superimposing over positive excursions, once for negative. In the coin flip used as example, the observed value of x is at about the 65th percentile of the theoretical distribution: We see how typical a random walk it is, in spite of its apparent "features" – the sharp trend at the outset, the jump some 30% of the way along, the near-stasis through the last two-thirds. Random walks fool the innocent observer with epiphenomena of this sort all the time (Feller, 1957).

Let me emphasize the delicacy of this construct: It is the distribution of the computed maximum sample excursion (the horizontal band in Figure A.3.3), a value observed once per random walk, over the *very* high dimensional space of all long random walks having a step of finite variance. That this distribution is essentially unique is a consequence of the central limit theorem; but, as is plain in the figure, the distribution of x is far from normal. The precise distribution, graphed here, is a deduction from the formula for the same probability in cumulative form, as given by Spitzer (1964) and tabulated in Bookstein (1987c). That shape is the subject of the following:

Theorem of the scaled maximum. For any $x > 0$, define $F(x)$ as the infinite series

$$F(x) = 1 - \frac{4}{\pi} \sum_{k=0}^{\infty} \frac{(-1)^k}{2k + 1} \exp\left[-\frac{\pi^2}{8}(2k + 1)^2 x \right].$$

Then for any symmetric random walk for which the elementary step X has finite variance σ^2, for any $x > 0$ we have

$$\lim_{n \to \infty} \text{prob}\left(\max_{1 \leq k \leq n} |S_k| \leq \sigma x \sqrt{n} \right) = 1 - F(x^{-2}).$$

In practice one must ignore the caveat about limiting behavior ("$n \to \infty$").

The statistic x has mean 1.27 and variance 0.269, and hence a coefficient of variation (as observed over replicate random walks) of 0.40. Because x is so long-tailed, the coefficient of variation of its square is 0.88, much larger.

397

The principal property of this statistic x that will give it immense power to block evolutionary inference is the fact that *it is not n-limited*. As an ordinary population sample becomes larger and larger, for example, the error of estimate for most familiar population parameters – mean, variance, slope of a regression on time or other covariate – becomes smaller and smaller. The more extensive the data, the more precisely their parameters can be estimated. But in random walk, there is only one single true parameter, the step variance; only this quantity σ^2 gains in precision with the length of the series. The statistic x, normalized to the expected "scale" of the data, does not do so: It retains its finite confidence interval, 0.62 to 2.25, no matter how large the sample becomes.

> **The standardized range of a random walk has a coefficient of variation of about 0.40; the squared range, 0.88. These do not drop as sample size increases.**

A.3.2. The coefficient of variation of "distance"

From the unexpected stubbornness of this coefficient of variation there follows a very serious objection to most current studies of evolutionary tempo and mode and to most current applications of morphological "distance" to classification and to ordination. The objection can be disabled only in the presence of conjoint information about the putative causes of the processes under study. Even a single exogenous variable, perhaps ecological or paleoclimatological, would be sufficient to wrest the analysis out of the domain of the random-walk hypothesis and into the much more tractable realm of linearly modeled dependence on a noncumulative causal *factor*. But in the absence of direct measurement of the causes of selective change, studies of evolution based purely on the morphology of single species over time are going to prove useless, in the main, for *any* insights about process and *any* reliable or phylogenetically valid taxonomies. Unless the hypothesis of random walk can be rejected, distributions in morphological space are devoid of measurable parameters, and *all* of the following forms of evolutionary "inference" are automatically blocked in most applications.

1. The interpretation of within-group covariance matrices. As is plain in Figure A.3.2, the eigenstructure of the observed trajectory of a random walk is meaningless. Any within-group covariance matrix combines a true underlying factor structure of phenotypic covariance with the contribution of random walk as it applies to the generational means. The longer the period covered by the data "within groups," the larger this second component. Re-

sponse to an exogenous cause executing a random walk inflates this matrix equally destructively.

2. Standardizing group differences to the within-group covariance matrix, as in computation of D^2 or discriminant functions. If the random-walk hypothesis is valid, the matrices whose quotient is to be diagonalized – the between-group and within-group covariance structures – have no meaning either separately or together. (Consider the meaninglessness of the "discrimination" between the first and last halves of the walks in Figure A.3.2.) If groups share a factor structure, canonical analysis under conditions of random walk will continue to conceal it (recall Section 4.3.3), while at the same time distorting the description of intergroup relationships. That D^2 is proportional to time is scant comfort when its value is rendered unreliable by so many other factors. For the first one or two canonical variates extracted, the distribution of x is even more long-tailed, as they are computed in the direction of multivariate space for which the between-group variance (approximately equivalent to range) is as great a fraction as possible of that within group, thus biasing the "findings" even more in the direction of trend.

3. Optimistic notions of character sampling underlying "net" dissimilarities. Suppose we accept the null hypothesis that most of our morphometric characters are undergoing independent random walk, so that the vectors of their interstratum differences may be used as measures of factor-free evolutionary divergence. We would then average ranges, in the form of x or x^2, over a suite of characters. Now, at last, we are in the context of the precise model governed by the scaled-maximum theorem; but its implications are devastating. Recall that, on the null hypothesis, the coefficient of variation of x is 0.40; of x^2, 0.88. *It is not a function of population size.* We can hope to reduce it only by increasing the number of characters. But it requires the averaging of 64 characters (for Euclidean distance, 310 characters!) to reduce the coefficient of variation of net dissimilarity measures even to the value 0.05; and most interesting questions in numerical taxonomy deal with discriminations of similarity well below that limen. It is not necessary to accept the computed distribution of the range statistic x to support this conclusion; even the χ^2 generated by the use of $|S_n|$ rather than $\max_{1 \le k \le n}|S_k|$ has a coefficient of variation high enough to prove impractical. Any such computation further assumes that characters are not correlated by virtue of any common factors, an assertion that is contradicted by everything we know about pleiotropy.

The conclusion that emerges is distinctly pessimistic. Morphological distance measures arrived at as the result of reasonable amounts of human effort are unlikely *ever* to support phylogenetic inference. Stable distances arise only in the domain of character sets as large as the count of base pairs used in DNA-based reconstructions. These explicitly accept the Markov model for conversion of transition probabilities into elapsed time; they compensate for the coefficient of variation of these estimates by aggregating evidence over huge numbers of putatively independent characters – and even here there are problems of nonindependence interfering with inferences from likelihood-based "distances."

The empirically oriented morphometrician should not despair. All the techniques that crumple against the probable finding of random walk are those for which morphology is the *independent variable* of the evolutionary analysis, *with no other measurements taken*. Analyses escape this critique when morphology is the *dependent* variable, when form is explained by means of forces and exogenous factors: not "time," but age, temperature, feeding behavior, climate, coenosis. That is to say, the biologist must measure the factors that underlie evolutionary explanation, not merely their shadows as conceivably encoded in form. It is unreasonable to expect the measurement of form to lead to firm quantitative findings about the processes that lead to it when those processes are not adumbrated as part of the same data base. The arena for interplay between morphometrics and evolutionary biology is the study of effects on form.

A.4. DATA SETS

In this appendix are listed several of the data sets used for the running examples of this book. The author will dump an electronic copy of any of these to readers who send him a message via electronic mail. As of this writing (December 1990), the author's electronic addresses are

Fred_L._Bookstein@um.cc.umich.edu

and

usersm7n@umichum.bitnet

A.4.1. The University School Study subsample

Listed here are the coordinates of eight craniofacial landmarks for 36 normal Ann Arbor boys and 26 girls observed near the ages of 8 and 14 years. The fields of the following records are, left to right: identification number of the subject; age of the record, in months; sex (1 for boys, 2 for girls); and Cartesian coordinates, in inches, of Sella, Nasion, Basion, Gonion, Menton, Ethmoid registration, Anterior nasal spine, and Posterior nasal spine in a coordinate system with Sella set to $(6, 6)$ and Nasion directly in front of it. For operational definitions of these landmarks, see Section 3.4.2. The coordinates are digitized directly from x-rays and thus represent a magnification of some 12.7% with respect to true anatomical scale at the midsagittal plane, upon which the bilateral landmarks Gonion and SER have been averaged. The history of the data set of which these are a very small part has been set down in Riolo et al. (1974). These data are analyzed in Sections 6.5.1 (three landmarks) and 7.4.3.

```
1872  96 1 6.000 6.000 9.018 6.000 4.941 4.710 5.356 3.229 7.528 1.739 7.007
      6.069 8.823 4.159 6.740 4.265
1872 168 1 6.000 6.000 9.268 6.000 4.876 4.604 5.165 2.772 7.836 1.160 7.049
      6.121 9.043 3.802 6.826 3.997
1890  96 2 6.000 6.000 9.142 6.000 5.082 4.685 5.776 3.414 7.441 1.898 7.110
      5.961 8.749 3.984 6.883 4.359
1890 170 2 6.000 6.000 9.385 6.000 5.036 4.587 5.580 3.128 7.549 1.259 7.185
      6.017 8.906 3.672 6.816 4.108
1953  96 1 6.000 6.000 8.870 6.000 4.817 4.591 5.433 3.407 7.494 1.522 6.959
      5.945 8.736 4.122 6.754 4.241
1953 168 1 6.000 6.000 9.086 6.000 4.607 4.242 5.199 3.037 7.676  .905 7.047
      6.077 9.050 3.718 6.742 3.954
1956  94 2 6.000 6.000 8.789 6.000 4.800 4.622 5.546 3.175 7.859 1.917 7.036
      5.972 8.599 3.972 6.701 4.293
1956 173 2 6.000 6.000 8.999 6.000 4.654 4.459 5.493 2.713 8.303 1.269 7.048
      5.972 8.776 3.678 6.767 4.086
2000  96 1 6.000 6.000 8.920 6.000 4.872 4.867 5.442 3.560 7.368 1.779 6.947
      6.137 8.678 4.051 6.702 4.228
2000 167 1 6.000 6.000 9.121 6.000 4.696 4.677 5.118 3.240 7.358 1.220 7.074
      6.098 8.908 3.700 6.522 4.014
2002  92 1 6.000 6.000 8.893 6.000 5.028 4.822 5.609 3.359 7.609 1.714 6.818
      5.908 8.781 4.052 6.620 4.349
2002 167 1 6.000 6.000 9.099 6.000 4.933 4.450 5.821 2.812 8.192  .948 6.873
      5.960 9.219 3.730 6.817 3.988
2007  97 1 6.000 6.000 8.723 6.000 4.984 4.748 5.375 3.554 7.323 1.757 6.897
      6.003 8.443 4.230 6.679 4.425
2007 162 1 6.000 6.000 8.941 6.000 4.877 4.541 5.199 3.234 7.448 1.289 6.928
      5.983 8.708 3.922 6.636 4.166
2026  96 1 6.000 6.000 8.886 6.000 4.975 5.099 5.605 3.829 7.601 2.278 7.059
      5.942 8.732 4.250 6.779 4.518
2026 168 1 6.000 6.000 9.079 6.000 4.805 5.049 5.355 3.314 7.861 1.579 7.086
      5.906 9.014 3.880 6.761 4.310
2101  96 1 6.000 6.000 9.082 6.000 4.969 4.400 5.622 3.042 7.562 1.260 7.020
      5.923 9.117 3.959 6.842 3.989
2101 167 1 6.000 6.000 9.319 6.000 4.808 4.186 5.540 2.434 7.775  .403 7.033
      5.960 9.383 3.544 6.884 3.664
2102  96 2 6.000 6.000 8.809 6.000 4.828 4.769 5.338 3.495 7.298 2.010 6.988
      5.933 8.593 4.114 6.333 4.413
2102 168 2 6.000 6.000 8.959 6.000 4.511 4.571 5.062 3.193 7.311 1.453 6.962
      6.000 8.761 3.679 6.398 4.224
2108  96 1 6.000 6.000 9.049 6.000 5.000 4.708 5.392 3.438 7.066 1.645 7.161
      6.066 8.794 3.964 6.689 4.333
2108 167 1 6.000 6.000 9.286 6.000 4.809 4.438 5.111 2.802 7.193  .750 7.227
      6.028 9.058 3.483 6.750 4.048
2109  96 2 6.000 6.000 8.694 6.000 4.992 4.814 5.396 3.624 7.353 1.970 7.072
      6.116 8.415 4.079 6.543 4.417
2109 172 2 6.000 6.000 8.872 6.000 4.762 4.464 5.234 3.130 7.727 1.319 7.080
      6.154 8.622 3.809 6.480 4.197
2113  95 1 6.000 6.000 8.924 6.000 5.029 4.624 5.577 3.275 7.556 1.823 7.059
      5.997 8.820 3.967 6.754 4.270
2113 172 1 6.000 6.000 9.219 6.000 5.005 4.555 5.446 2.668 8.001  .845 7.056
      5.974 9.214 3.686 6.754 3.994
2123  96 2 6.000 6.000 8.926 6.000 5.122 4.510 5.640 3.345 7.862 2.003 7.109
      6.044 8.705 4.109 6.845 4.313
```

```
2123 168 2 6.000 6.000 9.151 6.000 5.007 4.471 5.381 3.209 7.803 1.401 7.205
         6.129 8.744 3.864 6.761 4.152
2124  96 1 6.000 6.000 8.939 6.000 4.809 4.959 5.563 3.302 7.628 1.656 7.157
         6.118 8.756 4.138 6.844 4.400
2124 167 1 6.000 6.000 9.157 6.000 4.714 4.731 5.492 2.902 7.986 1.190 7.261
         6.098 9.062 3.880 6.860 4.143
2135  96 1 6.000 6.000 8.642 6.000 4.881 4.954 5.350 3.535 7.239 1.960 6.947
         6.032 8.323 4.172 6.486 4.406
2135 168 1 6.000 6.000 8.827 6.000 4.840 4.806 5.137 3.097 7.150 1.226 7.009
         6.009 8.368 3.757 6.397 4.144
2190  90 2 6.000 6.000 8.834 6.000 5.012 4.916 5.699 3.557 7.797 1.952 7.122
         5.993 8.760 4.150 6.702 4.465
2190 162 2 6.000 6.000 9.041 6.000 4.864 4.820 5.590 3.046 8.301 1.404 7.186
         5.932 9.069 3.842 6.788 4.169
2191  96 1 6.000 6.000 8.917 6.000 4.954 4.407 5.504 3.294 7.681 1.699 7.110
         5.891 8.641 4.194 6.447 4.309
2191 171 1 6.000 6.000 9.092 6.000 4.739 4.457 5.298 2.967 7.749 1.184 7.154
         5.941 8.837 3.925 6.385 4.154
2192  90 2 6.000 6.000 8.777 6.000 5.021 4.695 5.588 3.565 7.424 2.061 7.005
         6.042 8.644 4.196 6.719 4.384
2192 162 2 6.000 6.000 8.988 6.000 4.922 4.562 5.485 3.136 7.708 1.391 7.053
         6.162 8.835 3.892 6.704 4.201
2196  96 2 6.000 6.000 8.687 6.000 4.917 4.887 5.374 3.578 7.265 2.000 7.067
         6.041 8.453 4.241 6.445 4.516
2196 172 2 6.000 6.000 8.866 6.000 4.872 4.891 5.193 3.182 7.454 1.361 7.098
         6.015 8.644 3.938 6.422 4.250
2197  95 2 6.000 6.000 8.810 6.000 4.929 4.587 5.552 3.588 7.455 2.035 7.161
         6.086 8.741 4.236 6.732 4.371
2197 170 2 6.000 6.000 9.046 6.000 4.774 4.399 5.322 3.200 7.630 1.362 7.203
         6.133 8.843 3.877 6.626 4.084
2198  90 2 6.000 6.000 8.785 6.000 5.040 4.756 5.693 3.538 7.532 2.140 7.125
         6.019 8.772 4.117 6.743 4.369
2198 163 2 6.000 6.000 8.976 6.000 4.928 4.651 5.682 3.154 8.008 1.575 7.099
         6.053 9.034 3.790 6.789 4.121
2245  95 1 6.000 6.000 9.085 6.000 5.043 4.790 5.435 3.274 7.399 1.659 7.119
         6.036 8.955 3.911 6.783 4.247
2245 168 1 6.000 6.000 9.257 6.000 4.901 4.695 5.172 2.757 7.627  .865 7.102
         6.065 9.111 3.581 6.604 3.964
2257  97 1 6.000 6.000 8.863 6.000 4.816 4.757 5.378 3.546 7.379 1.992 7.021
         5.956 8.590 4.192 6.446 4.311
2257 168 1 6.000 6.000 8.951 6.000 4.699 4.615 5.363 2.995 7.901 1.445 7.044
         5.985 8.938 4.016 6.552 3.887
2259  96 1 6.000 6.000 9.116 6.000 4.748 4.760 5.303 3.407 7.196 1.569 7.042
         6.019 8.707 4.010 6.590 4.291
2259 168 1 6.000 6.000 9.339 6.000 4.739 4.553 5.160 2.939 7.306  .781 7.088
         5.965 8.960 3.555 6.557 4.055
2271  96 2 6.000 6.000 8.837 6.000 5.091 4.731 5.546 3.320 7.703 1.834 7.094
         6.035 8.773 4.072 6.839 4.331
2271 167 2 6.000 6.000 9.031 6.000 4.919 4.507 5.404 2.783 7.786  .989 7.095
         6.004 9.026 3.699 6.776 4.036
2276  95 2 6.000 6.000 8.838 6.000 5.016 4.529 5.795 3.115 8.319 1.972 7.078
         5.981 8.848 4.218 6.961 4.331
2276 168 2 6.000 6.000 9.037 6.000 4.844 4.391 5.646 2.664 8.553 1.440 7.146
         6.001 9.041 3.954 6.853 4.207
2279  96 2 6.000 6.000 8.805 6.000 4.773 4.817 5.432 3.586 7.151 1.917 7.070
         6.134 8.502 4.029 6.611 4.373
2279 168 2 6.000 6.000 8.928 6.000 4.719 4.640 5.095 3.358 7.165 1.406 7.072
         6.129 8.705 3.820 6.423 4.163
2286  90 2 6.000 6.000 8.873 6.000 4.770 4.722 5.408 3.502 7.237 1.777 7.019
         6.085 8.612 4.086 6.626 4.340
```

```
2286 166 2 6.000 6.000 9.057 6.000 4.658 4.620 5.180 3.220 7.272 1.192 7.034
         6.100 8.701 3.780 6.524 4.155
2367  96 1 6.000 6.000 9.015 6.000 4.779 4.715 5.448 3.086 7.637 1.544 7.046
         5.943 8.711 3.954 6.594 4.212
2367 168 1 6.000 6.000 9.289 6.000 4.675 4.445 5.339 2.495 7.935  .754 7.116
         5.963 8.957 3.600 6.570 3.887
2373  96 1 6.000 6.000 8.884 6.000 5.113 4.601 5.718 3.362 7.799 1.920 7.146
         6.102 8.789 4.176 6.812 4.308
2373 167 1 6.000 6.000 9.025 6.000 5.187 4.466 5.697 2.873 8.320 1.385 7.176
         6.105 9.009 4.081 6.863 4.094
2377  90 1 6.000 6.000 9.034 6.000 5.099 4.647 5.695 3.348 7.631 1.935 7.087
         5.995 8.913 4.112 6.855 4.278
2377 170 1 6.000 6.000 9.335 6.000 4.954 4.365 5.601 2.713 7.991 1.266 7.137
         6.020 9.332 3.721 6.847 4.036
2378  97 2 6.000 6.000 8.726 6.000 4.953 4.789 5.431 3.627 7.618 1.980 6.973
         5.989 8.679 4.075 6.759 4.275
2378 168 2 6.000 6.000 8.928 6.000 4.859 4.675 5.328 3.173 7.990 1.513 7.026
         5.979 8.971 3.774 6.755 4.071
2392  96 1 6.000 6.000 9.029 6.000 5.065 4.641 5.722 3.166 7.788 1.830 7.084
         5.923 9.052 4.118 6.842 4.238
2392 167 1 6.000 6.000 9.378 6.000 5.002 4.411 5.697 2.567 8.319 1.180 7.103
         5.972 9.507 3.781 6.954 3.991
2398  96 1 6.000 6.000 9.007 6.000 4.918 4.760 5.479 3.324 7.451 1.768 7.050
         6.104 8.801 4.065 6.781 4.258
2398 168 1 6.000 6.000 9.235 6.000 4.627 4.780 5.098 2.791 7.530  .827 7.155
         6.050 8.935 3.548 6.619 3.970
2399  90 1 6.000 6.000 9.084 6.000 5.000 4.707 5.636 3.206 7.989 1.798 7.244
         6.115 8.973 4.012 6.967 4.319
2399 173 1 6.000 6.000 9.257 6.000 4.791 4.440 5.422 2.425 8.305  .837 7.225
         6.190 9.092 3.710 6.805 4.101
2400  90 1 6.000 6.000 8.961 6.000 4.822 4.645 5.318 3.332 7.582 1.717 7.052
         5.943 8.732 4.024 6.768 4.225
2400 162 1 6.000 6.000 9.092 6.000 4.680 4.427 5.202 2.817 7.758 1.132 7.083
         5.976 8.962 3.819 6.718 4.030
2406  95 2 6.000 6.000 8.964 6.000 4.838 4.827 5.397 3.217 7.550 1.777 7.211
         6.032 8.900 4.048 6.792 4.253
2406 168 2 6.000 6.000 9.183 6.000 4.662 4.762 5.359 2.749 7.896 1.167 7.122
         6.043 9.176 3.773 6.725 4.038
2407  96 1 6.000 6.000 8.763 6.000 5.024 4.415 5.553 3.099 7.733 1.827 6.966
         6.019 8.641 3.995 6.650 4.274
2407 169 1 6.000 6.000 8.941 6.000 4.744 4.217 5.448 2.482 7.943 1.007 6.914
         5.989 8.966 3.610 6.760 3.998
2410  96 1 6.000 6.000 9.183 6.000 4.894 4.806 5.681 3.314 7.732 2.014 7.328
         6.054 8.922 3.996 6.761 4.422
2410 167 1 6.000 6.000 9.396 6.000 4.766 4.737 5.425 3.001 7.796 1.609 7.376
         6.034 9.146 3.639 6.733 4.196
2411  91 1 6.000 6.000 9.152 6.000 5.178 4.670 5.807 3.211 7.971 1.763 7.126
         5.956 8.854 3.999 6.869 4.277
2411 162 1 6.000 6.000 9.328 6.000 5.068 4.565 5.600 2.910 8.072 1.230 7.186
         6.015 9.151 3.651 6.818 4.034
2429  91 1 6.000 6.000 9.004 6.000 5.028 4.715 5.703 3.381 8.090 1.797 7.022
         6.217 8.943 4.242 6.924 4.410
2429 162 1 6.000 6.000 9.230 6.000 4.966 4.550 5.498 2.878 8.043 1.142 7.085
         6.237 9.099 4.054 6.937 4.194
2437  91 2 6.000 6.000 8.814 6.000 4.843 4.613 5.218 3.421 7.380 1.809 6.876
         6.104 8.843 4.106 6.678 4.299
2437 163 2 6.000 6.000 8.990 6.000 4.632 4.413 5.083 3.026 7.480 1.321 6.884
         6.148 8.900 3.718 6.537 4.133
2449  91 2 6.000 6.000 9.100 6.000 5.069 4.859 5.931 3.259 8.253 1.826 7.205
         6.009 9.161 4.172 7.001 4.297
```

```
2449 162 2 6.000 6.000 9.269 6.000 4.888 4.759 5.810 2.996 8.528 1.534 7.193
         6.067 9.332 3.986 6.979 4.171
2539  96 2 6.000 6.000 8.835 6.000 4.844 4.572 5.543 3.081 7.571 1.615 7.047
         5.951 8.928 3.971 6.810 4.197
2539 168 2 6.000 6.000 8.976 6.000 4.631 4.333 5.358 2.650 7.819  .988 7.049
         5.974 9.001 3.804 6.701 3.951
2541  96 1 6.000 6.000 8.985 6.000 4.882 4.565 5.501 3.151 7.910 1.862 7.129
         6.007 8.789 4.053 6.847 4.114
2541 168 1 6.000 6.000 9.137 6.000 4.816 4.329 5.421 2.702 8.235 1.308 7.129
         5.995 9.029 3.726 6.773 3.833
2545  95 1 6.000 6.000 9.017 6.000 5.053 4.517 5.571 3.131 7.738 1.718 7.166
         6.019 8.930 3.962 7.017 4.202
2545 168 1 6.000 6.000 9.185 6.000 4.977 4.456 5.492 2.790 8.058 1.235 7.187
         6.040 9.127 3.703 6.954 3.969
2548  90 2 6.000 6.000 8.618 6.000 5.291 4.654 5.741 3.004 7.764 1.873 7.140
         6.248 8.735 4.171 6.761 4.339
2548 162 2 6.000 6.000 8.754 6.000 5.178 4.422 5.698 2.409 8.160 1.341 7.132
         6.242 8.872 3.817 6.801 4.078
2549  95 1 6.000 6.000 8.960 6.000 5.015 4.707 5.468 3.137 7.721 1.746 7.174
         6.045 8.872 4.032 6.765 4.159
2549 168 1 6.000 6.000 9.170 6.000 4.781 4.527 5.104 2.711 7.796  .980 7.239
         6.167 9.024 3.661 6.671 3.930
2561  96 2 6.000 6.000 8.657 6.000 5.045 5.063 5.574 3.581 7.376 2.094 7.158
         6.135 8.586 4.221 6.759 4.537
2561 168 2 6.000 6.000 8.777 6.000 4.810 4.861 5.394 3.227 7.529 1.510 7.149
         6.112 8.735 3.890 6.626 4.263
2572  90 2 6.000 6.000 8.964 6.000 4.894 4.524 5.415 3.406 7.372 1.500 7.057
         5.972 8.946 3.832 6.775 4.159
2572 168 2 6.000 6.000 9.110 6.000 4.906 4.462 5.209 2.991 7.647  .888 7.015
         5.912 9.019 3.586 6.616 3.971
2578  96 1 6.000 6.000 8.968 6.000 4.801 4.664 5.461 3.423 7.289 1.693 6.969
         5.925 8.823 4.080 6.844 4.292
2578 168 1 6.000 6.000 9.221 6.000 4.590 4.358 5.314 2.680 7.874  .778 7.032
         5.924 9.312 3.631 6.957 3.925
2580  96 1 6.000 6.000 9.018 6.000 4.991 4.493 5.472 2.890 7.747 1.393 7.129
         5.989 8.907 3.897 6.866 4.068
2580 168 1 6.000 6.000 9.170 6.000 4.844 4.243 5.405 2.396 8.113  .736 7.137
         6.123 9.103 3.683 6.981 3.816
2594  90 1 6.000 6.000 8.867 6.000 5.009 4.636 5.442 3.272 7.560 1.705 7.022
         6.159 8.885 3.975 6.815 4.183
2594 168 1 6.000 6.000 9.068 6.000 4.839 4.500 5.046 2.726 7.851  .911 7.077
         6.115 8.965 3.480 6.597 3.815
2595  95 1 6.000 6.000 8.676 6.000 4.780 4.748 5.517 3.233 7.688 1.895 6.920
         6.008 8.868 4.048 6.655 4.222
2595 167 1 6.000 6.000 8.799 6.000 4.475 4.459 5.042 2.585 7.963 1.022 6.930
         6.015 8.995 3.618 6.630 3.937
2596  90 2 6.000 6.000 8.712 6.000 5.162 4.908 5.587 3.512 7.464 2.108 7.083
         6.039 8.696 4.213 6.714 4.374
2596 162 2 6.000 6.000 8.925 6.000 4.995 4.786 5.544 3.045 7.967 1.673 7.102
         6.019 9.011 3.928 6.721 4.182
2603  99 1 6.000 6.000 8.807 6.000 5.120 4.541 5.669 3.150 7.679 1.730 6.939
         6.140 8.821 4.081 6.741 4.241
2603 168 1 6.000 6.000 8.986 6.000 5.009 4.334 5.424 2.617 7.713 1.016 6.961
         6.135 8.982 3.700 6.671 3.923
2680  95 2 6.000 6.000 8.898 6.000 4.585 4.800 5.272 3.517 7.280 1.790 7.077
         5.949 8.593 3.970 6.622 4.328
2680 168 2 6.000 6.000 8.995 6.000 4.563 4.710 5.167 3.090 7.705 1.284 7.099
         5.955 8.785 3.742 6.554 4.156
2726  96 2 6.000 6.000 8.715 6.000 4.925 4.741 5.468 3.446 7.569 1.829 6.981
         6.102 8.731 4.104 6.791 4.366
```

```
2726 168 2 6.000 6.000 8.863 6.000 4.708 4.721 5.017 3.051 7.559 1.204 6.999
         6.121 8.777 3.801 6.627 4.110
2779 101 1 6.000 6.000 9.011 6.000 4.822 4.572 5.216 3.504 7.230 1.530 7.104
         6.073 8.730 3.802 6.773 4.240
2779 162 1 6.000 6.000 9.241 6.000 4.589 4.353 5.047 3.008 7.457  .798 7.192
         6.092 8.965 3.426 6.723 3.980
2781  96 2 6.000 6.000 8.828 6.000 4.866 4.777 5.580 3.792 7.267 2.253 6.975
         6.002 8.491 4.143 6.650 4.423
2781 167 2 6.000 6.000 8.964 6.000 4.763 4.666 5.525 3.448 7.502 1.810 6.967
         6.122 8.708 4.005 6.635 4.259
2802  90 1 6.000 6.000 8.891 6.000 4.952 4.877 5.823 3.300 7.827 1.951 7.078
         6.074 8.832 4.150 6.838 4.378
2802 168 1 6.000 6.000 9.085 6.000 4.796 4.718 5.607 2.898 8.103 1.405 7.034
         6.044 9.001 3.808 6.749 4.184
```

A.4.2. Apert syndrome

The following are the data underlying the example of Section 7.5.
Alternate pairs of lines list coordinates for the Ann Arbor age-
and sex-specific subsample means and for 14 cases of Apert
syndrome from the Institute for Reconstructive Plastic Surgery,
New York University, Joseph G. McCarthy, Director. The landmarks (Section 3.4.2) are Anterior nasal spine, Sella, Spheno-
ethmoid registration, Nasion, Orbitale, Inferior zygoma, Pterygo-
maxillary fissure, and Posterior nasal spine. One landmark is
missing for the ninth case; its coordinates are coded -0.

```
Fem.  9  8.72  4.03  6.00  6.00  7.06  6.04  8.86  6.00
          8.04  5.02  7.53  4.29  6.65  4.65  6.72  4.29
         12.59  8.90  9.74  9.70 11.07 10.16 12.13 10.67
         11.85  9.49 11.53  8.72 10.80  8.86 11.08  8.64
Male  7  8.77  4.12  6.00  6.00  7.07  6.03  8.91  6.00
          8.06  5.00  7.55  4.32  6.69  4.63  6.76  4.33
         12.34  8.58 10.04 10.04 11.36  9.98 12.69 10.12
         11.74  9.09 11.30  8.50 10.74  9.01 10.75  8.67
Fem.  6  8.63  4.20  6.00  6.00  7.04  6.05  8.77  6.00
          7.98  5.08  7.49  4.45  6.64  4.74  6.72  4.45
         12.19  9.43  9.76 10.31 11.00 10.59 12.12 10.96
         11.67  9.99 11.28  9.47 10.50  9.52 10.66  9.28
Male  6  8.77  4.20  6.00  6.00  7.06  6.03  8.86  6.00
          8.07  5.04  7.58  4.39  6.71  4.70  6.80  4.38
         12.29  8.31 10.53  9.79 11.29  9.75 12.70  9.70
         12.08  8.95 11.56  8.54 10.89  8.78 11.15  8.68
Male 15  9.07  3.68  6.00  6.00  7.12  6.05  9.20  6.00
          8.26  4.84  7.69  3.93  6.69  4.39  6.74  3.97
         12.11  9.39  9.70 10.24 11.05 10.47 12.21 11.00
         11.58  9.77 11.26  8.80 10.38  9.03 10.29  8.80
Male 13  9.01  3.77  6.00  6.00  7.10  6.03  9.13  6.00
          8.22  4.88  7.69  4.04  6.70  4.47  6.75  4.06
         12.23  9.09  9.57  9.87 10.84 10.18 11.96 10.99
         11.51  9.46 11.13  8.80 10.34  8.92 10.39  8.69
Fem. 11  8.79  3.94  6.00  6.00  7.07  6.05  8.92  6.00
          8.09  4.99  7.58  4.23  6.64  4.62  6.69  4.22
         12.46  8.16 10.12  9.14 11.39  9.31 12.56  9.79
         11.99  8.43 11.59  7.83 10.73  7.91 10.93  7.90
```

```
Fem. 15   8.92   3.83   6.00   6.00   7.08   6.04   9.03   6.00
                 8.15   4.95   7.62   4.14   6.64   4.59   6.70   4.13
          10.97   8.49   8.92   9.97  10.13  10.06  11.45  10.01
                 10.65   9.13  10.15   8.38   9.42   8.84   9.57   8.48
Fem. 12   8.81   3.88   6.00   6.00   7.08   6.03   8.95   6.00
                 8.11   4.97   7.60   4.18   6.64   4.56   6.71   4.19
          11.73   9.17   9.48  10.35  10.66  10.44  12.00  10.62
                 11.38   9.59  10.98   8.99  -0.    -0.     9.99   9.14
Fem. 15   8.92   3.83   6.00   6.00   7.08   6.04   9.03   6.00
                 8.15   4.95   7.62   4.14   6.64   4.59   6.70   4.13
          12.66   9.14  10.00  10.33  11.45  10.39  12.77  10.83
                 11.98   9.61  11.59   8.95  10.88   8.90  10.86   9.09
Fem. 15   8.92   3.83   6.00   6.00   7.08   6.04   9.03   6.00
                 8.15   4.95   7.62   4.14   6.64   4.59   6.70   4.13
          12.31   8.94   9.75   9.51  10.93  10.09  12.15  10.44
                 11.54   9.16  11.33   8.49  10.43   8.99  10.72   8.71
Male 10   8.90   3.95   6.00   6.00   7.09   6.03   9.02   6.00
                 8.16   4.94   7.63   4.18   6.70   4.54   6.77   4.18
          12.12   9.36   9.82  10.68  11.16  10.82  12.39  10.77
                 11.62   9.91  11.23   9.27  10.47   9.43  10.49   9.33
Male 15   9.07   3.68   6.00   6.00   7.12   6.05   9.20   6.00
                 8.26   4.84   7.69   3.93   6.69   4.39   6.74   3.97
          11.97   8.88   9.86  10.51  10.87  10.48  12.71  10.52
                 11.37   9.52  11.13   8.93  10.46   9.25  10.34   9.17
Fem. 15   8.92   3.83   6.00   6.00   7.08   6.04   9.03   6.00
                 8.15   4.95   7.62   4.14   6.64   4.59   6.70   4.13
          11.79   9.71   9.42  11.36  10.80  11.18  12.03  11.49
                 11.32  10.12  10.77   9.65   9.98   9.96  10.07   9.85
```

A.4.3. *Globorotalia*

The following are latitude, longitude, area (in units of 0.001 mm^2), and coordinates (in μm) of landmarks #1, #2, and #3 and pseudolandmarks #12, #23, and #31 (see Section 3.4.3.4) for 20 mean forms of *Globorotalia truncatulinoides* as computed by Lohmann's method (1983) of mean eigenshapes. The data were digitized by Fred Bookstein from outlines supplied by Lohmann.

```
16.3   66  151  -18   45  379  212  428-339  166  164  490  -64  200-175
17.8   63   87   -8   35  279  162  326-220  122  129  368  -20  141-108
20.6   68  200    0  -56  407  283  562-288  164  178  584   16  276-187
21.7   68  153  -10  -33  338  259  509-230  132  158  503   38  243-155
22.5   68  153    0    0  355  258  464-267  154  161  510    8  222-146
23.7   70  195  -24   76  450  217  425-382  200  195  544  -96  189-181
24.3   71  152  -24   56  408  190  370-331  175  176  475  -85  164-160
26.5   67  156  -15   34  405  203  404-303  171  180  493  -58  182-161
29.5   47  112  -19   37  332  166  376-269  140  147  419  -50  161-153
30.9  -38  134  -13   32  369  188  447-282  155  163  488  -38  207-160
30.9   58  110  -14   49  340  170  366-259  148  154  408  -47  153-138
32.3   -5   92   -2  -18  275  188  450-165  114  123  410   30  212-134
32.1   -9   99    0    0  300  191  444-205  129  128  434   10  213-132
32.3   51   95    0    0  295  186  420-194  126  129  409    7  195-139
34.0  -14   86    0    9  274  163  423-173  121  118  396   11  198-139
36.2   46  136   -3   23  381  206  461-268  169  163  482  -26  213-161
42.6   46  107   -8   29  320  155  412-226  138  147  435  -27  175-153
45.6   48   92    0    0  256  159  424-148  102  122  398   33  195-154
51.0  -46   91    1    9  245  156  438-144  102  119  412   43  196-143
51.4  -44   76   -4   17  234  130  403-135   99  112  369   23  180-148
```

406

A.4.4. *Brizalina*

The following are coordinates of six landmarks for 50 specimens of *Brizalina*: 10 in each of five strata. The *Brizalina* example in the text uses the second and fourth of these strata; the others are analyzed in Bookstein and Reyment (1989). The organisms were collected and photographed by Richard and Eva Reyment, and landmarks were digitized by Fred Bookstein. The first field is stratum number; the second is a relative magnification factor (which takes two values); then six Cartesian-coordinate pairs. The first landmark is Proloculus; the others follow clockwise. For operational definitions, see Section 3.4.3.1.

```
1 100    20 -350 -150   110  -60   380  100   310  210   230  230   130
1 100    15 -330 -160   100  -40   350  130   270  260   120  215    20
1 100   -30 -330 -195   100  -80   340   90   270  210   160  180     0
1 100    50 -350 -150    80  -30   335  150   230  280    80  255   -25
1 100     0 -400 -230    50 -160   310   70   250  205   190  220     0
1 100     0 -445 -180    35 -100   300   65   215  170   130  190   -25
1 100   -20 -310 -230    90 -150   320   40   250  170   140  150   -20
1 100    70 -440 -160   -30 -150   240   90   215  250   120  250   -40
1 100   -40 -325 -150    70  -30   300  120   210  190   120  170   -40
1 100    20 -435 -150     0  -15   255  150   170  250    90  250  -100
2 171    50 -330  -50    95    0   185  100   130  155    55  180   -30
2 171   -20 -205 -140   120  -65   270   20   220   90   150  100    65
2 100   -50 -400 -210    10 -125   255   40   180  130   110  155     0
2 171   -10 -280 -110   200  -40   240   25   185  100   100  100    20
2 171    50 -250  -70   100  -15   255  105   215  165   175  165    60
2 100   -60 -375 -220    20 -160   270   20   240  160   100  150   -50
2 171    40 -260  -70   160  -60   290   50   270  120   230  150   110
2 171    50 -210  -60    90  -20   185   90   160  170   110  175    30
2 171    30 -215  -65    40   65   240  120   150  160    90  150     0
2 171    30 -430 -100   100  -40   215   60   140  110    60  110    10
3 171    25 -270  -80    60  -20   195   80   170  145   125  160    30
3 171   -20 -220  -95    70  -40   215   65   170   95   140  105    75
3 171   -30 -250 -120    50  -50   165   40   140  120    90  120    10
3 171   -40 -275 -150   110  -90   240    0   210   70   140   80    40
3 171    70 -360  -55   130   10   300  120   260  190   190  200    40
3 171    45 -240  -70    40  -45   165   75   155  160   120  175    20
3 171   -10 -330 -120    90  -40   250   80   170  140    90  140     0
3 100    30 -550 -160   -20  -45   200  120   140  270   -10  230  -150
3 100   -20 -370 -210   -20 -130   220   55   175  190    80  180  -100
3 171   -30 -425 -250     0 -180   210    0   230  170   150  190   -30
4 100    20 -360 -115   -35  -90   190  100   170  225    85  230   -50
4 100   -10 -300 -185     0  -80   210   40   130  130    30  130   -80
4 100    25 -210 -120   -20  -80   140   70   140  155   100  185     0
4 100    65 -315 -160    40  -70   270  160   230  285   145  310     5
4 100    40 -410 -130    30  -70   300  120   220  270    70  250   -50
4 100    60 -380 -170   130  -25   315  130   260  270   150  260    10
4 171   -50 -355 -160    40  -40   215   70   160  130    80  140   -40
4 171   -40 -285 -170    30  -70   210   65   130  130   100  115    10
4 100    20 -475 -240    95 -110   330   70   260  120   245  185   185
4 171    50 -380 -265   125  -30   390  135   285  280    50  260   -30
5 171   -45 -190 -135   100  -70   245   50   200  130   150  140    50
5 171    50 -365  -40    70    0   245  120   180  165   135  160    15
5 171    80 -350 -100    70  -50   250   90   230  215   150  230   -20
5 171   -30 -300 -105    60  -60   180   30   150   90    95   90    20
5 100    40 -360 -140    -5  -65   280  145   260  270   170  270    10
```

```
5 100   30 -330 -100  230   25  315  140  245  250  120  230  -10
5 100   30 -405 -185   25 -120  230   90  230  210  150  240    0
5 171   40 -200 -150  -30 -120  180   60  170  185   85  175  -75
5 171  -30 -340 -250   50  -95  230   60  180  125  130  140   10
5 171  -10 -390 -100  155   10  280  100  220  180  150  180   10
```

A.4.5. Rat calvarial growth

The text's example of the single-factor model for size allometry involved a data set of eight landmark locations for 21 male laboratory rats observed at eight ages. The data were examined again in Chapter 7 in four separate contexts, as they showed a nearly uniform shape change at one stage, a residual from that change that was nearly purely inhomogeneous, and, for the full interval of the data, a trend that could be expressed either as an interesting quadratic term or as a composite of a two-dimensional uniform factor with one relative warp. Following is a listing of the complete data set as kindly sent to me in 1982 by Melvin Moss of Columbia University. Each line indicates animal sequence number, age of record, and eight Cartesian-coordinate pairs, corresponding to landmarks Basion, Opisthion, Interparietal suture, Lambda, Bregma, Spheno-ethmoid synchondrosis, Intersphenoidal synchondrosis, and Spheno-occipital synchondrosis. Operational definitions of these landmarks may be found in Section 3.4.1. The landmarks were originally taken to a Bregma–Lambda registration, a circumstance that has no effect whatsoever on our analyses. Four landmarks showed signs of substantial error in relation to their own earlier or later images. The coordinates of these four locations are indicated by 9999's in the file, and they have been omitted from all analyses.

```
1    7 -450 -475 -590 -280 -515 -120 -330    0    0    0  145 -395  -45 -420
    -260 -465
1   14 -530 -555 -685 -320 -625 -120 -400    0    0    0  230 -425   -5 -480
    -265 -525
1   21 -560 -570 -700 -335 -670 -120 -425    0    0    0  300 -440   15 -495
    -270 -540
1   30 -590 -580 -745 -355 -700 -100 -435    0    0    0  330 -445   30 -505
    -285 -565
1   40 -650 -580 -800 -340 -715  -90 -450    0    0    0  360 -445   40 -515
    -300 -580
1   60 -710 -580 -845 -340 -750  -65 -465    0    0    0  395 -450   50 -525
    -335 -590
1   90 -795 -565 -920 -315 -800  -50 -490    0    0    0  395 -450   50 -510
    -380 -590
1  150 -790 -555 -920 -305 -810  -25 -495    0    0    0  430 -455   70 -520
    -395 -585
2    7 -460 -475 -585 -285 -520 -140 -330    0    0    0  125 -380  -65 -415
    -265 -445
2   14 -495 -515 -655 -325 -635 -145 -380    0    0    0  245 -440   -5 -480
    -270 -505
2   21 -570 -555 -730 -340 -690 -130 -450    0    0    0  280 -445    5 -495
    -300 -535
```

```
2  30 -595 -545 -750 -320 -705 -110 -460   0   0   0  310 -450   25 -505
   -305 -545
2  40 -680 -550 -800 -310 -730  -70 -485   0   0   0  325 -455    0 -515
   -340 -560
2  60 -730 -545 -855 -295 -765  -55 -495   0   0   0  375 -465   15 -520
   -380 -580
2  90 -790 -535 -895 -285 -810  -35 -510   0   0   0  380 -465   25 -500
   -405 -565
2 150 -825 -505 -945 -265 -835  -10 -515   0   0   0  395 -470   35 -500
   -420 -545
3   7 -470 -460 -590 -280 -560 -115 -330   0   0   0  125 -400  -65 -420
   -275 -445
3  14 -505 -520 -660 -350 -620 -145 -395   0   0   0  225 -415   -5 -470
   -260 -510
3  21 -560 -540 -715 -335 -660 -130 -420   0   0   0  280 -430   10 -490
   -275 -535
3  30 -600 -555 -740 -315 -685 -100 -425   0   0   0  320 -440   15 -515
   -280 -550
3  40 -670 -565 -790 -325 -720  -85 -460   0   0   0  330 -455   15 -510
   -335 -560
3  60 -740 -570 -860 -340 -780  -80 -480   0   0   0  380 -455   15 -520
   -395 -580
3  90 -800 -555 -915 -330 -825  -55 -505   0   0   0 9999 9999   20 -515
   -425 -565
3 150 -810 -545 -940 -315 -840  -35 -495   0   0   0  420 -460   55 -520
   -415 -570
4   7 -495 -460 -615 -280 -565 -120 -350   0   0   0  130 -410  -75 -425
   -290 -455
4  14 -555 -545 -710 -340 -660 -125 -420   0   0   0  200 -450  -40 -500
   -300 -530
4  21 -565 -565 -745 -340 -690 -110 -440   0   0   0  250 -470  -15 -510
   -310 -550
4  30 -610 -560 -780 -315 -710  -90 -460   0   0   0  295 -480    0 -520
   -325 -560
4  40 -675 -575 -795 -315 -730  -95 -475   0   0   0  320 -505    5 -535
   -330 -580
4  60 -755 -580 -865 -325 -770  -70 -480   0   0   0  360 -510    5 -550
   -385 -615
4  90 -790 -580 -900 -320 -800  -45 -500   0   0   0  370 -505   35 -535
   -390 -615
4 150 -810 -550 -915 -280 -805  -20 -510   0   0   0  390 -500   30 -550
   -425 -600
5   7 -495 -465 -625 -275 -565 -115 -360   0   0   0  145 -395  -70 -405
   -290 -445
5  14 -555 -535 -690 -330 -640 -130 -395   0   0   0  200 -470  -25 -490
   -295 -515
5  21 -570 -560 -725 -335 -670 -120 -415   0   0   0  255 -485  -10 -510
   -305 -545
5  30 -605 -560 -770 -330 -715 -100 -445   0   0   0  295 -480    0 -510
   -320 -550
5  40 -670 -555 -800 -315 -730  -95 -455   0   0   0  330 -480   10 -515
   -335 -570
5  60 -730 -555 -855 -305 -755  -65 -480   0   0   0  345 -490    5 -520
   -365 -575
5  90 -785 -550 -900 -310 -790  -40 -495   0   0   0  360 -485   10 -515
   -395 -575
5 150 -835 -540 -955 -280 -820  -10 -495   0   0   0  365 -485   10 -520
   -440 -580
6   7 -475 -430 -605 -225 -550  -80 -345   0   0   0  115 -375  -85 -395
   -290 -420
```

```
6  14 -535 -515 -680 -305 -650 -135 -410   0   0   0  175 -445  -50 -470
      -290 -500
6  21 -570 -545 -720 -300 -680 -130 -440   0   0   0  240 -465  -20 -500
      -295 -530
6  30 -610 -540 -755 -295 -710 -105 -470   0   0   0  270 -465    0 -515
      -310 -545
6  40 -640 -525 -790 -280 -720  -70 -490   0   0   0  305 -475    0 -515
      -330 -555
6  60 -705 -560 -835 -295 -755  -65 -490   0   0   0  330 -485   10 -530
      -360 -580
6  90 -775 -570 -910 -325 -800  -65 -510   0   0   0  340 -480    5 -535
      -400 -600
6 150 -795 -570 -905 -310 -815  -45 -505   0   0   0  365 -490    5 -540
      -425 -605
7   7 -485 -465 -595 -280 -545 -135 -340   0   0   0  120 -410  -90 -415
      -280 -450
7  14 -520 -530 -660 -325 -615 -135 -390   0   0   0  200 -450  -45 -485
      -285 -515
7  21 -560 -540 -705 -315 -655 -110 -420   0   0   0  235 -460  -15 -495
      -295 -530
7  30 -600 -525 -745 -290 -700  -90 -425   0   0   0  280 -465    0 -490
      -320 -535
7  40 -625 -535 -755 -295 -690  -75 -435   0   0   0  330 -465   10 -500
      -320 -545
7  60 -695 -565 -810 -305 -730  -60 -455   0   0   0  380 -470   20 -525
      -350 -580
7  90 -750 -560 -845 -280 -755  -40 -470   0   0   0  390 -470   35 -520
      -375 -580
7 150 -770 -520 -885 -265 -760   -5 -480   0   0   0  400 -470   50 -520
      -410 -555
8   7 -450 -460 -570 -280 -540 -120 -335   0   0   0  110 -395  -70 -420
      -265 -440
8  14 -520 -530 -660 -335 -610 -125 -380   0   0   0  195 -435  -30 -460
      -280 -510
8  21 -580 -530 -720 -310 -660 -100 -410   0   0   0  250 -460  -10 -480
      -300 -525
8  30 -610 -525 -755 -295 -700  -75 -440   0   0   0  280 -450    5 -490
      -310 -525
8  40 -645 -540 -780 -295 -705  -70 -445   0   0   0  325 -450   20 -490
      -325 -535
8  60 -710 -560 -840 -310 -720  -55 -470   0   0   0  365 -455   35 -500
      -360 -555
8  90 -770 -535 -890 -280 -790  -35 -490   0   0   0  375 -455   10 -510
      -400 -550
8 150 -820 -535 -920 -270 -820  -15 -500   0   0   0  380 -455   10 -510
      -430 -550
9   7 -475 -445 -590 -260 -535 -120 -350   0   0   0  100 -390  -90 -410
      -275 -430
9  14 -530 -520 -670 -320 -630 -140 -410   0   0   0  185 -425  -25 -460
      -290 -490
9  21 -540 -535 -690 -330 -640 -130 -415   0   0   0  235 -440   -5 -480
      -280 -530
9  30 -640 -535 -750 -320 -695  -90 -430   0   0   0  250 -485   -5 -520
      -335 -545
9  40 -660 -535 -780 -300 -700  -70 -455   0   0   0  285 -465   -5 -505
      -345 -550
9  60 -735 -570 -825 -310 -720  -65 -470   0   0   0  330 -490   10 -510
      -375 -585
9  90 -810 -575 -880 -310 -765  -55 -495   0   0   0  340 -490    5 -520
      -420 -590
```

9	150	-810	-560	-920	-310	-780	-40	-510	0	0	0	365	-495	5	-525
		-435	-595												
10	7	-460	-460	-585	-270	-520	-115	-315	0	0	0	155	-395	-65	-415
		-255	-450												
10	14	-500	-510	-675	-320	-630	-125	-410	0	0	0	170	-420	-50	-460
		-285	-490												
10	21	-560	-520	-700	-300	-650	-105	-440	0	0	0	220	-430	-15	-485
		-290	-510												
10	30	-610	-525	-770	-285	-680	-90	-470	0	0	0	255	-435	-15	-495
		-320	-525												
10	40	-670	-520	-795	-275	-695	-55	-470	0	0	0	290	-460	-20	-510
		-350	-540												
10	60	-735	-505	-840	-260	-730	-30	-475	0	0	0	305	-465	-30	-505
		-400	-545												
10	90	-780	-520	-870	-265	-775	-35	-490	0	0	0	320	-485	-25	-500
		-425	-550												
10	150	-825	-530	-910	-270	-805	-25	-505	0	0	0	330	-485	-5	-495
		-450	-560												
11	7	-495	-480	-585	-285	-540	-115	-330	0	0	0	130	-395	-85	-425
		-295	-460												
11	14	-555	-535	-705	-325	-650	-125	-430	0	0	0	185	-460	-60	-495
		-305	-530												
11	21	-595	-565	-740	-330	-695	-125	-460	0	0	0	230	-490	-30	-520
		-310	-560												
11	30	-610	-565	-775	-320	-720	-95	-480	0	0	0	290	-465	-5	-515
		-320	-560												
11	40	-660	-580	-810	-310	-735	-90	-485	0	0	0	325	-475	5	-535
		-340	-585												
11	60	-720	-605	-860	-355	-755	-85	-500	0	0	0	350	-475	10	-545
		-365	-610												
11	90	-780	-575	-920	-320	-825	-65	-520	0	0	0	370	-475	10	-545
		-415	-595												
11	150	-830	-565	-940	-310	-860	-55	-520	0	0	0	400	-495	10	-560
		-430	-590												
12	7	-470	-460	-605	-260	-535	-105	-335	0	0	0	105	-370	-75	-400
		-270	-430												
12	14	-540	-520	-690	-300	-630	-115	-410	0	0	0	200	-460	-40	-490
		-295	-515												
12	21	-575	-545	-755	-315	-700	-100	-460	0	0	0	230	-450	-20	-505
		-305	-540												
12	30	-625	-545	-790	-290	-725	-80	-470	0	0	0	285	-450	0	-500
		-320	-555												
12	40	-690	-555	-845	-310	-750	-80	-480	0	0	0	325	-485	-15	-525
		-350	-575												
12	60	-755	-565	-890	-330	-775	-60	-495	0	0	0	365	-490	-5	-540
		-380	-580												
12	90	-800	-560	-935	-315	-840	-55	-510	0	0	0	380	-490	10	-540
		-415	-585												
12	150	-820	-575	-935	-315	-850	-45	-510	0	0	0	425	-495	45	-535
		-415	-590												
13	7	-465	-435	-585	-240	-520	-100	-340	0	0	0	120	-350	-45	-380
		-270	-420												
13	14	-535	-515	-670	-300	-610	-120	-400	0	0	0	190	-440	-45	-465
		-290	-490												
13	21	-575	-520	-695	-295	-640	-90	-430	0	0	0	240	-460	-20	-475
		-300	-520												
13	30	-600	-550	-750	-305	-660	-85	-450	0	0	0	295	-445	-5	-485
		-305	-535												
13	40	-660	-545	-780	-295	-685	-70	-460	0	0	0	315	-455	9999	9999
		-335	-550												

```
13  60 -710 -555 -830 -310 -710  -55 -460    0    0    0  360 -475   -5 -520
       -365 -565
13  90 -780 -530 -870 -265 -760  -30 -475    0    0    0  390 -485    0 -515
       -420 -565
13 150 -820 -520 -920 -260 -790   -5 -495    0    0    0  405 -490 9999 9999
       -450 -555
14   7 -495 -455 -615 -270 -575 -115 -365    0    0    0   80 -390 -105 -410
       -295 -435
14  14 -525 -535 -670 -325 -615 -125 -400    0    0    0  190 -435  -50 -475
       -290 -510
14  21 -590 -545 -740 -325 -685 -125 -460    0    0    0  235 -460  -25 -495
       -305 -535
14  30 -590 -545 -760 -320 -695 -110 -465    0    0    0  290 -475    0 -500
       -305 -545
14  40 -650 -555 -785 -310 -700  -90 -470    0    0    0  320 -465   15 -505
       -320 -570
14  60 -730 -595 -855 -335 -750  -75 -475    0    0    0  345 -490   25 -525
       -380 -595
14  90 -780 -575 -895 -320 -795  -60 -500    0    0    0  355 -480   25 -515
       -395 -590
14 150 -840 -570 -940 -290 -825  -35 -510    0    0    0  360 -490   25 -525
       -435 -585
15   7 -465 -446 -590 -285 -540 -110 -350    0    0    0   90 -370  -90 -400
       -280 -440
15  14 -525 -525 -690 -320 -620 -125 -400    0    0    0  180 -455  -45 -470
       -280 -505
15  21 -605 -540 -740 -315 -675 -105 -445    0    0    0  210 -470  -40 -495
       -320 -530
15  30 -645 -555 -780 -300 -705  -80 -445    0    0    0  270 -490  -40 -500
       -345 -545
15  40 -675 -545 -810 -300 -715  -70 -470    0    0    0  295 -490  -20 -510
       -355 -555
15  60 -730 -570 -835 -300 -730  -60 -475    0    0    0  335 -485    0 -505
       -370 -570
15  90 -765 -555 -865 -290 -755  -40 -480    0    0    0  350 -485   -5 -530
       -405 -565
15 150 -830 -555 -920 -295 -800  -25 -495    0    0    0  385 -490   15 -525
       -440 -585
16   7 -485 -465 -605 -270 -540 -115 -340    0    0    0  110 -385  -80 -405
       -290 -440
16  14 -560 -530 -700 -320 -650 -125 -445    0    0    0  190 -420  -40 -455
       -305 -510
16  21 -615 -540 -750 -320 -680  -95 -465    0    0    0  220 -455  -40 -490
       -330 -530
16  30 -620 -550 -765 -320 -690  -90 -475    0    0    0  275 -470  -20 -490
       -330 -550
16  40 -680 -580 -800 -320 -705  -80 -480    0    0    0  320 -470    5 -515
       -335 -575
16  60 -735 -615 -860 -355 -750  -80 -485    0    0    0  355 -460   10 -530
       -370 -595
16  90 -780 -585 -900 -330 -775  -55 -500    0    0    0  355 -465   15 -520
       -405 -580
16 150 -820 -560 -925 -305 -800  -25 -500    0    0    0  355 -470   15 -525
       -425 -575
17   7 -505 -475 -650 -275 -570 -125 -360    0    0    0  145 -365  -65 -405
       -285 -455
17  14 -575 -520 -700 -305 -650 -125 -430    0    0    0  210 -440  -40 -475
       -300 -510
17  21 -625 -535 -755 -305 -675 -100 -455    0    0    0  240 -460  -35 -500
       -320 -540
```

```
17  30 -645 -555 -785 -315 -710  -85 -480    0    0    0   280 -475  -20 -525
       -350 -565
17  40 -675 -565 -815 -325 -725  -75 -490    0    0    0   310 -485   -5 -515
       -360 -585
17  60 -750 -580 -855 -330 -735  -65 -480    0    0    0   350 -490  -15 -540
       -395 -605
17  90 -835 -565 -915 -305 -795  -40 -495    0    0    0   375 -505    0 -540
       -440 -605
17 150 -870 -540 -935 -255 -820  -10 -510    0    0    0   390 -510    5 -535
       -460 -595
18   7 -535 -485 -645 -275 -575 -125 -380    0    0    0   120 -415 -100 -445
       -310 -465
18  14 -570 -555 -725 -325 -675 -140 -430    0    0    0   170 -470  -50 -500
       -320 -545
18  21 -655 -560 -805 -325 -745 -125 -495    0    0    0   205 -505  -70 -525
       -350 -565
18  30 -670 -590 -825 -335 -760 -110 -500    0    0    0   250 -510  -70 -525
       -355 -580
18  40 -740 -600 -870 -335 -785  -95 -510    0    0    0   270 -515  -30 -545
       -385 -600
18  60 -790 -605 -910 -350 -805  -85 -525    0    0    0   315 -515  -30 -560
       -410 -620
18  90 -830 -585 -945 -330 -845  -55 -540    0    0    0   340 -510  -20 -555
       -445 -600
18 150 -865 -570 -975 -325 -850  -50 -540    0    0    0   360 -525    0 -550
       -470 -605
19   7 -500 -500 -625 -300 -570 -130 -350    0    0    0   115 -405  -75 -435
       -300 -480
19  14 -550 -550 -720 -330 -655 -125 -425    0    0    0   195 -475  -50 -505
       -305 -540
19  21 -615 -580 -790 -350 -715 -115 -470    0    0    0   245 -470  -40 -520
       -330 -565
19  30 -655 -575 -810 -325 -730 -105 -475    0    0    0   305 -495  -10 -535
       -340 -580
19  40 -720 -555 -850 -305 -770  -75 -505    0    0    0   315 -510  -20 -555
       -380 -585
19  60 -770 -590 -905 -345 -780  -75 -510    0    0    0   365 -520    0 -560
       -405 -600
19  90 -820 -605 -935 -345 -830  -60 -520    0    0    0   395 -520   20 -560
       -430 -605
19 150 -875 -600 -995 -350 -890  -45 -555    0    0    0   405 -525   20 -560
       -475 -620
20   7 -510 -475 -630 -260 -585 -115 -370    0    0    0   110 -415  -90 -445
       -295 -465
20  14 -550 -555 -705 -320 -645 -125 -430    0    0    0   205 -460  -30 -505
       -295 -540
20  21 -595 -560 -755 -330 -695 -105 -460    0    0    0   220 -475  -35 -510
       -320 -555
20  30 -600 -560 -780 -335 -720  -95 -465    0    0    0   290 -480  -15 -515
       -325 -555
20  40 -630 -575 -800 -320 -720  -80 -480    0    0    0   310 -495    0 -520
       -330 -565
20  60 -730 -590 -870 -330 -760  -70 -490    0    0    0   355 -505   10 -540
       -370 -600
20  90 -765 -585 -910 -325 -790  -60 -495    0    0    0   380 -505   25 -530
       -400 -600
20 150 -830 -575 -940 -315 -830  -40 9999 9999    0    0   400 -510   25 -535
       -440 -610
21   7 -515 -485 -615 -275 -560 -120 -365    0    0    0   120 -410  -90 -430
       -310 -455
```

413

```
21  14 -555 -560 -705 -315 -640 -140 -425    0    0    0  210 -465  -10 -505
       -300 -535
21  21 -595 -565 -740 -345 -695 -125 -445    0    0    0  245 -480  -15 -515
       -305 -550
21  30 -625 -560 -780 -330 -705  -90 -485    0    0    0  290 -485    0 -520
       -315 -560
21  40 -665 -560 -800 -320 -715  -80 -480    0    0    0  320 -485   15 -515
       -325 -570
21  60 -765 -580 -875 -335 -760  -70 -495    0    0    0  345 -505    0 -555
       -400 -610
21  90 -825 -580 -935 -330 -805  -50 -515    0    0    0  350 -505    5 -550
       -430 -600
21 150 -840 -585 -960 -325 -850  -35 -520    0    0    0  395 -505   20 -525
       -450 -595
```

Bibliography

This listing omits the readings in morphometrics, statistics, and geometry that were annotated *en bloc* in Section 2.5. Following each entry is a list of the sections in which it is cited.

Abe, K., R. Reyment, F. L. Bookstein, A. Honigstein, and O. Hermalin. 1988. Microevolutionary changes in *Veenia fawwarensis* (Ostracoda, Crustacea) from the Cretaceous (Santonian) of Israel. *Historical Biology* 1:303–22. (*3.4.3*)

Anderson, T. W. 1958. *An Introduction to Multivariate Statistical Analysis*. New York: Wiley. (*5.4.2*)

Avery, G. S., Jr. 1933. Structure and development of the tobacco leaf. *American Journal of Botany* 20:565–92. (*2.4.3*)

Baer, M. J., J. Bosma, and J. Ackerman. 1983. *The Postnatal Development of the Rat Skull*, 2 vols. Ann Arbor: University of Michigan Press. (*3.4.1*)

Blackith, R. E. 1965. Morphometrics. In T. H. Waterman and H. J. Morowitz, eds., *Theoretical and Mathematical Biology*, pp. 225–49. New York: Blaisdell. (*2.1, 4.4*)

Blackith, R. E., and R. Reyment. 1971. *Multivariate Morphometrics*. London: Academic. (*2.1, 2.5.1*)

Blum, H. 1973. Biological shape and visual science (Part I). *Journal of Theoretical Biology* 38:205–87. (*3.5*)

Blum, H. 1974. A geometry for biology. *Proceedings of the New York Academy of Sciences* 231:19–30. (*7.0*)

Blum, H., and R. N. Nagel. 1978. Shape description using weighted symmetric axis features. *Pattern Recognition* 10:167–80. (*3.5.2*)

Bookstein, F. L. 1978. *The Measurement of Biological Shape and Shape Change. Lecture Notes in Biomathematics*, vol. 24. Berlin: Springer. (*2.1, 2.4, 3.1.1, 3.2, 3.4.3, 3.5.4, 5.0, 6.6, 7.1*)

Bookstein, F. L. 1979. The line-skeleton. *Computer Graphics and Image Processing* 11:123–37. (*3.5.2*)

Bookstein, F. L. 1980*a*. When one form is between two others: an application of biorthogonal analysis. *American Zoologist* 20:627–41. (*6.2.3*)

Bookstein, F. L. 1980*b*. From biostereometrics to the comprehension of form. In A. Coblentz and R. Herron, eds., *Applications of Human Biostereometrics*, pp. 74–9. *Proceedings of the SPIE*, vol. 166. (*3.5.4*)

Bookstein, F. L. 1981*a*. Looking at mandibular growth: some new geometrical methods. In D. Carlson, ed., *Craniofacial Biology*, pp. 83–103. Ann Arbor: Center for Human Growth and Development, University of Michigan. (*3.5.2*)

Bookstein, F. L. 1981*b*. Comment on "Issues related to the prediction of craniofacial growth." *American Journal of Orthodontics* 79:442–8. (*7.4.3*)

Bookstein, F. L. 1982*a*. Foundations of morphometrics. *Annual Reviews of Ecology and Systematics* 13:451–70. (*2.1*)

Bookstein, F. L. 1982b. On the cephalometrics of skeletal change. *American Journal of Orthodontics* 82:177–98. (*2.1*)

Bookstein, F. L. 1983. The geometry of craniofacial growth invariants. *American Journal of Orthodontics* 83:221–34. (*3.4.1, 6.3, 7.3.1*)

Bookstein, F. L. 1984a. A statistical method for biological shape comparisons. *Journal of Theoretical Biology* 107:475–520. (*2.1, 5.3.1, 6.5.1*)

Bookstein, F. L. 1984b. Tensor biometrics for changes in cranial shape. *Annals of Human Biology* 11:413–37. (*2.1, 6.5, 7.5.5*)

Bookstein, F. L. 1985a. A geometric foundation for the study of left ventricular motion: some tensor considerations. In A. Buda and E. Delp, eds., *Digital Cardiac Imaging*, pp. 65–83. The Hague: Martinus Nijhoff. (*3.3.1*)

Bookstein, F. L. 1985b. Transformations of quadrilaterals, tensor fields and morphogenesis. In P. Antonelli, ed., *Mathematical Essays on Growth and the Emergence of Form*, pp. 221–65. Edmonton: University of Alberta. (*6.6, 7.4.2*)

Bookstein, F. L. 1986a. Size and shape spaces for landmark data in two dimensions (with discussion and rejoinder). *Statistical Science* 1:181–242. (*2.1, 3.4.3, 4.1, 5.0, 5.2.2, 5.5.2, 6.4, 8.2, A.2.1*)

Bookstein, F. L. 1986b. The elements of latent variable models: a cautionary lecture. *Advances in Developmental Psychology* 4:203–30. (*2.3.2*)

Bookstein, F. L. 1986c. From medical imaging to the biometrics of form. In S. L. Bacharach, ed., *Proceedings of the Ninth International Conference on Information Processing in Medical Imaging*, pp. 1–18. Dordrecht: Martinus Nijhoff. (*6.2.6*)

Bookstein, F. L. 1987a. Describing a craniofacial anomaly: finite elements and the biometrics of landmark location. *American Journal of Physical Anthropology* 74:495–509. (*2.1, 3.4.1, 6.6, 7.3.1, 7.5.5*)

Bookstein, F. L. 1987b. Morphometrics for functional imaging studies. In J. C. Mazziotta and S. H. Koslow, eds., Assessment of goals and obstacles in data acquisition and analysis from emission tomography: report of a series of international workshops. *Journal of Cerebral Blood Flow and Metabolism* 7:S23–7. (*2.2.4*)

Bookstein, F. L. 1987c. Random walk and the existence of evolutionary rates. *Paleobiology* 13:446–64. (*A.3*)

Bookstein, F. L. 1988a. Toward a notion of feature extraction for plane mappings. In C. de Graaf and M. Viergever, eds., *Proceedings of the Tenth International Conference on Information Processing in Medical Imaging*, pp. 23–43. New York: Plenum. (*2.2.4, 3.5.1, 3.5.4, 7.5*)

Bookstein, F. L. 1988b. Random walk and the biometrics of morphological characters. *Evolutionary Biology* 23:369–98. (*A.3*)

Bookstein, F. L. 1989a. Principal warps: thin-plate splines and the decomposition of deformations. *IEEE Transactions on Pattern Analysis and Machine Intelligence* 11:567–85. (*2.2, 7.5, A.1.2*)

Bookstein, F. L. 1989b. Comment on D. G. Kendall, "A survey of the statistical theory of shape." *Statistical Science* 4:99–105. (*2.1, 3.4.1, 7.6.3*)

Bookstein, F. L. 1989c. "Size and shape": a comment on semantics. *Systematic Zoology* 38:173–80. (*1.3, 4.3.3*)

Bookstein, F. L. 1990a. Four metrics for image variation. In D. Ortendahl and J. Llacer, eds., *Proceedings of the XI International Conference on Information Processing in Medical Imaging*, pp. 227–40. New York: Alan R. Liss. (*2.2, 7.6.4*)

Bookstein, F. L. 1990b. Least squares and latent variables. *Multivariate Behavioral Research* 25:73–8. (*2.3.2*)

Bookstein, F. L. 1990c. Soft modeling and the measurement of biological shape. In H. Wold, ed., *Theoretical Empiricism*, pp. 235–64. New York: Paragon. (*6.5.1*)

Bookstein, F. L. 1990d. Introduction to methods for landmark data. In F. J. Rohlf and F.

Bookstein, eds., *Proceedings of the Michigan Morphometrics Workshop*, pp. 215–26. Ann Arbor: University of Michigan Museums. (*3.4*)

Bookstein, F. L. 1990*e*. Higher-order features of shape change. In F. J. Rohlf and F. Bookstein, eds., *Proceedings of the Michigan Morphometrics Workshop*, pp. 237–50. Ann Arbor: University of Michigan Museums. (*1.3, 7.6.4*)

Bookstein, F. L. 1990*f*. Visualizing biological shape differences. In *Proceedings of the First Conference on Visualization in Biomedical Computing*, pp. 410–17. Los Alamitos, CA: IEEE Computer Society Press. (*7.5.2*)

Bookstein, F. L. 1990*g*. Distortion correction. In A. W. Toga, ed., *Three-Dimensional Neuroimaging*, pp. 235–49. New York: Raven. (*2.2, 2.4.3, 6.6, 7.5.1*)

Bookstein, F. L. 1991. Thin-plate splines and the atlas problem for biomedical images. In A. Colchester and D. Hawkes, eds., *Proceedings of the XII International Conference on Information Processing in Medical Imaging*, pp. 326–42. *Lecture Notes in Computer Science*, vol. 511. Berlin: Springer-Verlag. (*A.1.3*)

Bookstein, F. L., B. Chernoff, R. Elder, J. Humphries, G. Smith, and R. Strauss. 1982. A comment on the uses of Fourier analysis in systematics. *Systematic Zoology* 31:85–92. (*2.4.1*)

Bookstein, F. L., B. Chernoff, R. Elder, J. Humphries, G. Smith, and R. Strauss. 1985. *Morphometrics in Evolutionary Biology. The Geometry of Size and Shape Change, with Examples from Fishes*. Academy of Natural Sciences of Philadelphia. (*2.3, 2.4, 2.5, 3.1.1, 3.2, 3.3.3, 3.5.2, 4.1.4, 4.2, 4.4, 5.4.1, 5.5, 6.2.1, 6.6, 7.1.4, 8.1*)

Bookstein, F. L., and C. Cutting. 1988. A proposal for the apprehension of curving craniofacial form in three dimensions. In K. W. Vig and A. Burdi, eds., *Craniofacial Morphogenesis and Dysmorphogenesis*, pp. 127–40. Ann Arbor: Center for Human Growth and Development, University of Michigan. (*3.3.2, 3.5.4, 8.1*)

Bookstein, F. L., B. Grayson, C. Cutting, H.-C. Kim, and J. McCarthy. 1991. Landmarks in three dimensions: reconstruction from cephalograms versus direct observation. *American J. of Orthodontics and Dentofacial Orthopedics* 100:133–40. (*4.1.4, 5.4.4*)

Bookstein, F. L., and W. Jaynes. 1990. Thin-plate splines and the analysis of biological shape. Videotape, 20 minutes. (*8.4.2*)

Bookstein, F. L., and R. Reyment. 1989. Microevolution in *Brizalina* studied by canonical variate analysis and analysis of landmarks. *Bulletin of Mathematical Biology* 51:657–79. (*2.1, 3.2, 3.4.3, 5.3.4*)

Bookstein, F. L., and P. Sampson. 1987. Statistical models for geometric components of shape change. In *Proceedings of the Section on Statistical Graphics, 1987 Annual Meeting of the American Statistical Association*, pp. 18–27. Alexandria, VA: American Statistical Association. (*2.1, 3.4.4, 5.4.3*)

Bookstein, F. L., and P. Sampson. 1990. Statistical models for geometric components of shape change. *Communications in Statistics: Theory and Methods* 19:1939–72. (*2.1, 3.4.4, 5.4.3, 7.2.4*)

Bookstein, F. L., P. Sampson, A. Streissguth, and H. Barr. 1990. Measuring "dose" and "response" with multivariate data using Partial Least Squares techniques. *Communications in Statistics: Theory and Methods* 19:765–804. (*2.3.2*)

Burnaby, T. P. 1966. Growth-invariant discriminant functions and generalized distances. *Biometrics* 22:96–110. (*4.4*)

Busemann, H., and P. Kelly. 1953. *Projective Geometry and Projective Metrics*. New York: Academic. (*A.2.1*)

Campbell, N. A. 1982. Robust procedures in multivariate analysis. II. Robust canonical variates analysis. *Applied Statistics* 31:1–8. (*4.3.1*)

Capowski, J. J. 1989. *Computer Techniques in Neuroanatomy*. New York: Plenum. (*2.4.3*)

Cheverud, J. M., and J. Richtsmeier. 1986. Finite-element scaling applied to sexual dimorphism in rhesus macaque (*Macaca mulatta*) facial growth. *Systematic Zoology* 35:381–99. (*2.1, 6.6*)

Clarren, S., P. Sampson, J. Larsen, D. Donnell, H. Barr, D. Martin, F. L. Bookstein, and A. Streissguth. 1987. Facial effects of fetal alcohol exposure: assessment by photographs and morphometric analysis. *American Journal of Medical Genetics* 26:651–66. (*1.2.2, 2.1, 3.4.4*)

Coolidge, J. L. 1940. *A History of Geometrical Methods*. Oxford University Press. (*2.5.3, 4.1.2*)

Coxeter, H. S. M. 1965. *Non-Euclidean Geometry*, 5th ed. University of Toronto Press. (*2.5.3, A.2*)

Crespi, B. J., and F. L. Bookstein. 1989. A path-analytic model for the measurement of selection on morphology. *Evolution* 43:18–28. (*2.3.1, 2.4.2, 3.5.3*)

Darroch, J. H., and J. Mosimann. 1985. Canonical and principal components of shape. *Biometrika* 72:241–52. (*3.5.3*)

Diewart, V. M., and S. Lozanoff. 1988. Finite element methods applied to analysis of facial growth during primary palate formation. In K. W. Vig and A. Burdi, eds., *Craniofacial Morphogenesis and Dysmorphogenesis*, pp. 53–71. Ann Arbor: Center for Human Growth and Development, University of Michigan. (*6.6*)

Duchon, J. 1976. Interpolation des fonctions de deux variables suivant le principe de la flexion des plaques minces. *RAIRO Analyse Numérique* 10:5–12. (*2.2.4*)

Farkas, L. G. 1981. *Anthropometry of the Head and Face in Medicine*. Amsterdam: Elsevier–North Holland. (*1.2.2*)

Feldkamp, L. A., S. Goldstein, A. Parfitt, G. Jesion, and M. Kleerkoper. 1989. The direct examination of three-dimensional bone architecture in vitro by computed tomography. *Journal of Bone and Mineral Research* 4:3–11. (*2.4.3*)

Feller, W. 1957. *An Introduction to Probability Theory and Its Applications*, 2nd ed., vol. 1. New York: Wiley. (*A.3.1*)

Felsenstein, J. 1985. Confidence limits on phylogenies. *Evolution* 39:783–91. (*4.4*)

Ferson, S., F. J. Rohlf, and R. Koehn. 1985. Measuring shape variation of two-dimensional outlines. *Systematic Zoology* 34:59–68. (*2.4.2*)

Fink, W. L. 1990. Data acquisition in systematic biology. In F. J. Rohlf and F. Bookstein, eds., *Proceedings of the Michigan Morphometrics Workshop*, pp. 9–20. Ann Arbor: University of Michigan Museums. (*5.4.4*)

Frobin, W., and E. Hierholzer. 1982. Analysis of human back shape using surface curvatures. *Journal of Biomechanics* 15:379–90. (*3.3.2*)

Goodall, C. R. 1983. The statistical analysis of growth in two dimensions. Doctoral dissertation, Department of Statistics, Harvard University. (*2.1, 6.6*)

Goodall, C. R. 1986. Comment on F. L. Bookstein, "Size and shape spaces for landmark data in two dimensions." *Statistical Science* 1:234–8. (*6.2.1*)

Goodall, C. R. 1991. Procrustes methods in the statistical analysis of shape (with discussion and rejoinder). *Journal of the Royal Statistical Society*, Series B 53:285–339. (*2.1, 3.4.1, 5.6, 7.1, 7.2.3, 8.2*)

Goodall, C. R., and A. Bose. 1987. Procrustes techniques for the analysis of shape and shape change. In R. Heiberger, ed., *Computer Science and Statistics: Proceedings of the 19th Symposium on the Interface*, pp. 86–92. Alexandria, VA: American Statistical Association. (*3.4.1, 7.1*)

Goodall, C. R., and N. Lange. 1990. Growth-curve models for repeated triangular shapes. Unpublished manuscript. (*5.6, 8.3*)

Goodall, C. R., and K. Mardia. 1990. The noncentral Bartlett decomposition, and shape densities in the rank 2 and rank 3 cases. Unpublished manuscript. (*5.6.3, 7.2.3*)

Gower, J. C. 1970. Statistical methods of comparing different multivariate analyses of the same data. In F. R. Hudson et al., eds., *Mathematics in the Archaeological and*

Historical Sciences, pp. 138–49. Edinburgh University Press. (*7.1*)

Gower, J. C. 1975. Generalized Procrustes analysis. *Psychometrika* 40:33–50. (*7.1*)

Grayson, B., F. L. Bookstein, H.-C. Kim, C. Cutting, and J. McCarthy. 1990. Characterizing mandibular shape in Apert and Crouzon syndrome. Unpublished manuscript. (*3.5*)

Grayson, B., F. L. Bookstein, and J. McCarthy. 1986. The mandible in mandibulofacial dysostosis: a cephalometric study. *American Journal of Orthodontics* 89:393–8. (*3.5*)

Grayson, B., F. L. Bookstein, J. McCarthy, and T. Mueeddin. 1987. Mean tensor cephalometric analysis of a patient population with clefts of the palate and lip. *Cleft Palate Journal* 24:267–77. (*2.1*)

Grayson, B., C. Cutting, F. L. Bookstein, H.-C. Kim, and J. McCarthy. 1988. The three-dimensional cephalogram: theory, technique, and clinical application. *American Journal of Orthodontics* 94:327–37. (*2.1, 3.3.3, 5.4.4, 6.5.4*)

Grayson, B., N. Weintraub, F. L. Bookstein, and J. McCarthy. 1985. A comparative cephalometric study of the cranial base in craniofacial syndromes. *Cleft Palate Journal* 22:75–87. (*2.1, 5.4.3, 7.3.3*)

Gunderson, H. J. G. 1988. The nucleator. *Journal of Microscopy* 151:3–21. (*2.4.3*)

Gunderson, H. J. G., and 10 others. 1988*a*. Some new, simple and efficient stereological methods and their use in pathological research and diagnosis. *APMIS* 96:379–94. (*2.4.3*)

Gunderson, H. J. G., and 12 others. 1988*b*. The new stereological tools: disector, fractionator, nucleator and point sampled intercepts and their use in pathological research and diagnosis. *APMIS* 96:857–81. (*2.4.3*)

Hilbert, D., and S. Cohn-Vossen. 1952. *Geometry and the Imagination*. New York: Chelsea. (*2.5.3, 6.2.3*)

Hopkins, J. W. 1966. Some considerations in multivariate allometry. *Biometrics* 22:747–60. (*4.2.3*)

Humphries, J. H., F. Bookstein, B. Chernoff, G. Smith, R. Elder, and S. Poss. 1981. Multivariate discrimination by shape in relation to size. *Systematic Zoology* 30:291–308. (*2.4.2, 4.4*)

Huxley, J. 1932. *Problems of Relative Growth*. London: Methuen. (*2.1, 2.3, 3.2, 7.4.2*)

Karger, A., and J. Novák. 1985. *Space Kinematics and Lie Groups*. New York: Gordon & Breach. (*1.3, 2.5.1*)

Kass, M., A. Witkin, and D. Terzopoulos. 1987. Snakes: active contour models. *International Journal of Computer Vision* 1:321–31. (*2.2.2*)

Kendall, D. G. 1984. Shape-manifolds, procrustean metrics and complex projective spaces. *Bulletin of the London Mathematical Society* 16:81–121. (*2.1, 5.6, 8.3*)

Kendall, D. G. 1986. Comment on F. L. Bookstein, "Size and shape spaces for landmark data in two dimensions." *Statistical Science* 1:222–6. (*5.6*)

Kendall, D. G. 1989. A survey of the statistical theory of shape (with discussion and rejoinder). *Statistical Science* 4:87–120. (*5.6*)

Kent, J. 1990. Presentation at S. S. Wilks Workshop on Shape Theory, Princeton, NJ. (*5.3.2*)

Ketterlinus, R. D., F. L. Bookstein, P. Sampson, and M. Lamb. 1989. Partial Least Squares analysis in developmental psychopathology. *Development and Psychopathology* 1:351–71. (*2.3.2*)

Klein, F. 1928. *Vorlesungen über nicht-euklidische Geometrie*. Berlin: Springer. (*2.5.3, A.2.1*)

Koenderink, J. 1990. *Solid Shape*. Cambridge, MA: MIT Press. (*2.5.3, 8.1*)

Kuhn, J. L., S. Goldstein, L. Feldkamp, R. Goulet, and G. Jesion. 1990. Evaluation of a microcomputed tomography system to study trabecular bone structure. *Journal of Orthopedic Research* 8:833–42. (*2.4.3*)

Lanczos, C. 1970. *Space through the Ages*. New York: Academic. (*2.5.3, 6.2.5*)

Lele, S. 1989. Some comments on coordinate free and scale invariant methods in morphometrics. Mimeo #2006,

Department of Statistics, University of North Carolina at Chapel Hill. (*6.4.3*)

Lewis, J. L., W. Lew, and J. Zimmerman. 1980. A nonhomogeneous anthropometric scaling method based on finite element principles. *Journal of Biomechanics* 13:815–24. (*6.6*)

Lohmann, G. P. 1983. Eigenshape analysis of microfossils: a general morphometric procedure for describing changes in shape. *Mathematical Geology* 15:659–72. (*2.4.1, 3.4.3, 6.5.2, A.4.3*)

Lohmann, G. P., and P. Schweitzer. 1990. On eigenshape analysis. In F. J. Rohlf and F. Bookstein, eds., *Proceedings of the Michigan Morphometrics Workshop*, pp. 147–66. Ann Arbor: University of Michigan Museums. (*2.4.1*)

MacLeod, N., and J. Kitchell. 1990. Morphometrics and evolutionary inference: a case study involving ontogenetic and developmental aspects of foraminiferal evolution. In F. J. Rohlf and F. Bookstein, eds., *Proceedings of the Michigan Morphometrics Workshop*, pp. 283–300. Ann Arbor: University of Michigan Museums. (*7.6*)

Mandelbrot, B. 1982. *The Fractal Geometry of Nature*. San Francisco: Freeman. (*7.6*)

Marcus, L. F. 1990. Traditional morphometrics. In F. J. Rohlf and F. Bookstein, eds., *Proceedings of the Michigan Morphometrics Workshop*, pp. 77–122. Ann Arbor: University of Michigan Museums. (*2.1, 3.2*)

Mardia, K. V., and I. Dryden. 1989*a*. The statistical analysis of shape data. *Biometrika* 76:271–82. (*2.1, 5.4.2, 5.6, 7.2, A.2.2*)

Mardia, K. V., and I. Dryden. 1989*b*. Shape distributions for landmark data. *Advances in Applied Probability* 21:742–55. (*5.6, 8.2*)

Mardia, K. V., and I. Dryden. 1990. Presentations at S. S. Wilks Workshop on Shape Theory, Princeton, NJ. (*5.6.4, 7.2.3*)

Mardia, K. V., J. Kent, and J. Bibby. 1979. *Multivariate Analysis*. London: Academic. (*2.5.2, 5.6.3*)

Meinguet, J. 1979*a*. Multivariate interpolation at arbitrary points made simple. *Zeitschrift für Angewandte Mathematik und Physik* (*ZAMP*) 30:292–304. (*2.2.4*)

Meinguet, J. 1979*b*. An intrinsic approach to multivariate spline interpolation at arbitrary points. In B. Sahney, ed., *Polynomial and Spline Approximation*, pp. 163–90. Dordrecht: D. Reidel. (*2.2.4*)

Meinguet, J. 1984. Surface spline interpolation: basic theory and computational aspects. In S. P. Singh et al., eds., *Approximation Theory and Spline Functions*, pp. 127–42. Dordrecht: D. Reidel. (*2.2.4*)

Metz, C. E., and L. Fencil. 1989. Determination of three-dimensional structure in biplane radiography without prior knowledge of the relationship between the two views: theory. *Medical Physics* 16:45–51. (*3.3.3*)

Misner, C. W., K. Thorne, and J. A. Wheeler. 1973. *Gravitation*. San Francisco: Freeman. (*6.2.5*)

Morrison, D. F. 1990. *Multivariate Statistical Methods*, 3rd ed. New York: McGraw-Hill. (*2.5.2, 5.4.2, 7.2.4*)

Mosimann, J. E. 1970. Size allometry: size and shape variables with characterizations of the log-normal and generalized gamma distributions. *Journal of the American Statistical Association* 65:930–45. (*1.3, 4.3.3, 5.0, 5.5.2*)

Mosimann, J. E. 1975. Statistical problems of size and shape. I. Biological applications and basic theorems. In G. P. Patil et al., eds., *Statistical Distributions in Scientific Work*, vol. 2, pp. 187–217. Dordrecht: D. Reidel. (*5.0*)

Mosimann, J. E., and F. C. James. 1979. New statistical methods for allometry with application to Florida red-winged blackbirds. *Evolution* 33:444–59. (*3.5.3*)

Moss, M. L., R. Skalak, H. Patel, K. Sen, L. Moss-Salentijn, M. Shinozuka, and H. Vilmann. 1985. Finite element method modeling of craniofacial growth. *American Journal of Orthodontics* 87:453–74. (*3.4.1, 6.6, 7.2.4*)

Moss, M. L., H. Vilmann, L. Moss-Salentijn, K. Sen, H. Pucciarelli, and R. Skalak. 1987.

Studies on orthocephalization: growth behavior of the rat skull in the period 13–49 days as described by the finite element method. *American Journal of Physical Anthropology* 72:323–42. (*3.4.1, 6.6*)

Mosteller, F., and J. Tukey. 1977. *Data Analysis and Regression*. Reading, MA: Addison-Wesley. (*6.3.1*)

Moyers, R. E., F. L. Bookstein, and W. Hunter. 1988. Analysis of the facial skeleton: cephalometrics. In R. E. Moyers, ed., *Handbook of Orthodontics*, 4th ed., pp. 247–301. Chicago: Year Book Medical Publishers. (*3.4.2*)

Mulaik, S. A. 1972. *The Foundations of Factor Analysis*. New York: McGraw-Hill. (*4.2.2*)

Oxnard, C. E. 1978. One biologist's view of morphometrics. *Annual Reviews of Ecology and Systematics* 9:219–41. (*2.1*)

Palmer, A. R., and C. Strobeck. 1986. Fluctuating asymmetry: measurement, analysis, patterns. *Annual Reviews of Ecology and Systematics* 17:391–421. (*7.1.4*)

Pedoe, D. 1970. *A Course of Geometry for Colleges and Universities*. Cambridge University Press. (*2.5.3, 4.1.1, 5.5.1*)

Rao, C. R. 1973. *Linear Statistical Inference and Its Applications*, 2nd ed. New York: Wiley. (*2.3.2, 2.5.2, 5.4, 5.6.3, 7.2.4*)

Raup, D. M. 1966. Geometric analysis of shell coiling: general problems. *Journal of Paleontology* 40:1178–90. (*7.4.4*)

Reyment, R. A. 1990. Reification of classical multivariate statistical analysis in morphometry. In F. J. Rohlf and F. Bookstein, eds., *Proceedings of the Michigan Morphometrics Workshop*, pp. 123–44. Ann Arbor: University of Michigan Museums. (*2.4.2, 3.2, 4.2.3*)

Reyment, R. A. 1991. *Multidimensional Palaeobiology*. Oxford: Pergamon. (*2.4.2, 2.5.1, 3.4.3*)

Reyment, R. A., R. Blackith, and N. Campbell. 1984. *Multivariate Morphometrics*, 2nd ed. London: Academic. (*2.1, 2.5.1, 3.1.1, 6.5*)

Reyment, R. A., F. L. Bookstein, K. G. McKenzie, and S. Majoran. 1988.

Ecophenotypic variation in *Mutilus pumilis* (Ostracoda) from Australia, studied by canonical variate analysis and tensor biometrics. *Journal of Micropalaeontology* 7:11–20. (*3.4.3, 4.3.1*)

Richards, O. W., and A. J. Kavanagh. 1943. The analysis of the relative growth gradients and changing form of growing organisms: illustrated by the tobacco leaf. *American Naturalist* 77:385–99. (*2.1, 2.4.3*)

Richards, O. W., and A. J. Kavanagh. 1945. The analysis of growing form. In W. E. Le Gros Clark and P. B. Medawar, eds., *Essays on Growth and Form presented to D'Arcy Wentworth Thompson*, pp. 188–230. Oxford: Clarendon Press. (*2.4.3*)

Richtsmeier, J. T. 1988. Craniofacial growth in Apert syndrome as measured by finite-element scaling analysis. *Acta Anatomica* 133:50–6. (*6.6*)

Riolo, M. L., R. E. Moyers, J. S. McNamara, and W. S. Hunter. 1974. *An Atlas of Craniofacial Growth*. Ann Arbor: Center for Human Growth and Development, University of Michigan. (*3.4.2, 3.5.1, A.4.1*)

Rohlf, F. J. 1986. The relationships among eigenshape analysis, Fourier analysis, and the analysis of coordinates. *Mathematical Geology* 18:845–54. (*2.4.1*)

Rohlf, F. J. 1990*a*. Fitting curves to outlines. In F. J. Rohlf and F. Bookstein, eds., *Proceedings of the Michigan Morphometrics Workshop*, pp. 167–78. Ann Arbor: University of Michigan Museums. (*2.1, 2.4.1*)

Rohlf, F. J. 1990*b* Rotational fit (Procrustes) methods. In F. J. Rohlf and F. Bookstein, eds., *Proceedings of the Michigan Morphometrics Workshop*, pp. 227–36. Ann Arbor: University of Michigan Museums. (*7.1*)

Rohlf, F. J., and F. L. Bookstein. 1987. A comment on shearing as a method of "size correction." *Systematic Zoology* 36:356–67. (*2.4.2, 4.2.1, 4.3.1, 4.4*)

Rohlf, F. J., and F. L. Bookstein, eds. 1990. *Proceedings of the Michigan Morphometrics Workshop*. Ann Arbor: University of

Michigan Museums. (*2.1, 2.2.4, 2.4.2, 7.2.4, 7.4.2, 7.5, 7.6.2, 8.1, 8.3*)

Rohlf, F. J., and D. Slice. 1990. Methods for comparison of sets of landmarks. *Systematic Zoology* 39:40–59. (*7.1, 7.2.3, 7.5.4, 8.2*)

Rudnick, J., and G. Gaspari. 1987. The shapes of random walks. *Science* 237:384–9. (*A.3.1*)

Salmon, G. 1914. *A Treatise on the Analytic Geometry of Three Dimensions*, 6th ed., vol. 1. London: Longmans Green. (*4.1.2*)

Sampson, P. D. 1981. Dental arch shape: a statistical analysis using conic sections. *American Journal of Orthodontics* 79:535–48. (*2.4.1*)

Sampson, P. D. 1986. Comment on F. L. Bookstein, "Size and shape spaces for landmark data in two dimensions." *Statistical Science* 1:229–34. (*5.4, 5.5.3*)

Sampson, P. D., F. L. Bookstein, S. Lewis, C. Hurley, and P. Guttorp. 1991. Computation and application of deformations for landmark data in morphometrics and environmetrics. To appear in J. Kettenring, ed., *Proceedings of the 23rd Conference on the Interface Between Computer Science and Statistics*. New York: IEEE. (*6.6*)

Sampson, P. D., A. Streissguth, H. Barr, and F. L. Bookstein. 1989. Neurobehavioral effects of prenatal alcohol. Part II. Partial least squares analyses. *Neurotoxicology and Teratology* 11:477–91. (*2.3.2, 6.5.1, 7.4.4*)

Schönemann, P. H. 1970. On metric multidimension scaling. *Psychometrika* 35:349–66. (*7.1*)

Schüepp, O. 1966. *Meristeme*. Basel: Birkhauser. (*2.4.3*)

Schwerdtfeger, H. 1962. *Geometry of Complex Numbers*. University of Toronto Press. (*2.5.3, 5.1.2, 5.3.2, A.2*)

Serra, J. 1982. *Image Analysis and Mathematical Morphology*. London: Academic. (*2.4.3*)

Siegel, A. F., and R. H. Benson. 1982. A robust comparison of biological shapes. *Biometrics* 38:341–50. (*7.1.3*)

Skalak, R., G. Dasgupta, M. Moss, E. Otten, P.

Dullemeijer, and H. Vilmann. 1982. Analytical description of growth. *Journal of Theoretical Biology* 94:555–77. (*6.6*)

Small, C. G. 1988. Techniques of shape analysis on sets of points. *International Statistical Review* 56:243–57. (*2.1, 5.6*)

Smith, D., B. Crespi, and F. L. Bookstein. 1990. Asymmetry and morphological abnormality in the honey bee, *Apis mellifera*: effects of ploidy and hybridization. Unpublished manuscript. (*7.1.4*)

Sneath, P. H. A. 1967. Trend-surface analysis of transformation grids. *Journal of Zoology* 151:65–122. (*2.1*)

Sneath, P. H. A., and R. Sokal. 1973. *Principles of Numerical Taxonomy*, 2nd ed. San Francisco: Freeman. (*2.4.2, 4.4*)

Sokal, R. R., and F. J. Rohlf. 1981. *Biometry*, 2nd ed. San Francisco: Freeman. (*2.3*)

Spitzer, F. 1964. *Principles of Random Walk*. Princeton: Van Nostrand. (*A.3.1*)

Srivastava, M. S., and E. Carter. 1983. *An Introduction to Applied Multivariate Statistics*. Amsterdam: North Holland. (*7.2.4*)

Stigler, S. M. 1986. *The History of Statistics*. Cambridge, MA: Harvard University Press. (*2.3, 2.5.2*)

Stoyan, D. 1990. Estimation of distances and variances in Bookstein's landmark model. *Biometrical Journal* 32:843–9. (*5.3.1*)

Stoyan, D., W. Kendall, and J. Mecke. 1987. *Stochastic Geometry and Its Applications*. New York: Wiley. (*2.4.3*)

Straney, D. O. 1990. Median axis methods in morphometrics. In F. J. Rohlf and F. Bookstein, eds., *Proceedings of the Michigan Morphometrics Workshop*, pp. 179–200. Ann Arbor: University of Michigan Museums. (*2.1, 3.3.3, 3.5.2*)

Strauss, R. E., and F. L. Bookstein. 1982. The truss: body form reconstruction in morphometrics. *Systematic Zoology* 31:113–35. (*4.1.4*)

Tabachnick, R. E. 1988. Evolving entities in fossil populations: a morphometric analysis of Miocene planktonic foraminifera (*Globorotalia*). Doctoral dissertation,

Department of Geology, University of Michigan. (*3.4.3*)

Tabachnick, R. E., and F. L. Bookstein. 1990*a*. The structure of individual variation in Miocene *Globorotalia*, DSDP Site 593. *Evolution* 44:416–34. (*1.3, 3.4.3, 6.5.1, 7.4.4*)

Tabachnick, R. E., and F. L. Bookstein. 1990*b*. Resolving factors of landmark deformation: Miocene *Globorotalia*, DSDP Site 593. In F. J. Rohlf and F. Bookstein, eds., *Proceedings of the Michigan Morphometrics Workshop*, pp. 269–82. Ann Arbor: University of Michigan Museums. (*3.4.3, 7.2.3, 7.6.4*)

Terzopoulos, D. 1983. Multilevel computational processes for visual surface reconstruction. *Computer Vision, Graphics, and Image Processing* 24:52–96. (*2.2.2*)

Terzopoulos, D. 1986. Regularization of inverse visual problems involving discontinuities. *IEEE Transactions on Pattern Analysis and Machine Intelligence* 8:413–24. (*2.2.2*)

Thompson, D'A. W. 1961. *On Growth and Form*, abridged edition, J. T. Bonner, ed. (first published 1917). Cambridge University Press. (*2.1, 3.2*)

Toga, A., ed. 1990. *Three-Dimensional Neuroimaging*. New York: Raven. (*2.4.3*)

Van Valen, L. 1962. A study of fluctuating asymmetry. *Evolution* 16:125–42. (*7.1.4*)

Velicer, W. F., and D. Jackson. 1990. Component analysis vs. common factor analysis: some issues in selecting an appropriate procedure. *Multivariate Behavioral Research* 25:1–114. (*2.3.2*)

Wahba, G. 1990. *Spline Models for Observational Data*. Philadelphia: Society for Industrial and Applied Mathematics. (*2.2.2, A.1.2*)

Weibel, E. 1979–80. *Stereological Methods*, 2 vols. London: Academic. (*2.4.3*)

Widder, D. V. 1961. *Advanced Calculus*, 2nd ed. Englewood Cliffs, NJ: Prentice-Hall. (*5.0*)

Witkin, A., D. Terzopoulos, and M. Kass. 1987. Signal matching through scale space. *International Journal of Computer Vision* 1:133–44. (*2.2.2*)

Wolchonok, L. 1959. *The Art of Three-Dimensional Design*. New York: Harper & Brothers; reprinted Dover, 1969. (*8.1.2*)

Wolberg, G. 1990. *Digital Image Warping*. Los Alamitos, CA: IEEE Computer Society Press. (*2.4.1*)

Wold, H. 1975. Path models with latent variables: the NIPALS approach. In H. M. Blalock et al., eds., *Quantitative Sociology: International Perspectives on Mathematical and Statistical Modeling*, pp. 307–57. New York: Academic. (*2.3.2*)

Wright, S. 1932. General, group and special size factors. *Genetics* 17:603–19. (*2.3.2, 4.2.2*)

Wright, S. 1954. The interpretation of multivariate systems. In O. Kempthorne et al., eds., *Statistics and Mathematics in Biology*, pp. 11–33. Ames: Iowa State College Press. (*2.3.2, 4.2.2, 4.3.1*)

Wright, S. 1968. *Evolution and the Genetics of Populations. Vol. 1: Genetic and Biometric Foundations.* University of Chicago Press. (*2.3.2, 4.2.2, 4.3.1*)

Yaglom, I. M. 1979. *A Simple Non-Euclidean Geometry and Its Physical Basis*. New York: Springer. (*2.5.3, 7.6.1*)

Index

An *f* following a page number denotes a figure.

uniform components
  examples of, 10, 280–1, 354
  factor estimate of, 277–80, 362
  principal components of, 10, 279,
    353–7, 365, 366
  and relative warps, 15, 353–7
  standard errors of, 280
uniform distribution of shape, 181–2
uniform shear, *see* uniform
    transformations
uniform transformations, 9–10,
    270–87
  algebra of, 188–99, 272–3
  anisotropy as metric for, 26, 283–5
  basis for, 273
  and bending energy, 318f, 320, 321,
    353
  circle construction, assumed in, 202
  examples, 9–10, 283–7, 299
  factor estimation of, *see* uniform
    components
  and finite elements, 253–5
  fitting, 255, 274, 276–7
  formula for, 273
  geometry of, 271–3; *see also* square,
    transformations of, to
    parallelogram
  as polynomial, 273, 302
    versus quadratic model, 304
  and Procrustes superpositions,
    260–2, 266–7
  reporting, 284–5, 354f, 355–7, 366
  residuals, localizing, 292, 299
  versus rigid motion, 314
  as a subspace of shape space, 13,
    25, 273–4, 318f, 353

for symmetrized forms, 9–10
tests of, 255, 281–7, 299
in thin-plate spline analysis, 324,
  327f, 335, 339f
and triangles, 277, 283
visualizations of, 31, 189f, 206f, 272
University of Michigan University
  School Study (example)
  data listings, 400–6
  in deformity studies, 246
  growth findings, 73f, 166–7,
    228–41, 248–51, 309–10
  growth prediction, 238–9
  landmarks of, 68–72
  mandibular form in, 80–5, 166–7,
    248–51
  scatter of shape in, 133f, 229f
Upper vermilion (landmark), 7, 79
USS, *see* University of Michigan
  University School Study

variables
  from the circle construction, 201f,
    209f, 234, 243, 245, 247
  extents as, 57, 119–20
  from Fourier analysis, 46
  geometric ordering of, 59–60, 228;
    see also geometry, of shape space
  latent, 42–44
  from the medial axis, 82–3
  morphometric, 2–3, 17, 21, 23, 36,
    55–6; *see also* answers;
    multivariate analysis, reporting
  for purely inhomogeneous change,
    290

sampling of, 398–400
scale of, and log transformations,
  102
from tensor findings, 214–22
see also distances; multivariate
  analysis; ratios; shape
  coordinates; shape variables; size
  variables
variance
  of Cartesian coordinates, 149–50
  "explained," 39
    by projection onto shape
      subspaces, 282, 284, 299, 301,
      310, 311, 314
  and factors, 113–14, 153–5
  of shape coordinates, 142–50,
    153–5, 283
  of the uniform factor estimate, 280
  per unit bending, *see* relative warps
Veenia (example), 313–14
  landmarks for, 74–5
visualization, 370–72
volume, as variable, 57, 85
  formula for, 92

warps
  blur rigid motions, 330
  and fractals, 346
  see also partial warps; principal
    warps; relative warps; thin-plate
    spline
weight, as variable, 57
wings, insect, landmarks for, 268f
workstations, 19, 370–2

Printed in the United States
115164LV00007B/63-66/A

9 780521 585989